Antioxidants: Health and Healing

Antioxidants: Health and Healing

Editor: Nina Pegg

AMERICAN
MEDICAL PUBLISHERS
www.americanmedicalpublishers.com

AMERICAN
MEDICAL PUBLISHERS
www.americanmedicalpublishers.com

Cataloging-in-Publication Data

Antioxidants : health and healing / edited by Nina Pegg.
p. cm.
Includes bibliographical references and index.
ISBN 978-1-63927-537-3
1. Antioxidants. 2. Health. 3. Healing. 4. Antioxidants--Health aspects. 5. Antioxidants--Therapeutic use. I. Pegg, Nina.
RB170 .A58 2022
613.286--dc23

American Medical Publishers,
41 Flatbush Avenue,
1st Floor, New York,
NY 11217, USA

ISBN 978-1-63927-537-3 (Hardback)

Contents

Preface

This book has been a concerted effort by a group of academicians, researchers and scientists, who have contributed their research works for the realization of the book. This book has materialized in the wake of emerging advancements and innovations in this field. Therefore, the need of the hour was to compile all the required researches and disseminate the knowledge to a broad spectrum of people comprising of students, researchers and specialists of the field.

Compounds that inhibit oxidation are called antioxidants. Oxidation can produce free radicals and lead to chain reactions, which damage healthy cells. To prevent this from occurring, animals and plants maintain complex systems of overlapping antioxidants, such as vitamin C and E, glutathione and enzymes. Antioxidants are classified as hydrophilic and lipophilic. These may be synthesized in the body or obtained from diet. A certain proportion of antioxidant vitamins are needed in the diet for good health. However, the proportion and the antioxidant species with positive health effects are still debated. Research is being undertaken to investigate the potential effects of dietary antioxidants on neurodegenerative diseases, such as Parkinson's diseases, amyotrophic lateral sclerosis and Alzheimer's disease. This book is compiled in such a manner, that it will provide in-depth knowledge about the importance of antioxidants in health and disease. Different approaches, evaluations, methodologies and advanced studies on antioxidants have been included herein. A number of latest researches have been included to keep the readers up-to-date with the global concepts in this area of study.

At the end of the preface, I would like to thank the authors for their brilliant chapters and the publisher for guiding us all-through the making of the book till its final stage. Also, I would like to thank my family for providing the support and encouragement throughout my academic career and research projects.

Editor

1

Impact of Thermal Degradation of Cyanidin-3-*O*-Glucoside of Haskap Berry on Cytotoxicity of Hepatocellular Carcinoma HepG2 and Breast Cancer MDA-MB-231 Cells

Eric Pace [1], Yuanyuan Jiang [1,2], Amy Clemens [1], Tennille Crossman [1] and H.P. Vasantha Rupasinghe [1,*]

1 Department of Plant, Food, and Environmental Sciences, Faculty of Agriculture, Dalhousie University, Truro, NS B2N 5E3, Canada; pace.eric.arthur@gmail.com (E.P.); yyjiang@dal.ca (Y.J.); am661344@dal.ca (A.C.); tennille.crossman@dal.ca (T.C.)
2 College of Science, Sichuan Agricultural University, Yaan 625014, China
* Correspondence: vrupasinghe@dal.ca

Abstract: Cyanidin-3-*O*-glucoside (C3G), the predominant anthocyanin in haskap berries (*Lonicera caerulea* L.), possesses antioxidant and many other biological activities. This study investigated the impact of temperature and pH on the degradation of the C3G-rich haskap fraction. The effect of the thermal degradation products on the viability of hepatocellular carcinoma HepG2 and breast cancer MDA-MB-231 cells was also studied in vitro. Using column chromatography, the C3G-rich fraction was isolated from acetone extracts of haskap berries. The C3G stability in these fractions was studied under elevated temperatures (70 °C and 90 °C) at three different pH values (2.5, 4, and 7) by monitoring the concentration of C3G and its major degradation products, protocatechuic acid (PCA) and phloroglucinaldehyde (PGA), using liquid chromatography mass spectrometry. Significant degradation of C3G was observed at elevated temperatures and at neutral pH. Conversely, the PCA and PGA concentration increased at higher pH and temperature. Similar to C3G, neutral pH also has a prominent effect on the degradation of PGA, which is further accelerated by heating. The C3G-rich fraction exhibited dose-dependent inhibitory effects on cell metabolic activity when the HepG2 cells were exposed for 48 h. Interestingly, PGA but not PCA exhibited cytotoxic effects against both MDA-MB-231 and HepG2 cells. The results suggest that thermal food processing of haskap could influence its biological properties due to the degradation of C3G.

Keywords: anthocyanin; food processing; antioxidant; cancer; cell viability; phenolic compounds

---

1. Introduction

Haskap (*Lonicera caerulea* L.) berries, also known as blue honeysuckle and honeyberry, are a relatively new crop in North America. Berries of this genus have been used for medicinal purposes in Russia and some Asian countries for thousands of years [1,2]. There are three major cultivars of this berry being produced in Canada, and they have attracted interest due to their relatively high concentration of health-promoting anthocyanins when compared with other commonly consumed fruit [1,3,4]. Many studies have indicated that anthocyanins have the potential to be effective in cancer chemoprevention. Anti-proliferative effects on multiple cancer cell types in vitro, pro-apoptotic effects on cancer cell lines, reduction in inflammatory pathway expression, anti-angiogenesis effects, and induced differentiation have been observed [5–12]. Anthocyanins administered in vivo have reduced cancer development in animals treated with carcinogens, and in animals with the common hereditary development of colon, lung, skin and esophageal cancers [13–15]. Anthocyanins, which degrade rapidly, are the least stable class of flavonoids. The stability of anthocyanins is affected by pH, light exposure, oxidation, enzymatic action, and the presence of metal ions [16]. Under acidic conditions (pH < 3), anthocyanins exist in their most stable form, red flavylium cations. When the pH is between four and five, anthocyanins undergo hydroxylation and form a colorless pseudo base. At a higher pH (pH > 6), anthocyanins exist as a quinoidal base and exhibit a blue color. Under alkaline conditions, anthocyanins can also form chalcones, which exhibit a yellow color, and can degrade to produce phenolic acids [17].

Cyanidin-3-*O*-glucoside (C3G), which is the predominant anthocyanin in haskap berries [18,19], thermally degrades into protocatechuic acid (PCA) and phloroglucinaldehyde (PGA) [20]. PCA has exhibited anti-inflammatory and anti-oxidative effects and has reduced liver toxicity in vivo [21]. PCA may also possess anti-tumoral properties, inducing apoptosis in human leukemia cells, as well as in human salivary gland carcinoma (HSG1) cells [22]. Conversely, PCA has also been shown to increase proliferation in 12-*O*-tetradecanoylphorbol-13-acetate (TPA)-induced mouse skin tumors [23]. Currently, limited studies are showing the antiproliferative effects of PGA, with only two studies suggesting anti-proliferative effects against colon cancer cells Caco-2 [24,25]. Recent studies investigating the pharmacokinetics of C3G in humans have identified the presence of both PCA and PGA in the blood serum of individuals who have ingested labeled C3G [26,27]. Therefore, this study aims to characterize C3G degradation, PCA and PGA formation in the haskap extract, and the antiproliferative properties of C3G and its major degradation products against hepatocellular carcinoma HepG2 and breast adenocarcinoma MDA-MB-231 cells.

2. Materials and Methods

2.1. Plant Material

Haskap berries of the Tundra cultivar (TN) were obtained from LaHave Natural Farm, Blockhouse, Nova Scotia, Canada and stored at −20 °C.

2.2. Chemicals and Reagents

High performance liquid chromatography (HPLC) grade methanol, ethyl acetate, 88% formic acid, acetone, phosphate buffered saline (PBS), dimethyl sulfoxide (DMSO), Eagle Minimum Essential Growth Medium (EMEM), Dulbecco's Modified Eagle's Medium (DMEM), penicillin-streptomycin, fetal bovine serum (FBS), PCA, PGA, doxorubicin (DOX), and all other chemical reagents were purchased from Sigma-Aldrich (Oakville, ON, Canada). C3G was purchased from Extrasynthese (Genay Cedrix, France). Trisodium citrate and anhydrous dibasic sodium phosphate were purchased from Fisher Scientific (Ottawa, ON, Canada). Sorafenib was purchased from Cayman Chemicals (Cedarlane, Burlington, ON, Canada). 5-[3-(Carboxymethoxy) phenyl]-3-(4,5-dimethyl-2-thiazolyl)-2-(4-sulfophenyl)-2H-tetrazolium inner salt (MTS) was purchased from Promega (Madison, WI, USA).

2.3. Preparation of Extracts

2.3.1. Preparation of Crude Extract

The crude extract (CE) was prepared using frozen haskap berries (500 g) extracted in semi-dark conditions. Berries were ground in a blender (Model HBB909, Hamilton Beach Brands Inc., Glen Allen, VA, USA) in a solution of 70:28:2 acetone:deionized water (DI H_2O):formic acid. For every 1 g of frozen berries, 4 mL of solvent was used. The blended berries and solvent were filtered through six layers of cheese cloth, then vacuum filtered through Whatman # 8 filter paper (Fisher Scientific, Ottawa, ON, Canada). Samples were subjected to rotary evaporation to remove the solvent, then frozen at −80 °C and freeze-dried. Crude extracts were then stored at −80 °C.

2.3.2. Preparation of C3G-Rich Fraction

C3G-rich fraction (PE) was prepared in the same manner as crude extracts with additional steps, as described in a previous method [28]. Following rotary evaporation to remove acetone, the resultant liquid was added to equal volumes of ethyl acetate in a separatory funnel under dark conditions and was allowed to separate for 12 h before the aqueous phase was collected. Trace amounts of ethyl acetate were removed from the aqueous phase via rotary evaporation. A column (3.8 × 45 cm, Sati International Scientific Inc., Dorval, QC, Canada) was packed with 600 g adsorbent (Sorbent SP207-05 Sepabeads Resin Brominated Styrenic Adsorbent: particle size 250 µm, surface area 630 m^3/g, Sorbent Technologies, Atlanta, GA, USA) and conditioned with methanol followed by DI H_2O acidified to pH 2.5 with hydrochloric acid (HCl). The crude extract was applied to the column and washed with 1 L DI H_2O acidified to pH 2.5 with HCl. C3G-rich fraction was eluted with about 500 mL of methanol. Methanol was removed using rotary evaporation and then freeze-dried to prepare dried PE, which was stored at −80 °C.

2.4. *Degradation Kinetics*

2.4.1. Sample Preparation

PE was prepared at a concentration of 40 mg/mL in a citrate–phosphate buffer (0.2 M tri-sodium citrate, 0.3 M dibasic sodium phosphate). Portions of this solution were acidified to pH 2.5, 4, and 7 with citric acid and stored in 2-mL aliquots in 2-mL sealed amber glass vials. Samples were incubated in triplicate, in a water bath at either 70 °C or 90 °C, for periods of 0, 0.5, 1, 2, 4, or 8 h. After incubation, samples were immersed in an ice bath to limit further degradation. Samples were then stored at −80 °C until analysis. Pure PGA solutions (50 µg/mL, 2 mL) were incubated in a 90 °C water bath for 0, 0.5, 1, 2, 4, and 8 h periods in 2-mL sealed amber glass vials at pH of 2.5, 4, and 7. Each of the heated solutions was diluted with 2 mL MeOH and filtered before HPLC analysis.

2.4.2. Quantification of Total Monomeric Anthocyanins, C3G, PCA, and PGA

Total monomeric anthocyanin concentration (TAC) was determined using a spectrophotometric pH differential method [29]. The TAC is expressed as milligrams (mg) C3G equivalent with a molar extinction coefficient 26,900 and a molecular weight of 449.2 g/mol. C3G, PGA, and PCA were quantified as described before by [28] using ultra HPLC electrospray ionization tandem mass spectrometry (UPLC-ESI-MS/MS) on a Waters H-class UPLC separations module (Waters, Milford, MA, USA) coupled with a Micromass Quattro micro API MS/MS system and MassLynx V4.0 control software (Micromass, Cary, NC, USA). The column used was an Aquity BEH C18 (100 mm × 2.1 mm × 1.7 µm) (Waters, Milford, MA, USA). PCA and PGA were analyzed using single ion monitoring mode (SIM) with electrospray ionization in negative mode (ESI−) with a capillary voltage of 3000 V, a nebulizer gas temperature (N_2) of 375 °C, and a flow rate of 0.35 mL/min. C3G was analyzed using electrospray ionization in positive ion mode (ESI+), with a capillary voltage of 3500 V, a nebulizer gas temperature (N_2) of 375 °C, and a flow rate of 0.35 mL/min. Samples were diluted 1:1 with methanol, then filtered through 0.22 µm nylon filters into amber glass UPLC vials.

2.4.3. Statistical Analysis

Repeated measures analysis ($p \leq 0.05$) was performed using the statistical analysis system software (SAS Institute, Cary, NC, USA). The data for C3G incubated at 90 °C was normalized using a $\log_{10}$ transformation.

2.5. *Antiproliferative Activity*

2.5.1. Preparation of Extracts

PE was prepared for cell-based assays by dissolving freeze-dried PE to a concentration of 60 mg/mL in deionized water (DI H_2O). Degraded extracts were prepared by subjecting aliquots of this PE solution to thermal degradation at 90 °C in a shaking water bath for 2 h (HPE2) or 8 h (HPE8). The crude extract (CE) was prepared by dissolving freeze-dried CE to a concentration of 60 mg/mL in DI H_2O.

2.5.2. Cell Culture

Breast adenocarcinoma (MDA-MB-231; American Type Culture Collection (ATCC) # HTB 26) cells were obtained from the American Type Culture Collection (ATCC, Manassas, VA, USA) and cultured at 37 °C with 5% CO_2, in DMEM with 2 mM L-glutamine, 10% heat-inactivated FBS, 1% 4-(2-hydroxyethyl)-1-piperazineethanesulfonic acid (HEPES), and 1% penicillin–streptomycin. Hepatocellular carcinoma (HepG2; ATCC # 8065) cells were also obtained from the ATCC and cultured in EMEM with 2 mM L-glutamine, 10% FBS, and 1% penicillin-streptomycin at 37 °C with 5% CO_2.

2.5.3. Cell Viability MTS Assay

A CellTiter 96® AQ$_{ueous}$ One Solution Cell Proliferation Assay (Promega, Madison, WI, USA) was used to determine cell viability. Cells were seeded in 96-well plates at a density of 5×10^3 cells per well and incubated for 24 h to promote cell adhesion. Cells were treated with PE, HPE2, HPE8, or CE. For HepG2 cells, treatments were added at concentrations of 75, 150, and 300 µg/mL with a positive control of sorafenib in DMSO with a final concentration of 10 µg/mL and negative controls consisting of either EMEM with: 0.5% DI H_2O for PE, HPE2, HPE8, or CE treatments, or 0.5% DMSO for PCA or PGA treatments. For MDA-MB-231 cells, treatments were added at concentrations of 50, 100, and 200 µg/mL with a positive control of doxorubicin in DMSO at a final concentration of 50 µM, and negative controls of DMEM with either 0.5% DI H_2O (PE, HPE2, HPE8, or CE) or 0.5% DMSO (PCA, PGA). After either a 24 or 48 h incubation, 20 µL of MTS was added to each well. Plates were incubated for three hours at 37 °C in a 5% CO_2 atmosphere before absorbance was measured at 490 nm using a FLUOstar Optima microplate reader (BMG Labtech, Ortenberg, Germany). Cell viability calculated with treated cells being expressed as a percent of cells treated with vehicle only.

2.5.4. Acid Phosphatase Assay

Acid phosphatase buffer was prepared with 0.1 M sodium acetate (NaAc), 0.1% *v*/*v* Triton X-100, and 4 mg/mL phosphatase substrate (Sigma-Aldrich, Oakville, ON, Canada), adjusted to a pH of 5.5 with HCl, and stored at 4 °C. HepG2 cells were treated with PE, PCA, and PGA at concentrations of 75, 150, and 300 µg/mL with a positive control of sorafenib in DMSO with a final concentration of 10 µg/mL, and negative controls consisting of EMEM with either: 0.5% DI H_2O for PE treatments, or 0.5% DMSO for PCA or PGA treatments. After incubation for a period of 48 h, plates were centrifuged at 2000 rpm for 10 min before the supernatant was removed and 100 µL of PBS added to each well. Plates were again centrifuged before PBS was removed and 100 µL of assay buffer was added to each well. Plates were then incubated for two hours at 37 °C in a 5% CO_2 atmosphere. After incubation, 10 µL of 1 N sodium hydroxide was added to each well, and absorbance was measured at 405 nm using a FLUOstar Optima microplate reader (BMG Labtech, Ortenberg, Germany). Cell viability was calculated as described in Section 2.5.3.

2.5.5. Adenosine Triphosphate (ATP) Assay

The CellTiter-Glo® Luminescent Cell Viability Assay (Promega, Madison, WI, USA) was used to determine cell viability and ATP levels. HepG2 cells were treated under the same conditions as those in the acid phosphatase assay. The CellTiter-Glo® reagent was prepared as directed by the manufacturer from CellTiter-Glo® substrate and the CellTiter-Glo® buffer, and 100 μL of reagent was added to each well. Plates were shaken for 2 min at 60 rpm using a VWR orbital shaker (Troemner LLC, Mini Shaker, Thorofare, NJ, USA) to induce cell lysis followed by a 10-min room-temperature incubation. Luminescence was measured using a FLUOstar Optima microplate reader (BMG Labtech, Ortenberg, Germany). Cell viability was calculated as described in Section 2.5.3.

2.5.6. Statistical Analysis

All experiments were designed using completely randomized design. Assays were performed in triplicate ($n = 3$), and all results were expressed as the mean ± standard deviation (SD). Analyses were compared using one-way analysis of variance (ANOVA) and Tukey's test ($p \leq 0.05$). Statistical analyses were carried out using the Minitab v.17 software (Minitab, State College, PA, USA) package.

3. Results

3.1. C3G Degradation

Monomeric anthocyanins' degradation was more pronounced in extracts incubated at 90 °C than at 70 °C (Figure 1A,E). Also, extracts incubated at the pH of 7.0 exhibited significantly greater anthocyanin degradation than extracts incubated in acidic pH conditions. As demonstrated in Figure 1B,F, at incubation temperatures of 70 °C and 90 °C, the breakdown of C3G in haskap PE was significantly affected ($p \leq 0.05$) by both incubation time and pH.

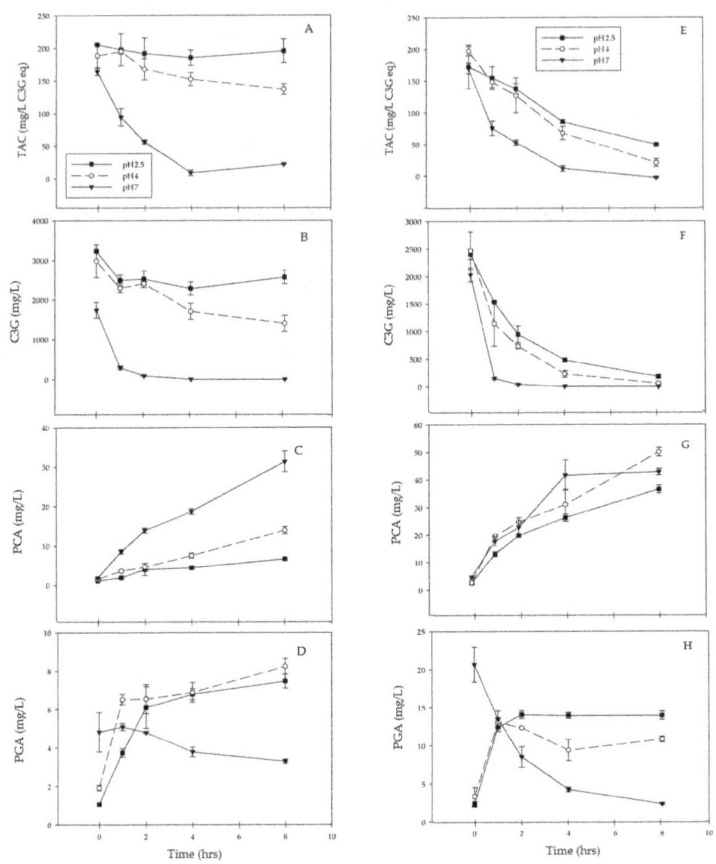

Figure 1. Total monomeric anthocyanin (TAC), cyanidin-3-*O*-glucoside (C3G), protocatechuic acid (PCA) and phloroglucinaldehyde (PGA) content at 70 °C (**A–D**) and 90 °C (**E–H**). TAC was measured using pH differential spectrophotometric assay and quantification of C3G, PCA, and PGA by ultra HPLC electrospray ionization tandem mass spectrometry (UPLC-ESI-MS/MS).

As the pH increased, C3G degraded more readily, with extracts incubated at 90 °C degrading more quickly than those incubated at 70 °C. Extracts incubated for 8 h at pH 2.5, lost 21% of the initial C3G content at 70 °C, and lost 95% of the initial C3G content at 90 °C. Extracts at pH 4.0 followed a similar trend losing 53% of the C3G content at 70 °C versus a 98% loss at 90 °C. At pH 7.0, C3G was almost completely lost at both 70 °C and 90 °C. C3G is the least stable at pH 7 when compared to pH 2.5 and pH 4.0 (Figure 1B,F).

3.2. Formation of PCA

The accumulation of PCA, one of C3G's major breakdown products, was quantified in the thermally degraded purified extracts. PCA concentration increased as C3G degraded under all tested conditions. Time and pH both significantly ($p \leq 0.05$) affected the accumulation of PCA as C3G degraded. The highest concentration of accumulated PCA, 50.0 mg/L, was observed over an 8-h incubation at pH 4 and 90 °C. As with C3G degradation, at 70 °C the largest differences in PCA concentrations were found when comparing pH 7.0 to an acidic pH of 2.5 or 4.0. At 90 °C variations were less dramatic, suggesting that the presence of PCA in C3G-rich extracts is an indicator of C3G degradation (Figure 1C,G).

3.3. Formation of PGA

PGA concentration (Figure 1D,H) showed less of an association to C3G degradation than PCA concentration. At 70 °C and 90 °C, and pHs of 2.5 and 4.0, extracts showed an increase in PGA concentration, with most of the accumulation occurring during the first 2 h of the 8-h incubation. Depending on incubation conditions, after the initial 2 h, PGA accumulation decelerated, stabilized, or for pH 7.0 at both 70 °C and 90 °C PGA concentration decreased.

To understand whether the PGA can be further degraded at pH 7 after 2 h, the second experiment was performed using pure PGA (Figure 2). PGA heated at pH of 2.5 and 4 showed minimal degradation over the 8 h period. However, at pH 7, the PGA experienced rapid degradation and exhibited over 90% loss after 8 h of heating. This is in agreement with the previous experiment, which found that PGA accumulated from C3G degradation had decreased concentrations at pH 7. A visible color change could be seen with PGA solutions mixed with the pH 7 buffer; PGA solutions at pH 2.5 and 4 remained colorless, while pH 7 solutions became increasingly yellow with longer heating times.

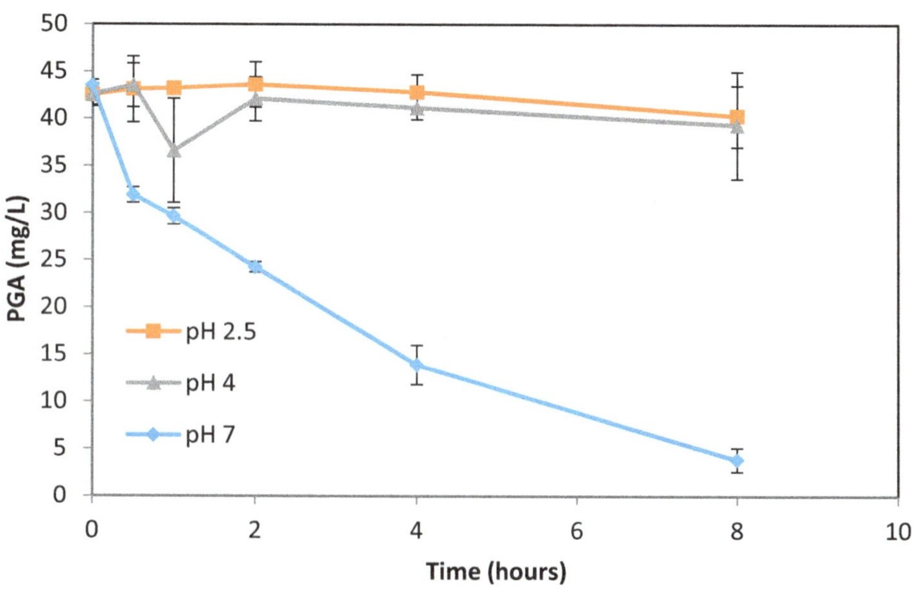

Figure 2. Phloroglucinaldehyde (PGA) concentration at 90° C at pH 2.5, 4, and 7, respectively.

3.4. *Breast Adenocarcinoma MDA-MB-231 Viability*

The viability of treated MDA-MB-231 cells was assessed using an MTS assay. PE, HPE2, HPE8, CE, PCA, and PGA were used to treat the cells. The concentrations of C3G, PCA, and PGA in each extract are displayed in Table 1. Cellular viability was measured by comparing cells treated with extracts and commercially purchased PCA and PGA, at concentrations of 50, 100, and 200 μg/mL, to negative and positive controls. The negative control consisted of DMEM growth medium with 0.5% DMSO, and the positive control was 0.5% DMSO with the chemotherapy drug doxorubicin at a concentration of 50 μM.

Table 1. The composition of the C3G-rich extracts and thermally-challenged extracts (500 μg/mL) used for the cell viability analyses.

Treatment	C3G (μg/mL)	PCA (μg/mL)	PGA (μg/mL)
PE	59.92 ± 1.6	0.28 ± 0.001	0.023 ± 0.0002
HPE2	34.23 ± 3.3	0.77 ± 0.04	0.29 ± 0.01
HPE8	5.76 ± 0.5	2.02 ± 0.2	0.467 ± 0.01
CE	11.35 ± 0.1	N/A	N/A

C3G, Cyanidin-3-*O*-glucoside; PCA, protocatechuic acid; PGA, phloroglucinaldehyde; PE, C3G-rich fraction; HPE2, the PE subjected to 90 °C for 2 h; HPE8, the PE subjected to 90 °C for 8 h; CE, crude extract.

None of the haskap-derived treatments affected cellular viability except PGA (Table 2). At concentrations of 100 μg/mL and above, PGA significantly reduced MDA-MB-231 viability over periods of 24 and 48 h. In both cases, a cell viability of 35% was observed; with a strong dose-dependent trend but no clear time-dependence.

3.5. *Hepatocellular Carcinoma HepG2 Cell Viability*

The viability of HepG2 cells, after exposure to haskap berry extracts containing C3G and its metabolites, was assessed using an MTS assay, an acid phosphatase assay, and an ATP assay. Cellular viability was compared to a negative control consisting of EMEM growth medium with 0.5% DMSO, and a positive control containing 10 μg/mL of the chemotherapy drug sorafenib. Cells were treated with PE, HPE2, HPE8, CE, PCA, and PGA at concentrations of 75, 150, and 300 μg/mL.

MTS-based viability determination (Table 2) showed a dose- and time-dependent reduction in cell viability for PE and PGA. After a 24-h incubation, cell viability was 52% with a PGA concentration of 75 μg/mL, and only 20.2% with a concentration of 300 μg/mL, when compared to the negative control. For PE at 300 μg/mL after a 24-h incubation, cell viability was 64% compared to the negative control. PCA treatments showed no effect on HepG2 viability as determined via MTS assay. Treatments showing dose-dependent inhibition (PE & PGA), along with PCA due to conflicting reports of its anti-tumorigenic activity, were selected for further testing over 48-h incubations.

Cell viability, as determined in an acid phosphatase assay, showed that PE (Figure 3A) induced a strong dose-dependent reduction in cellular viability. This reduction ranged from 84.5% at a dosage of 75 μg/mL, to 21.2% at 300 μg/mL, as seen in Figure 3A. PGA also induced a significant reduction in cell viability, with all three treatments exhibiting similar activity to the positive control. PCA showed no significant dose-dependent reduction in cellular viability.

Table 2. Cell viability measured using the MTS assay.

Treatment	Concentration (μg/mL)	24 h (% Viability ± SD)	48 h (% Viability ± SD)
		MDA-MB-231	
PE	50	97.43 ± 2.04 [ab]	103.10 ± 10.17 [a]
	100	107.02 ± 6.71 [ab]	105.15 ± 5.29 [a]
	200	109.86 ± 1.50 [ab]	106.52 ± 6.50 [a]
HPE2	50	100.22 ± 2.14 [cd]	98.34 ± 0.91 [a]
	100	104.96 ± 1.42 [ab]	106.43 ± 4.20 [a]
	200	108.38 ± 4.16 [ab]	94.13 ± 8.44 [a]
HPE8	50	103.82 ± 2.48 [ab]	107.68 ± 6.24 [a]
	100	104.19 ± 4.13 [ab]	104.78 ± 4.45 [a]
	200	100.55 ± 3.11 [ab]	85.10 ± 11.13 [a]
CE	50	103.31 ± 4.98 [ab]	105.37 ± 3.46 [a]
	100	99.33 ± 3.24 [ab]	98.99 ± 12.10 [a]
	200	98.73 ± 2.18 [ab]	99.16 ± 3.86 [a]
PCA	50	101.18 ± 11.40 [ab]	94.43 ± 6.65 [a]
	100	101.08 ± 8.12 [ab]	81.96 ± 13.33 [a]
	200	107.89 ± 10.21 [ab]	86.96 ± 29.52 [a]
PGA	50	78.22 ± 2.37 [bc]	80.35 ± 5.54 [a]
	100	35.30 ± 26.66 [d]	36.25 ± 5.11 [bc]
	200	7.09 ± 8.93 [e]	17.71 ± 13.55 [c]
Dox	27.2	53.30 ± 13.56 [cd]	7.89 ± 7.29 [c]
		HepG2	
PE	75	89.26 ± 11.01 [bc]	72.9 ± 3.07 cd
	150	88.39 ± 2.43 [bc]	70.97 ± 7.32 d
	300	64.32 ± 14.33 [cd]	35.57 ± 11.55 e
HPE2	75	105.92 ± 7.78 [ab]	92.09 ± 4.61 [abc]
	150	104.28 ± 9.19 [ab]	91.26 ± 5.18 [abcd]
	300	97.34 ± 8.48 [ab]	81.58 ± 6.69 [bcd]
HPE8	75	105.64 ± 8.35 [ab]	90.15 ± 7.96 [abcd]
	150	102.85 ± 5.86 [ab]	81.65 ± 10.15 [bcd]
	300	103.35 ± 5.08 [ab]	80.07 ± 6.22 [bcd]
CE	75	102.92 ± 3.59 [ab]	95.2 ± 5.03 [ab]
	150	102.59 ± 7.62 [ab]	94.67 ± 3.6 [ab]
	300	104.76 ± 4.90 [ab]	93.35 ± 3.29 [abc]
PCA	75	84.98 ± 4.04 [bc]	90.943 ± 1.6 [abcd]
	150	92.41 ± 8.27 [ab]	89.99 ± 7.21 [abcd]
	300	114.06 ± 7.53 [ab]	108.66 ± 7.77 [a]
PGA	75	52.85 ± 3.82 [de]	25.71 ± 7.07 [ef]
	150	18.34 ± 10.46 [f]	15.16 ± 7.36 [efg]
	300	20.23 ± 8.25 [f]	1.80 ± 1.70 [g]
Sorafenib	10	39.38 ± 5.48 [ef]	11.40 ± 9.22 [fg]

Results represent the mean ± SD, Letters (a–g) indicate significantly different means ($p \leq 0.05$) within temperature treatments. MTS: 5-[3-(Carboxymethoxy) phenyl]-3-(4,5-dimethyl-2-thiazolyl)-2-(4-sulfophenyl)-2H-tetrazolium inner salt.

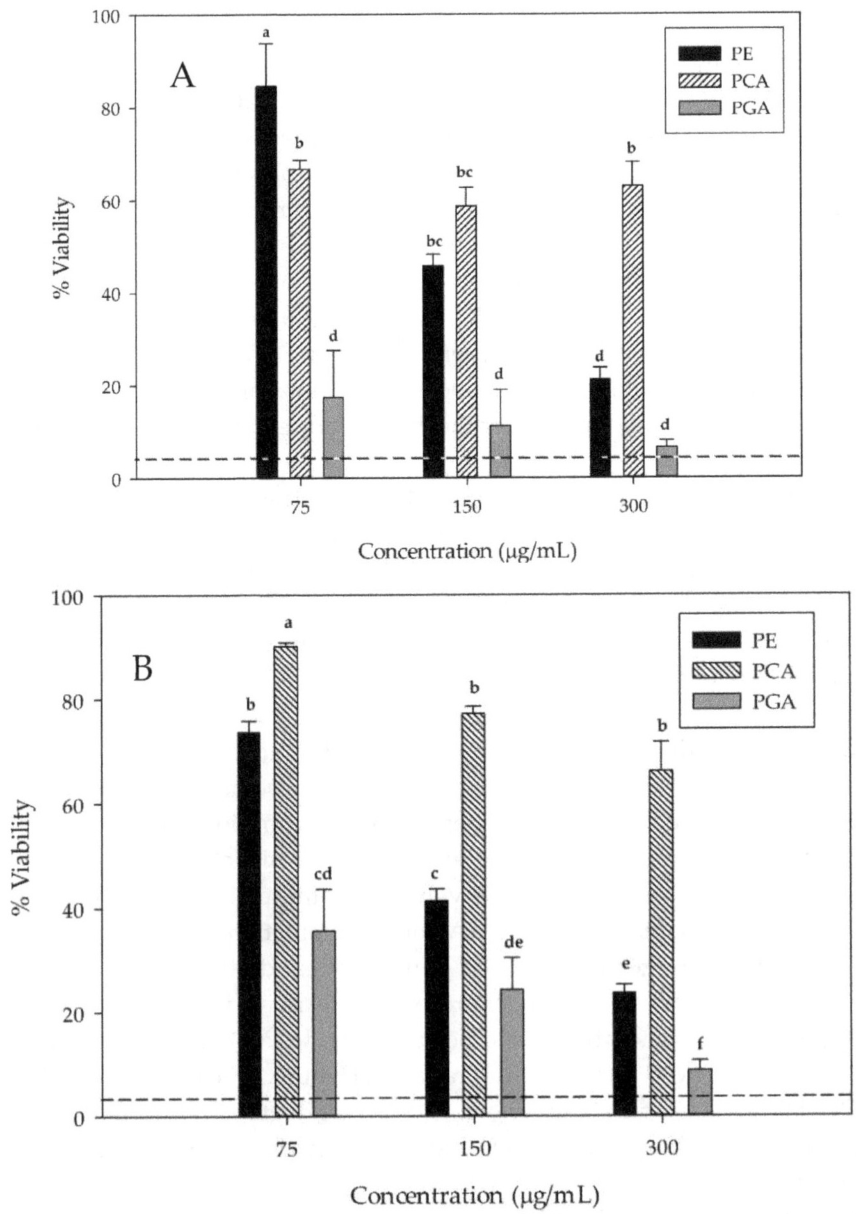

Figure 3. Cellular viability (% relative to the control) as determined by an acid phosphatase assay (**A**) and ATP content (**B**) of HepG2 cells incubated with C3G-rich fraction (PE), PCA, and PGA for 48 h. Dashed line represents positive control sorafenib at a concentration of 10 μg/mL. Letters (a–f) on the bars indicate significantly different means ($p \leq 0.05$). PE, C3G-rich fraction; PCA, protocatechuic acid; PGA, phloroglucinaldehyde.

It was determined via an ATP assay that PE-induced a dose-dependent reduction in ATP activity after an incubation of 48 h (Figure 3B). PE added at a concentration of 75 μg/mL did not generate a value that was significantly different from the vehicle control ($p \leq 0.05$); however, PE added at a concentration of 300 μg/mL induced an ATP reduction to 23.5%. PGA induced a strong reduction in detectable ATP, ranging from 35.6% of luminescence at a concentration of 75 μg/mL, to 8.8% at a concentration of 300 μg/mL (Figure3B). PCA induced a slight dose-dependent reduction in luminescence with 150 μg/mL and 300 μg/mL being significantly different than the negative control, but not significantly different from each other.

4. Discussion

Numerous studies and reviews have investigated and confirmed that anthocyanins undergo first-order kinetic degradation [30–34]. At a neutral pH, anthocyanins are liable to undergo spontaneous degradation, making the treatment temperature less significant for samples at neutral pH [16,30,35]. As demonstrated in Figures 1 and 2, for samples degraded at both 70 °C and 90 °C at time 0, samples at pH 7.0 showed a C3G reduction of almost 50% compared to the samples at pH 2.5. Within a given pH, C3G degradation accelerates at higher temperatures. This indicates that for C3G containing products, lower-temperature processing may preserve anthocyanin content compared to higher temperature methods. A study by Khattab et al. [36] monitored anthocyanin degradation in the drying of whole haskap berries at temperatures of 60, 100, and 140 °C. The study found that reductions of 74–76%, 79–81%, and 91–95%, respectively, of total anthocyanins were observed at those temperatures. Among the five predominant anthocyanins present in haskap berries, C3G was the least thermally stable [36].

Along with affecting the rate of C3G degradation, solution pH may also affect the mechanism of degradation. For C3G at a pH of 3.5, it appears that the opening of the pyrylium ring initiates anthocyanin degradation, forming a glycosylated chalcone [37]. For C3G at a pH of 1, deglycosylation was proposed as the first step in the degradation pathway [20]. It has been determined that the addition of sugars could help prevent anthocyanin degradation under some storage and treatment conditions [38]. This could be valuable, especially at higher temperatures and both acidic and neutral pH.

As with C3G degradation, the widest variation in PCA concentration was observed between measurements taken at pH 2.5 and 7.0 at 70 °C, with there being slightly less variation at 90 °C. This could indicate an inverse relationship, where PCA concentration could potentially represent the level of C3G degradation (Figure 1). The value of PCA as a bioactive compound is still unknown and PCA does not impart vibrant color, so its value for commercial products is still undetermined. Further investigation into the bioactivity of PCA and its interactions is recommended.

For incubation times longer than 2 h, at both 70 °C and 90 °C, PGA accumulation slowed or stabilized. For all samples at pH 7.0, there was a decrease in PGA concentration over time. The decelerating of PGA accumulation could be attributed to PGA degradation. Incubation of pure PGA at 90 °C at pH 7.0 showed its further degradation (Figure 2). This indicates that, like its parent anthocyanin C3G, PGA is unstable at higher pH, and further degrades as the incubation time increases. High pH values appear to have a prominent effect on the degradation of PGA, which is further accelerated by heating.

Haskap extract did not significantly reduce MDA-MB-231 cell viability. This is likely due to differing anthocyanin profiles between haskap berries and blueberries. Interestingly, PGA significantly reduced the MDA-MB-231 viability, which has not previously been reported. PGA has been shown to be anti-proliferative when incubated with Caco-2 cells in vitro [24,25]. Further studies should be conducted to determine if this reduction in viability is selective, and to elucidate the underlying mechanism. For HepG2 cells exposed to haskap berry extracts, and C3G metabolites, CE reduced cell viability to 64% when treated at a level of 300 μg/mL. Based on the ATP assay, PCA caused a significant reduction in HepG2 viability. PCA has been reported to reduce HepG2 viability [39]. The results of the MTS, ATP, and acid phosphatase assays suggest that PCA and PGA in thermally degraded haskap extracts may not be present in high enough concentrations to induce cytotoxicity in both cancer cell lines. However, both PE and PGA caused dose-dependent inhibition of HepG2.

5. Conclusions

Solution pH, incubation time, and temperature affect anthocyanin stability. As these increase, the anthocyanin concentration decreases. C3G is more stable when treated at lower temperatures over longer incubations when compared to shorter incubations at higher temperatures. Incubation at pH 7.0 promotes rapid C3G degradation; therefore, maintaining an acidic pH during processing is favorable for C3G retention. Haskap juice is naturally acidic in nature, and this acidity should be preserved to maintain anthocyanin stability. Haskap berry extract with high levels of C3G produced a time- and dose-dependent inhibition of HepG2 cell proliferation and PGA generated dose-dependent inhibition of MDA-MB-231 cells. This preliminary in vitro study suggests that haskap berry anthocyanins could potentially have cancer chemopreventive properties. It also indicates that the inhibitory effects of haskap berry extracts are mediated, at least in part, by C3G. Further studies are required to determine the anti-cancer potential and mechanism of action of C3G. One of C3G's thermal degradation product and in vivo primary metabolites, PGA, also generated significant anti-proliferative effects on HepG2 cells. Processing of haskap berries and their storage could exacerbate anthocyanin degradation, which could lead to a reduction in putative health benefits for the consumer. Since there is growing interest in the use of fruit-derived C3G as a food additive, natural colorant, dietary antioxidant, and nutraceutical, further research is required to determine the toxicity and biological activity of PGA.

Acknowledgments: This study was supported by grants from the Beatrice Hunter Cancer Research Institute (to Eric Pace), the Natural Sciences and Engineering Research Council (NSERC) of Canada (to Eric Pace and H.P. Vasantha Rupasinghe) and the Chinese Scholarship Council (to Yuanyuan Jiang).

Author Contributions: Eric Pace performed the extractions and impact of temperature studies. Yuanyuan Jiang and Eric Pace conducted the cell culture experiments. Amy Clemens assessed the impact of temperature on PGA. Tennille Crossman assisted with the experiments and writing the manuscript. H.P. Vasantha Rupasinghe, the principal investigator of the project, designed all the experiments. All the co-authors contributed to writing the manuscript and have read and approved the final manuscript.

Conflicts of Interest: The authors have no conflict of interest to declare.

References

1. Rupasinghe, H.P.V.; Yu, L.J.; Bhullar, K.S.; Bors, B. Haskap (*Lonicera caerulea*): A new berry crop with high antioxidant capacity. *Can. J. Plant Sci.* **2012**, *92*, 1311–1317. [CrossRef]
2. Celli, G.B.; Ghanem, A.; Brooks, M.S.L. Haskap berries (*Lonicera caerulea* L.)—A critical review of antioxidant capacity and health-related studies for potential value-added products. *Food Bioprocess Technol.* **2014**, *7*, 1541–1554. [CrossRef]
3. Khattab, R.; Brooks, M.S.; Ghanem, A. Phenolic analyses of haskap berries (*Lonicera caerulea* L.): Spectrophotometry versus high performance liquid chromatography. *Int. J. Food Prop.* **2016**, *19*, 1708–1725. [CrossRef]
4. Chen, L.; Xin, X.; Yuan, Q.; Su, D.; Liu, W. Phytochemical properties and antioxidant capacities of various colored berries. *J. Sci. Food Agric.* **2014**, *94*, 180–188. [CrossRef] [PubMed]
5. Fan, Z.L.; Wang, Z.Y.; Liu, J.R. Cold-field fruit extracts exert different antioxidant and antiproliferative activities in vitro. *Food Chem.* **2011**, *129*, 402–407. [CrossRef]
6. Sun, C.; Zheng, Y.; Chen, Q.; Tang, X.; Jiang, M.; Zhang, J.; Li, X.; Chen, K. Purification and anti-tumour activity of cyanidin-3-*O*-glucoside from Chinese bayberry fruit. *Food Chem.* **2012**, *131*, 1287–1294. [CrossRef]
7. Liu, W.; Xu, J.; Wu, S.; Liu, Y.; Yu, X.; Chen, J.; Tang, X.; Wang, Z.; Zhu, X.; Li, X. Selective anti-proliferation of HER2-positive breast cancer cells by anthocyanins identified by high-throughput screening. *PLoS ONE* **2013**, *8*, e81586. [CrossRef] [PubMed]
8. Serra, D.; Paixão, J.; Nunes, C.; Dinis, T.C.P.; Almeida, L.M. Cyanidin-3-glucoside suppresses cytokine-induced inflammatory response in human intestinal cells: Comparison with 5-aminosalicylic acid. *PLoS ONE* **2013**, *8*, e73001. [CrossRef] [PubMed]
9. Zhao, J.G.; Yan, Q.-Q.; Lu, L.-Z.; Zhang, Y.-Q. In vivo antioxidant, hypoglycemic, and anti-tumor activities of anthocyanin extracts from purple sweet potato. *Nutr. Res. Pract.* **2013**, *7*, 359–365. [CrossRef] [PubMed]
10. Aboonabi, A.; Singh, I. Chemopreventive role of anthocyanins in atherosclerosis via activation of Nrf2–ARE as an indicator and modulator of redox. *Biomed. Pharmacother.* **2015**, *72*, 30–36. [CrossRef] [PubMed]
11. Rupasinghe, H.P.V.; Boehm, M.M.; Sekhon-Loodu, S.; Parmar, I.; Bors, B.; Jamieson, A.R. Anti-inflammatory activity of haskap cultivars is polyphenols-dependent. *Biomolecules* **2015**, *5*, 1079–1098. [CrossRef] [PubMed]
12. Roleira, F.M.F.; Tavares-da-Silva, E.J.; Varela, C.L.; Costa, S.C.; Silva, T.; Garrido, J.; Borges, F. Plant derived and dietary phenolic antioxidants: Anticancer properties. *Food Chem.* **2015**, *183*, 235–258. [CrossRef] [PubMed]

13. Duthie, S.J.; Gardner, P.T.; Morrice, P.C.; Wood, S.G.; Pirie, L.; Bestwick, C.C.; Milne, L.; Duthie, G.G. DNA stability and lipid peroxidation in vitamin E-deficient rats in vivo and colon cells in vitro: Modulation by the dietary anthocyanin, cyanidin-3-glycoside. *Eur. J. Nutr.* **2005**, *44*, 195–203. [CrossRef] [PubMed]
14. Fantini, M.; Benvenuto, M.; Masuelli, L.; Frajese, G.; Tresoldi, I.; Modesti, A.; Bei, R. In vitro and in vivo antitumoral effects of combinations of polyphenols, or polyphenols and anticancer drugs: Perspectives on cancer treatment. *Int. J. Mol. Sci.* **2015**, *16*, 9236–9282. [CrossRef] [PubMed]
15. Hui, C.; Bin, Y.; Xiaoping, Y.; Long, Y.; Chunye, C.; Mantian, M. Anticancer activities of an anthocyanin-rich extract from black rice against breast cancer cells in vitro and in vivo. *Nutr. Cancer* **2010**, *62*, 1128–1136. [CrossRef] [PubMed]
16. Kopjar, M.; Piližota, V. Prevention of thermal degradation of anthocyanins in blackberry juice with addition of different sugars. *CyTA-J. Food* **2011**, *9*, 237–242. [CrossRef]
17. Kamiloglu, S.; Capanoglu, E.; Grootaert, C.; Van Camp, J. Anthocyanin absorption and metabolism by human intestinal caco-2 cells—A review. *Int. J. Mol. Sci.* **2015**, *16*, 21555–21574. [CrossRef] [PubMed]
18. Chaovanalikit, A.; Thompson, M.M.; Wrolstad, R.E. Characterization and quantification of anthocyanins and polyphenolics in blue honeysuckle (*Lonicera caerulea* L.). *J. Agric. Food Chem.* **2004**, *52*, 848–852. [CrossRef] [PubMed]
19. Kusznierewicz, B.; Piekarska, A.; Mrugalska, B.; Konieczka, P.; Namies, J. Phenolic composition and antioxidant properties of polish blue-berried honeysuckle genotypes by HPLC-DAD-MS, HPLC postcolumn derivatization with ABTS or FC, and TLC with DPPH visualization. *J. Agric. Food Chem.* **2012**, *60*, 1755–1763. [CrossRef] [PubMed]
20. Sadilova, E.; Stintzing, F.C.; Carle, R. Thermal degradation of acylated and nonacylated anthocyanins. *J. Food Sci.* **2006**, *71*, 504–512. [CrossRef]
21. Liu, C.L.; Wang, J.M.; Chu, C.Y.; Cheng, M.T.; Tseng, T.H. In vivo protective effect of protocatechuic acid on *tert*-butyl hydroperoxide-induced rat hepatotoxicity. *Food Chem. Toxicol.* **2002**, *40*, 635–641. [CrossRef]
22. Babich, H.; Sedletcaia, A.; Kenigsberg, B. In vitro cytotoxicity of protocatechuic acid to cultured human cells from oral tissue: Involvement in oxidative stress. *Pharmacol. Toxicol.* **2002**, *91*, 245–253. [CrossRef] [PubMed]
23. Nakamura, Y.; Torikai, K.; Ohto, Y.; Murakami, A.; Tanaka, T.; Ohigashi, H. A simple phenolic antioxidant protocatechuic acid enhances tumor promotion and oxidative stress in female ICR mouse skin: Dose-and timing-dependent enhancement and involvement of bioactivation by tyrosinase. *Carcinogenesis* **2000**, *21*, 1899–1907. [CrossRef] [PubMed]
24. Forester, S.C.; Waterhouse, A.L. Gut metabolites of anthocyanins, gallic acid, 3-*O*-methylgallic proliferation of caco-2 cells. *J. Agric. Food Chem.* **2010**, *58*, 5320–5327. [CrossRef] [PubMed]
25. Forester, S.C.; Oteiza, P.; Waterhouse, A.L.; Forester, S.C.; Oteiza, P.; Waterhouse, A.L. The anthocyanin metabolites gallic acid, 3-*O*-methylgallic acid, and 2,4,6-trihydroxybenzaldehyde decrease human colon cancer cell viability by regulating pro-oncogenic signals. *Mol. Carcinog.* **2014**, *53*, 432–439. [CrossRef] [PubMed]
26. De Ferrars, R.M.; Czank, C.; Zhang, Q.; Botting, N.P.; Kroon, P.A.; Cassidy, A.; Kay, C.D. The pharmacokinetics of anthocyanins and their metabolites in humans. *Br. J. Pharmacol.* **2014**, *171*, 3268–3282. [CrossRef] [PubMed]
27. Czank, C.; Cassidy, A.; Zhang, Q.; Morrison, D.J.; Preston, T.; Kroon, P.A.; Botting, N.P.; Kay, C.D. Human metabolism and elimination of the anthocyanin, cyanidin-3-glucoside: A 13C-Tracer study. *Am. J. Clin. Nutr.* **2013**, *97*, 995–1003. [CrossRef] [PubMed]
28. Bhullar, K.S.; Rupasinghe, H.P.V. Antioxidant and cytoprotective properties of partridgeberry polyphenols. *Food Chem.* **2015**, *168*, 595–605. [CrossRef] [PubMed]
29. Lee, J.; Durst, R.W.; Wrolstad, R.E. Determination of total monomeric anthocyanin pigment content of fruit juices, beverages, natural colorants, and wines by the pH differential method: Collaborative study. *J. AOAC Int.* **2005**, *88*, 1269–1278. [PubMed]
30. Liu, L.; Cao, S.Q.; Pan, S.Y. Thermal degradation kinetics of three kinds of representative anthocyanins obtained from blood orange. *Agric. Sci. China* **2011**, *10*, 642–649. [CrossRef]
31. Nayak, B.; Liu, R.H.; Tang, J. Effect of processing on phenolic antioxidants of effect of processing on phenolic antioxidants of fruits, vegetables, and grains—A review. *Crit. Rev. Food Sci. Nutr.* **2015**, *55*, 887–918. [CrossRef] [PubMed]

32. Olivas-Aguirre, F.J.; Rodrigo-García, J.; Martínez-Ruiz, N.R.; Cárdenas-Robles, A.I.; Mendoza-Díaz, S.O.; Álvarez-Parrilla, E.; González-Aguilar, G.A.; de la Rosa, L.A.; Ramos-Jiménez, A.; Wall-Medrano, A. Cyanidin-3-*O*-glucoside: Physical-Chemistry, foodomics and health effects. *Molecules* **2016**, *21*, 1264. [CrossRef] [PubMed]
33. Patras, A.; Brunton, N.P.; Donnell, C.O.; Tiwari, B.K. Effect of thermal processing on anthocyanin stability in foods; mechanisms and kinetics of degradation. *Trends Food Sci. Technol.* **2010**, *21*, 3–11. [CrossRef]
34. Brenes, C.H.; Del Pozo-Insfran, D.; Talcott, S.T. Stability of copigmented anthocyanins and ascorbic acid in a grape juice model system. *J. Agric. Food Chem.* **2005**, *53*, 49–56. [CrossRef] [PubMed]
35. Zorić, Z.; Dragović-Uzelac, V.; Pedisić, S.; Kurtanjek, Ž.; Garofulić, I.E. Kinetics of the degradation of anthocyanins, phenolic acids and flavonols during heat treatments of freeze-dried sour cherry Marasca paste. *Food Technol. Biotechnol.* **2014**, *52*, 101–108.
36. Khattab, R.; Ghanem, A.; Brooks, M.S.-L. Stability of haskap berry (*Lonicera caerulea* L.) anthocyanins at different storage and processing conditions. *J. Food Res.* **2016**, *5*, 67. [CrossRef]
37. Sadilova, E.; Carle, R.; Stintzing, F.C. Thermal degradation of anthocyanins and its impact on color and in vitro antioxidant capacity. *Mol. Nutr. Food Res.* **2007**, *51*, 1461–1471. [CrossRef] [PubMed]
38. Arslan, D. Effects of degradation preventive agents on storage stability of anthocyanins in sour cherry concentrate. *Agron. Res.* **2015**, *13*, 892–899.
39. Yin, M.; Lin, C.-C.; Wu, H.; Tsao, S.; Hsu, C.-K. Apoptotic effects of protocatechuic acid in human breast, lung, liver, cervix, and prostate cancer cells: Potential mechanisms of action. *J. Agric. Food Chem.* **2009**, *57*, 6468–6473. [CrossRef] [PubMed]

2

Cytoprotective Activities of Milk Thistle Seed Oil used in Traditional Tunisian Medicine on 7-Ketocholesterol and 24S-Hydroxycholesterol-Induced Toxicity on 158N Murine Oligodendrocytes

Wiem Meddeb [1,2,3,4], Leila Rezig [5], Amira Zarrouk [6,7], Thomas Nury [1], Anne Vejux [1], Michel Prost [8], Lionel Bretillon [9], Mondher Mejri [2,3,10] and Gérard Lizard [1,*]

1 Team Bio-PeroxIL, Biochemistry of the Peroxisome, Inflammation and Lipid Metabolism (EA7270)/University Bourgogne Franche-Comté/Inserm, 21000 Dijon, France; wiem.meddeb7@gmail.com (W.M.); thomas.nury@u-bourgogne.fr (T.N.); anne.vejux@u-bourgogne.fr (A.V.)
2 Department of Biotechnology, Institut Préparatoire aux Etudes Scientifiques et Techniques (IPEST), La Marsa 2070, Tunisia; mondhermejri54@gmail.com
3 Laboratory Matériaux, Molécules et Applications (LMMA), University of Carthage, La Marsa, Tunis 2078, Tunisia
4 Faculty of Science of Bizerte, Zarzouna, Bizerte 7021, Tunisia
5 Food Conservation and Valorization Laboratory, High Institute of Food Industries, 58 Avenue Alain Savary, El Khadra City, Tunis 1003, Tunisia; l_rezig@yahoo.fr
6 Lab. NAFS, Nutrition—Functional Food & Vascular Diseases LR12-ES-05, University of Monastir, Monastir 5000, Tunisia; zarroukamira@gmail.com
7 Faculty of Medicine, University of Sousse, Sousse 4002, Tunisia
8 Laboratoire Spiral, 21560 Couternon, France; michelprost.spiral@wanadoo.fr
9 Eye & Nutrition Research Group, CSGA, UMR 1324 INRA, 6265 CNRS, 21000 Dijon, France; lionel.bretillon@inra.fr
10 Department of Biotechnology, University of Jendouba, Jendouba 8100, Tunisia
* Correspondence: gerard.lizard@u-bourgogne.fr

Abstract: The Asteraceae family is economically very important, because many of these plants are grown mainly for their food value, such as lettuce (Lactuca), chicory (Cichorium), and sunflower (Heliantus aminus). One of the typical properties of this family, which includes milk thistle (*Sylibum marianum*), is the richness of the oil in various compounds (flavonoids, alkaloids, tocopherols, and unsaturated fatty acids). Currently, and for the coming decades, age-related diseases, including neurodegenerative diseases, are a major public health problem. Preventing their appearance or opposing their evolution is a major objective. In this context, the cytoprotective activities of milk thistle seed oil produced in Tunisia were studied on the 158N model using 7-ketocholesterol (7KC) and 24S-hydroxycholesterol (24S) as cytotoxic agents. 7KC and 24S were used because they can be increased in the brain and body fluids of patients with major age-related neurodegenerative diseases, such as Alzheimer's and Parkinson's diseases. In order to evaluate the cytoprotective properties of milk thistle seed oil, complementary techniques of microscopy, flow cytometry, and biochemistry were used. The chemical composition of milk thistle seed oil has also been determined by various chromatography techniques. Milk thistle seed oils from different area of Tunisia are rich in tocopherols and are strongly antioxidant according to various biochemical tests (KRL (Kit Radicaux Libres), FRAP (Ferric Reducing Antioxidant Power), and DPPH (2,2-diphenyl-1-picrylhydrazyl)). The main fatty acids are linoleic acid (C18:2 n-6) and oleic acid (C18:1 n-9). The main polyphenols identified are homovanillic acid, p-coumaric acid, quercetin, and apigenin, with a predominance of vanillic acid. On 158N cells, milk thistle seed oil attenuates the cytotoxicity of 7KC and 24S including: loss of cell adhesion, increased plasma membrane permeability, mitochondrial dysfunction, overproduction of reactive oxygen species, induction of apoptosis, and autophagy. The attenuation of the cytotoxicity of 7KC and 24S observed with the milk thistle seed oil is in the order of that observed with α-tocopherol used as a positive control. In the presence of nigella seed oil, considered potentially cytotoxic, no cytoprotective effects were observed. Given the chemical characteristics, antioxidant properties, and cytoprotective activities of milk thistle seed oil, our results highlight the potential benefit of this oil for human health.

Keywords: 158N murine oligodentrocytes; milk thistle seed oil; *Silybum marianum*; 7-ketocholesterol; 24S-hydroxycholesterol; cytoprotection

---

1. Introduction

Ageing and age-related diseases, including neurodegenerative diseases, are dependent on genetic and epigenetic factors, including environmental and lifestyle parameters. In nerve cells, these factors can favor neurodegeneration and increase the risk of Alzheimer's disease and Parkinson disease which are age-related diseases [1]. It is therefore important to determine the main causes of these neurodegenerative diseases and to better understand their physiopathology. Indeed, this will permit further identification of natural or synthetic compounds that are capable of preventing neurodegeneration which has increased in developed and developing countries mainly due to the enhancement of life expectancy [2].

Among the potentially deleterious compounds present in the body, several oxysterols (which are cholesterol derivatives brought by the diet, formed by auto-oxidation and/or enzymatically) play important roles in cell metabolism, RedOx balance and inflammation, particularly in vascular and nerve cells which are strongly affected by the aging process [3–6].

In vitro data have shown that the oxysterols negatively affect many cell types: the brain, eyes, heart, bone, colon, and prostate cells [7]. Oxysterols have been identified as important actors in the pathophysiology of several age-related diseases, such as atherosclerosis, type 2 diabetes mellitus, Alzheimer's disease, age-related macular degeneration (ARMD) and cataract, osteoporosis, and some forms of cancer (colon carcinoma and prostate cancer) [4,6,7].

7-ketocholesterol (7KC), resulting from the auto-oxidation of cholesterol [8], is often present in enhanced levels in the tissues, plasma, and/or cerebrospinal fluid of patients with cardiovascular diseases, ARMD, and neurodegenerative diseases [9–13]. This oxysterol is a powerful inducer of oxidative stress, inflammation, cell death (apoptosis and autophagy (oxiapoptophagy: OXIdative stress + APOPTOsis + autoPHAGY) in different cell lines (monocytes, neurons, oligodendrocytes, retinal pigment epithelial cells). Another important oxysterol is 24S-hydroxycholesterol (24S). This oxysterol, also named cerebrosterol, which is synthesized in the brain by the neurons via the enzyme CYP46A1, is able to cross the blood–brain barrier for further degradation in the liver [11].

To prevent oxysterol-induced cytotoxic activities (oxidative stress, inflammation, and cell death) [4], it is important to identify natural and synthetic compounds, and mixture of compounds, that are capable of counteracting or attenuating their side effects.

Natural products are generally classified as primary or secondary metabolites. Among the primary metabolites that are widely distributed in nature are vegetable oils [14]. Several plant extracts are known for their preventive as well as curative effects for age-related diseases, including cardiovascular diseases, neurodegenerative diseases, ocular diseases, intestinal cancers, and cancer of the lungs, prostate and breast.

The extract of pistachio seeds induces a decrease in the proliferation of MCF-7 (Michigan Cancer Foundation–7) breast cancer cells and could be exploited as a "natural food additive" in combination with chemotherapy treatment [15]. Other plant extracts have also shown anti-proliferative effects, such as milk thistle seed extract and pumpkin seed extract which inhibit the proliferation of Human Colon Cancer Cells (HT-29) [16]. Work realized by Rahal et al. [17] highlighted the biological activity of milk thistle oil on a colon cancer cell line, Caco-2. These extracts contain bioactive components which could be responsible for their therapeutic effects, such as antioxidants, tocopherols, and carotenoids [16,18]. It has also been shown that black and red raspberry extracts and grapes, which have anti-proliferative activity against human HT-29 cancer cells, contain elevated concentrations of phenols and anthocyanins, tocopherols and carotenoids, and α-linolenic acid (C18:3 n-3) [16,18]. The α-linolenic acid found in these extracts can be converted to eicosapentaenoic acid (EPA: C20:5 n-3) and docosahexaenoic acid (DHA: C22:6 n-3) which can have cytoprotective activity against several chronic human diseases, including cardiovascular diseases and cancer [19,20].

Among the biologically active natural components present in milk thistle (*Silybum marianum*), silymarin is a polyphenol with antioxidant properties that has been reported to have anti-proliferative effects against several cancer cells [21,22]. The anti-proliferative effects of milk thistle seed components have been reported in several cancers: prostate [21,23], bladder [24,25], colon [26,27], lung [21,28], and breast cancer cells [22]; the associated mechanisms include cell cycle arrest, cyclin-dependent kinase and cyclin inhibition, and induction of apoptosis. However, one study on breast carcinogenesis in rats and mice demonstrated an increase in breast tumors with silymarin treatment compared to a control [29]. The use of silymarin as a molecule that can prevent cancer has been summarized by Vejux et al., exposing its effects on the process of carcinogenesis, oxidative stress, cell cycle arrest, kinase pathways, and cell death [30].

Work realized by Kittur et al. [31], which evaluated the effects of milk thistle extract on the differentiation and survival of neural cells, demonstrates that this extract can promote differentiation and neuronal survival (evocating neurotrophic activities), and protect the neurons of the rat hippocampus against cell death induced by oxidative stress. These latter data suggest a potential benefit of the chemicals present in milk thistle on the nervous system.

Other plant extracts of *Centella Asiatic*, which is known for its pharmacological effects in the central nervous system [32], have also shown neuroprotective effects, such as the prevention of mitochondrial dysfunction, increased expression of antioxidant enzymes, and decreased lipid peroxidation, which are the main causes of dopaminergic neurodegeneration in Parkinson's disease.

Altogether, these studies suggest that several plant extracts, including that of milk thistle, could be used to prevent neurodegenerative diseases. Indeed, some of these compounds, especially tocopherols and polyphenols, are capable to cross the blood–brain barrier. Currently, herbal products are increasingly being used as dietary supplements and therapeutic agents. Most of these natural products are used in traditional medicine due to their antioxidant properties. Among the oils that are the most well known for their pharmacological properties in traditional Arab herbal medicine, milk thistle seed oil is very rich in α-tocopherol. As α-tocopherol has been shown to have neuroprotective effects, milk thistle seed oil could be a useful candidate for preventing the cytotoxic effects induced by 7KC and 24S which can be observed at increased levels in the brains and plasma of patients with neurodegenerative diseases [6,11,13].

In the present study, the chemical compositions (fatty acids, polyphenols, phytosterols, tocopherols) of milk thistle seed oils from different area of Tunisia (Zaghouan, Bizete, Sousse) were determined as well as their antioxidant properties. The ability of milk thistle oil to attenuate 7KC- and 24S-induced side effects (inhibition of cell proliferation, mitochondrial dysfunction, oxidative stress, apoptosis, and autophagy) was also studied on 158N murine oligodendrocytes. As nigella seed oil is considered potentially cytotoxic based on popular empirical knowledge, the chemical characteristics of this oil were also determined as well as its ability to prevent, or not, 7KC- and 24S-induced side effects on 158N cells. It is noteworthy that, whereas no cytoprotective effects were observed with nigella seed oil, a marked attenuation of 7KC- and 24S-induced side effects was observed with milk thistle seed oil from different areas of Tunisia (Zaghouan, Bizerte, and Sousse).

2. Materials and Methods

2.1. Cold Extraction of Oils

2.1.1. Seed Materials

The present study mainly concerns milk thistle (*Silybum marianum*) seeds originating from three different area of Tunisia, namely Zaghouan (36°24′ N 10°09′ E), Bizerte (37°16′28″ N 9°52′26″ E), and Sousse (35°50′ N 10°38′ E). The plants were harvested in May and June 2014, during which time the plants reach maturity and senescence. Currently, as little is known about the effects of the environment (soil, climate) on the characteristics of milk thistle seed oils, the seed were collected in three different area of Tunisia.

Seeds of *Nigella sativa* (Asian origin, also named black cumin) were also used; they were bought from souk Blat (Tunisia).

2.1.2. Extraction of Oils

The seeds of milk thistle (*Silybum marianum* L.) and nigella (*Nigella sativa*) were obtained by cold pressing. This technique provides a cold extraction of the solid sample oil contained in a plant hopper. The oils obtained were stored at (−20 °C) for further analyses.

2.2. Cell Culture and Treatments

Murine oligodendrocytes (158N) [33] were cultured in Dulbecco's Modified Eagle's Medium (DMEM) (Lonza, Amboise, France) with 5% (v/v) heat-inactivated fetal bovine serum (FBS) (Dutscher, Brumath, France) and 1% antibiotics (penicillin, streptomycin) (Dutscher). The cells were inoculated at 30,000 cells/cm^2, either in petri dishes (100 × 20 mm, FALCON, Corning, NY, USA) with 10 mL of culture medium, or at 240,000 cells per well on six-well plates with 2 mL of culture medium.

7-Ketocholesterol (7KC; Ref: C2394) was from Sigma-Aldrich (St Quentin Fallavier, France) and 24S-hydroxycholesterol (24S) was provided by Mohammad Samadi (University of Lorraine, Metz, France). The stock solutions of 7KC and 24S were prepared at 800 μg/mL (2 mM), as described by Ragot et al. [34]. After 24 h of culture, treatments with 7KC and 24S (25 and 50 μM) were performed for 24 h with or without milk thistle seed oil. *Nigella sativa* seed oil, known for its potential cytotoxic effects, was simultaneously used, as well as α-tocopherol (Sigma-Aldrich: 400 μM) which is known to prevent 7KC-induced side effects [34]. The concentrations of 7KC, 24S, and α-tocopherol as well as the times of treatment were in accordance with those described with these compounds in previous studies [35–41].

Stock solutions of milk thistle seed oils (milk thistle oils from different area of Tunisia: Zaghouan, Bizerte, and Sousse) and nigella seed oil were prepared at 10% (v/v) in absolute ethanol. For cell processing, one volume of this stock solution was diluted into 100 volumes of culture medium; the final oil concentration was 0.1% (v/v).

When the cells were treated with 7KC and 24S, associated with milk thistle seed oil, nigella seed oil, or α-tocopherol, these compounds were added 2 h before 7KC and 24S. Based on the concentrations of 7KC and 24S used, it was assumed that the intracellular oxysterol content obtained in vitro was in the range of those that occur in vivo [34,42]. α-Tocopherol was used at the highest non-cytotoxic concentration (400 μM) capable of preventing 7KC and 24S-induced oxiapoptophagy in many cell types [35,36,38,39,43].

2.3. Determination of the Fatty Acid Profiles of Milk Thistle Oils and Nigella Oil by Gas Chromatography

The lipids were extracted from the various oils (milk thistle seed oils from different areas of Tunisia (Zaghouan, Bizerte, Sousse) and nigella oil) according to the method of Moilanen and Nikkari [44]. C19:0 was used as an internal standard. The lipids were transmethylated using boron trifluoride in methanol, in accordance with Morrison & Smith [45]. The fatty acid methyl esters were then analyzed under the same conditions as those described by Debbabi et al. [46] and Badreddine et al. [47]. The data were processed with EZChrom Elite software (Agilent Technologies, Massy, France) and are reported in mg/g total lipids.

2.4. Determination of the Tocopherol Profile of Milk Thistle Oils and Nigella Oil by High Pressure Liquid Chromatography

Before the high performance liquid chromatography (HPLC) analysis, 0.5 g of the seed oil was diluted with 5 mL of hexane, and 5 μL of the sample was then injected. The tocopherol composition of the seed oils was determined by HPLC in accordance with the standard [NF EN ISO 9936] [46,47]. The samples were then analyzed by HPLC (Agilent 1100, Palo Alto, CA, USA), as previously described by Debbabi et al. [46] and Badreddine et al. [47]. The quantification was based on an external standard method and the tocopherol standards were mixed in a solution of hexane (2 mg/mL) prepared on the basis of the standard compounds: α-, β-, γ- and δ-tocopherols.

2.5. Analysis of Polyphenols of Milk Thistle Oils and Nigella Oil

Three grams of each oil were dissolved in 6 mL of petroleum ether and then, were cleaned on a cartridge of silica for solide phase extraction (SPE) (conditioned with 6 mL of petroleum ether). The cartridge was then washed with 12 mL of petroleum ether and dried under a stream of nitrogen for 10 min. The polyphenolic compounds were eluted with 8 mL of methanol/distilled water 80/20 (*v*/*v*) and then with 8 mL of acetonitrile. The eluate was evaporated under reduced pressure at 50 °C. The residue was taken up in 1 mL of a mixture of methanol/distilled water 60/40 (*v*/*v*). The resulting extract was filtered through an 0.45 μm nylon membrane. The analysis of the polyphenols was done by the HPLC-MS method, as described by Badreddine et al. [47]. The phenolic compounds were identified using a combination of high performance liquid chromatography (HPLC) with Agilent 1100 diode array detection and electrospray ionization mass spectrometry (ESI-LC-MS) based on their ultraviolet (UV) spectra, comparing the spectra with those of the authentic standards available.

2.6. Analysis of Phytosterols of Milk Thistle Oils and Nigella Oil

The analysis of sterols was realized as described by Badreddine et al. [47], Mounts et al. [48], and Park et al. [49]. Quantitation of phytosterols and phytostanols was performed by adding cholestanol as an internal standard. The analyses were performed in triplicate.

2.7. KRL (Kit Radicaux Libres) Test

The antioxidant potential of milk thistle oils, nigella oil, α-tocopherol, silymarin, resveratrol, and ferrulic acid was evaluated with the KRL (Kit Radicaux Libres) test, as previously described [46,50]. The data are presented in Trolox equivalents. Hemolysis was recorded using a 96-well microplate reader by measuring the decay of the optical density at 450 nm on a spectrophotometer. For each well, absorbance measurements were made 75 times, once every 150 s.

2.8. Determination of Ferric Reducing Antioxidant Power (FRAP)

The Ferric Reducing Antioxidant Power (FRAP) test, which measures the antioxidant potential of compounds or mixtures of compounds by reducing ferric iron (Fe^{3+}) to ferrous iron (Fe^{2+}), was realized as previously described [51,52]. The absorbance of the reaction medium was read at 700 nm against a blank prepared by replacing the extract with distilled water to calibrate the spectrophotometer. An increase in absorbance corresponded to an increase in the reducing power of the extracts tested [53]. The reducing power of the extracts in mg of Trolox per g of dry matter (mg of Trolox/g of dry matter) was calculated as follows:

$$\text{Iron reduction power (\%)} = [\text{Absorbance control 700} - \text{Absorbance sample 700})/\text{Absorbance control 700}] \times 100.$$

For milk thistle oils, nigella oil, α-tocopherol, ferrulic acid, resveratrol, and silymarin (used as a positive control), the FRAP method was performed as described by Debbabi et al. [46]. For the various oils analyzed, the corresponding antioxidant power was expressed in Trolox equivalents for 1 mL of oil.

2.9. DPPH Assay

The DPPH assay for 2,2-diphenyl-1-picrylhydrazyl (C18H12N5O6) (Sigma-Aldrich) can be regarded as a free radical scavenger test. The DPPH assay is used to measure the anti-radical activity of compounds or mixtures of compounds. The absorbance was read at 517 nm (Sunrise spectrophotometer, Tecan, Lyon, France). The negative control contained 100 μL of water and 100 μL of the DPPH solution. The antioxidant potentials of α-tocopherol, silymarin, ferrulic acid, and resveratrol (used as positive controls) were estimated in Trolox equivalents (1 mole of α-tocopherol, silymarin, ferrulic acid, or resveratrol is equivalent to X mole of Trolox; the calibration curve was obtained with Trolox) [46,47]. For the milk thistle oils from the different areas of Tunisia and for the nigella oil, the corresponding antioxidant powers were expressed as the Trolox equivalent for 1 mL of oil.

2.10. Crystal Violet Test

Crystal violet staining (Sigma-Aldrich) is used to highlight cell proliferation by estimating the proportion of adherent cells [54]. After cell staining with violet crystal (Sigma-Aldrich) in 12-well plates, the absorbance was measured at 598 nm with a microplate reader (Sunrise spectrophotometer, Tecan, Lyon, France).

2.11. Measurement of Mitochondrial Activity with the MTT (Methylthiazolyldiphenyl-Tetrazolium Bromide) Test

To evaluate the mitochondrial activity, the MTT test was used. It is based on the reduction of MTT salt to formazan in metabolically active cells [55,56]. At the end of the treatment, the cells were incubated in the presence of MTT for 3 h, formazan was solubilized by the addition of dimethylsulfoxide (Sigma-Aldrich), and the optical density was measured at 570 nm with a microplate reader (Sunrise spectrophotometer).

2.12. Measurement of Superoxide Anions Production with Dihydroethidium

Dihydroethidium (DHE, Life Technologies) was used to detect overproduction of the superoxide anion ($O_2\bullet^-$) [57]. DHE (2 μM final concentration, incubation: 15 min, 37 °C) is rapidly oxidized in the cells in ethidium by reactive oxygen species, mainly $O_2\bullet^-$ [58]. The fluorescent signals were collected through a 590/20 nm bandpass filter on a logarithmic scale on a GALAXY flow cytometer (Partec); 10,000 cells were acquired. Flomax (Partec) or Flowjo (Tree Star Inc., Ashland, OR, USA) was used to analyze the data.

2.13. Measurement of Plasma Membrane Permeability with Propidium Iodide

The measurement of plasma membrane permeability was based on the property of propidium iodide (PI) to enter in dead cells and/or in cells with damaged plasma membranes [59]. The fluorescence of PI (used at 1 μg/mL) was collected with a 630 nm pass filter on a Galaxy flow cytometer (Partec). Ten thousand cells were acquired, and Flomax (Partec) or Flowjo (Tree Star Inc.) was used to analyze the data.

2.14. Quantification of Apoptotic Cells after Nuclei Staining with Hoechst 33342

The nuclear morphology of apoptotic cells can be determined after staining with Hoechst 33342 (2 μg/mL). Observations were performed by fluorescence microscopy under a UV light with an Axioskop microscop (Zeiss, Jena, Germany). The percentages of cells with condensed and/or fragmented nuclei, which are characteristic of apoptotic cells, were determined [59]. For each sample, 300 cells were observed. The cells were deposited on glass slides by cytocentrifugation (5 min, 1500 rpm) with a cytospin 2 (Shandon, Cheshire, UK).

2.15. Analysis of Caspase-3 and Microtubule-Associated Protein 1 Light Chain 3 (LC3) by Polyacrylamide Gel Electrophoresis and Western Blotb

The analysis of caspase-3 and LC3 was realized by polyacrylamide gel electrophoresis and Western blot analysis, as previously described by Nury et al. [39]. Briefly, cell lysis was performed in a Radioimmunoprecipitation assay buffer (RIPA buffer) containing protease inhibitors (Roche Diagnostics, Indianapolis, IN, USA) for 30 min on ice followed by centrifugation (20 min, 20,000× *g*) to remove cell debris. Seventy micrograms of protein were separated on a 14% SDS-PAGE gel for caspase-3 and LC3 and transferred to a nitrocellulose membrane (Bio-Rad, Marne La Coquette, France). After blocking nonspecific binding sites for 2 h with 5% milk powder in PBST (PBS, 0.1% Tween 20, pH 7.2), the membrane was incubated overnight at 4 °C with the primary antibody diluted in PBST—antibodies to caspase-3 (rabbit polyclonal antibody, Ozyme/Cell Signaling, ref: # 9662) and LC3-I/II (rabbit polyclonal antibody, Sigma-Aldrich, ref.: L8918)—at a final dilution of 1/1000. To standardize the results, an antibody directed against β-actin (mouse monoclonal antibody, ref: A2228, Sigma-Aldrich) was used at a final concentration of 1/10,000. After 2 washings with PBST, the membrane was incubated for 1 h at room temperature with a goat anti-rabbit antibody conjugated with horseradish peroxidase (Cell Signaling, No. 7074) diluted to 1/5000. The membrane was then revealed using an improved chemiluminescence detection kit (Supersignal West Femto Maximum Sensitivity Substrate, Thermo-Scientific) and ChemiDoc™ XRS+ (Bio-Rad). The (LC3-II/LC3-I) ratio was calculated and the levels of cleaved caspase-3 were normalized with actin with Image Lab software (Bio-Rad).

2.16. Statistical Analyses

The data are expressed as means ± standard deviations (SDs). Statistical analyses involved two-way ANOVAs (Tukey Multiple Comparison Test) with GraphPad Prism 6.07 software (GraphPad Software, La Jolla, CA, USA). p-Values less than or equal to 0.05 were considered statistically significant.

3. Results and Discussion

3.1. Profiles of Fatty Acids, Phytosterols, Tocopherols, and Polyphenols Cold-Extracted from Milk Thistle Seed Oils from Different Area of Tunisia

Milk thistle seed oil (MTSO) is known for its high level of secondary metabolites, such as phenolic acids, tocopherols, fatty acids, and phytosterols, which depend on many intrinsic (genetic) and extrinsic (environmental) parameters [60–62]. In the present study, we focused on the fatty acids, phytosterols, polyphenols and tocopherols present in MTSO. Data obtained were compared with nigella seed oil which is mainly empirically known for its toxic activity.

Milk thistle seed oil (MTSO; from Tunisia—Bizerte, Sousse and Zaghouan) and nigella seed oil (NSO; from Tunisia) were analyzed. The fatty acid compositions of these oils are given in Table 1. Linoleic acid (C18:2 n-6) was the most abundant polyunsaturated fatty acid (PUFA) detected in MTSO and NSO. The results show that the oils used in this experiment had high levels of linoleic acid. From a nutritional point of view, as for many other dietary oils, MTSO is a good source of essential fatty acids, especially linoleic acid. Another unsaturated fatty acid quantitatively high in MTSO was oleic acid (C18:1 n-9). Palmitic acid (C16:0) was the most abundant saturated fatty acid in MTSO and NSO, followed by stearic acid (C18:0). Very long-chain saturated fatty acids (C22:0 and C24:0) were found to have high amounts in MTSO. In addition to the fatty acid profiles, the composition of tocopherols is an important parameter to define the potential health benefits of vegetable oils. The tocopherol contents of the oils studied are given in Table 2. The results show that α- and β-tocopherols were the only ones detected in cold-pressed MTSO from Bizerte and represented 47.65 mg/kg and 1.91 mg/kg, respectively. In the oils from Zaghouan and Sousse, the four tocopherols were detected with a predominance of α-tocopherol which represented 98.92% and 88.59%, respectively. The amounts of α-tocopherol in the MTSO of Zaghouan and Sousse were in the same range as those reported by El-Mallah et al. [60] in MTSO extracted with chloroform-methanol (84.5%) and those reported by Fathi-Achachlouei and Azadmard-Damirchi [61] for Iranian varieties of Barak, and for MTSO extracted by hexane/isopropanol (84.9% and 86.36%, respectively). The amount of α-tocopherol was greater than that reported by Parry et al. [16] (78.78%) in cold-pressed MTSO, and by Hasanlou et al. [63] in MTSO (69.02%) extracted by petroleum ether (Soxhlet apparatus). In the MTSO from Sousse, the high content of α-tocopherol (considered to be the most biologically active tocopherol) [64] was followed by γ-tocopherol, β-tocopherol, and δ-tocopherol. The amounts of β- and γ-tocopherol were greater than those observed in the MTSO from Zaghouan. Thus, the cold pressed MTSO from Zaghouan is an ideal source of total α-tocopherol, while that of Sousse could serve as a source of γ-tocopherol. It is noteworthy that compared to olive and argan oils, the highest values of α-tocopherol were observed in MTSO [46,47].

Table 1. Saturated fatty acid and unsaturated fatty acid contents expressed as percentage of total fatty acids (FA) in milk thistle seed oil (MTSO) and nigella seed oil (NSO).

Fatty Acids	Origins of Milk Thistle Seed Oil (MTSO)			Nigella Seed Oil (NSO)
	Sousse	Zaghouan	Bizerte	
C12:0	0.00	0.00	0.11 ± 0.00	0.00
C14:0	0.08 ± 0.00	0.07 ± 0.02	0.13 ± 0.00	0.16 ± 0.001
C15:0	0.00	0.00	0.00	0.00
C16:0	13.06 ± 0.07	6.25 ± 2.00	8.89 ± 0.14	12.29 ± 0.043
C17:0	0.09 ± 0.00	0.08 ± 0.03	0.10 ± 0.00	0.07 ± 0.00
C18:0	3.35 ± 0.11	4.03 ± 1.32	5.21 ± 0.02	3.37 ± 0.05
C20:0	1.48 ± 0.06	2.33 ± 0.71	2.72 ± 0.09	0.22 ± 0.01
C22:0	0.76 ± 0.00	1.86 ± 0.59	1.99 ± 0.11	0.05 ± 0.00
C24:0	0.19 ± 0.00	0.40 ± 0.13	0.46 ± 0.03	0.00
C16:1 n-7	19.24 ± 0.17	18.98 ± 0.80	19.63 ± 0.10	0.22 ± 0.00
C16:1 n-9	0.00	0.00	0.00	0.00
C18:1n-9	21.39 ± 0.02	15.78 ± 4.95	19.03 ± 0.01	22.76 ± 0.02
C18:1 n-7	0.79 ± 0.01	0.40 ± 0.13	0.57 ± 0.01	1.09 ± 0.00
C18:2 n-6	56.77 ± 0.57	48.70 ± 14.94	58.47 ± 0.20	54.56 ± 0.14
C20:1 n-9	0.31 ± 0.00	0.72 ± 0.21	0.81 ± 0.01	0.32 ± 0.00
C18:3 n-3	0.49 ± 0.01	0.11 ± 0.03	0.16 ± 0.00	1.54 ± 0.02
C20:2 n-6	0.00	0.00	0.00	2.25 ± 0.02
C22:1 n-9	0.00	0.06 ± 0.04	0.00	0.11 ± 0.02
∑SFA	19.24 ± 0.17	18.98 ± 0.80	19.63 ± 0.10	16.18 ± 0.01
∑UFA	80.83 ± 1.86	83.30 ± 4.39	79.12 ± 0.20	82.85 ± 0.14

SFA: saturated fatty acids; UFA: unsaturated fatty acids. Values are the mean ± SD of three determinations.

Table 2. Tocopherol content (mg kg^{-1}) of milk thistle seed oil (MTSO).

Area from Tunisia	Bizerte	Zaghouan	Sousse
Tocopherol			
α	47.65 ± 3.54	286.22 ± 25.49	278.47 ± 24.64
β	1.91 ± 0.21	3.58 ± 0.37	6.66 ± 0.74
γ	0.0	14.24 ± 1.25	23.94 ± 2.14
δ	0.0	14.24 ± 1.22	5.23 ± 0.61
Total	49.57 ± 5.11	318.29 ± 28.45	314.31 ± 30.77

Values are the mean ± SD of three determinations.

As phytosterols are components that are present in the unsaponifiable lipid fraction of plant cell membranes [64] and are abundant in vegetable oils (nuts, cereals), it was important to determine the content and composition of the sterols in the MTSO studied (Table 3). β-Sitosterol was the main sterol in all oils. Schottenol was also detected at a high level in MTSO and, in particular, in Zaghouan MTSO. Campesterol was determined in appreciable amounts, especially in the MTSO from Sousse. The presence of cholesterol is in agreement with the results reported by Fathi-Achachlouei and Azadmard-Damirchi [61] as well as by Dabbour et al. [62]. Cholesterol could be formed by demethylation of sitosterol. The synthesis of cholesterol in plants remains to be clarified [65]. Cholesterol can be localized in the nucleus, chloroplasts, and microsomes in free or esterified form. Cholesterol is an important constituent of the leaf wall. It should be noted that high levels of cholesterol have been reported in palm, corn, and sunflower oils [66]. Cholesterol has never been identified, even at very low levels, in olive and argan oils, whatever the geographic origin of the oils [46,47].

Table 3. Sterol and phytosterol contents (% of total sterols) of milk thistle seed oil (MTSO) and nigella seed oil (NSO).

Sterols	Origins of Milk Thistle Seed Oil (MTSO)			Nigella Seed Oil (NSO)
	Bizerte	Zaghouan	Sousse	
Cholesterol	11.47 ± 0.04	4.53 ± 0.01	9.53 ± 0.03	0.55 ± 0.01
Campesterol	4.75 ± 0.01	4.77 ± 0.02	10.89 ± 0.03	6.97 ± 0.06
Δ7-Campesterol	4.14 ± 0.01	4.81 ± 0.02	2.73 ± 0.02	0.18 ± 0.03
Spinasterol	0	0	0	0
β-Sitosterol	31.96 ± 0.13	32.78 ± 0.05	42.33 ± 0.01	34.91 ± 0.30
Schotenol	20.97 ± 0.09	24.54 ± 0.12	6.86 ± 0.03	0.51 ± 0.03
Stigmasterol	20.97 ± 0.09	5.91 ± 0.03	4.88 ± 0.01	6.92 ± 0.09
β-amyrine	4.72 ± 0.01	5.14 ± 0.04	3.08 ± 0.01	1.29 ± 0.08
Δ5 avenasterol	2.83 ± 0.03	3.03 ± 0.02	4.59 ± 0.02	8.50 ± 0.05
cycloartenol	2.14 ± 0.07	1.67 ± 0.03	1.51 ± 0.05	18.34 ± 0.21
Δ7 avenasterol	3.82 ± 0.05	4.68 ± 0.06	3.98 ± 0.07	1.33 ± 0.06
24-Methylene cycloartenol	2.07 ± 0.03	2.40 ± 0.02	2.52 ± 0.01	12.55 ± 0.10
24-Methylene cholesterol	0.25 ± 0.01	0.20 ± 0.01	0.77 ± 0.00	0.82 ± 0.03
Campestanol	0.50 ± 0.01	0.54 ± 0.02	0.91 ± 0.02	0.79 ± 0.01
Δ7-Stigmasterol	0	0	0	0
Clerosterol	0	0	0	0.85 ±0.05
Graminasterol	1.31 ± 0.04	1.54 ± 0.06	1.39 ± 0.02	1.80 ± 0.04
Lupeol	0	0	0	0
Fucosterol	1.77 ± 0.01	2.03 ± 0.05	2.79 ± 0.00	0.91 ± 0.12
Citrostadienol	1.57 ±0.01	1.43 ± 0.00	1.24 ± 0.00	2.78 ± 0.11
Total content (mg/kg)	5206.13 ± 24.23	5088.54 ± 71.96	5891.82 ± 118.12	2659.29 ± 189.56

Values are the mean ± SD of three determinations.

The polyphenol compositions of the oils are given in Table 4. Homovanillic acid, vanillin, p-coumaric acid, quercetin-3β-glucoside, quercetin, and apigenin were identified in MTSO. In nigella seed oil, 2,6-dihydroxybenzoic acid, homovanillic thymoquinone acid, vanillin and some amounts of chlorogenic acid, ferulic acid, quercetin, and apigenin were detected.

As many compounds present in MTSO (phytosterols, polyphenols, tocopherols) are able to prevent nerve cell dysfunction and can cross the blood–brain barrier [67,68], these data reinforced our interest in evaluating the ability of MTSO to prevent the toxic effects of 7KC and 24S [68,69]. So, the ability of MTSO to prevent the side effects induced by 7KC and 24S was compared to α-tocopherol (used as a positive cytoprotective control) and to nigella seed oil (supposed as potentially cytotoxic).

Table 4. Polyphenol contents (mg equivalents quercetin/100 g of oil) of milk thistle seed oil (MTSO) and nigella seed oil (NSO).

Polyphenols	Origins of Milk Thistle Seed Oil (MTSO)			Nigella Seed Oil (NSO)
	Bizerte	Zaghouan	Sousse	
Homovanillic acid	ND	0.13	ND	0.19
Vanillin	ND	0.20	0.33	0.23
p-Coumaric acid	ND	0.07	ND	ND
Quercetine-3β-glucoside	ND	0.08	ND	ND
Quercetin	ND	0.12	ND	0.13
Apigenin	ND	0.09	ND	ND
2,6-Dihydroxybenzoïc acid	ND	ND	ND	1.27
Chlorogenic acid	ND	ND	ND	0.09
Ferrulic acid	ND	ND	ND	0.09
Thymoquinone	ND	ND	ND	0.70
Hydroxytyrosol	ND	ND	ND	ND
Tyrosol	ND	ND	ND	ND
Oleuropein	ND	ND	ND	ND
Luteoline	ND	ND	ND	ND
Protocatechic acid	ND	ND	ND	ND

ND: not detected. Values are the mean ± SD of three determinations.

3.2. Evaluation of the Antioxidant Properties of Milk Thistle Seed Oil from Different Area of Tunisia with the KRL, FRAP, and DPPH Tests

The antioxidant properties of α-tocopherol, silymarin, resveratrol, ferrulic acid, and milk thistle seed oil from different area of Tunisia (Zaghouan, Bizerte and Sousse) were determined by three complementary methods: the KRL (Kit Radicaux Libres), the Ferric Reducing Antioxidant Power (FRAP) test, and the DPPH test. These three tests provide similar information for the different compounds studied (Table 5). The α-tocopherol data were in the range of those previously reported and allowed us to validate our data [46,47]. According to the three tests, the antioxidant properties of MTSO and nigella seed oil were similar.

Table 5. Estimation of the antioxidant activities of milk thistle seed oil (MTSO) with the KRL (Kit Radicaux Libres), the ferric reducing antioxidant power (FRAP) test, and the (DPPH) test.

Compounds	Antioxidant Activities (Trolox Equivalent)		
	KRL	FRAP	DPPH
α-Tocopherol	0.94 ± 0.01	0.80 ± 0.06	1.33 ± 0.03
Resveratrol	7.90 ± 0.05	5.27 ± 0.03	4.52 ± 0.04
Silymarin	3.67 ± 0.03	3.47± 0.07	2.96 ± 0.02
Ferrulic acid	4.73 ± 0.05	2.02 ± 0.04	3.36 ± 0.03
Zaghouan MTSO	144.25 ± 0.58	211.06 ± 0.42	216.16 ± 0.45
Bizerte MTSO	180.48 ± 0.49	125.122 ± 0.35	139.480 ± 0.53
Sousse MTSO	160.173 ± 0.33	122.14 ± 0.47	98.54 ± 0.29
Nigella seed oil	ND	312.29 ± 0.35	227.53 ± 0.28

Data are presented in Trolox equivalents for the references (α-tocopherol, resveratrol, silymarin, ferrulic acid): one mole of α-tocopherol, resveratrol, silymarin, ferrulic acid is equivalent to X moles (values shown in the table) of Trolox. For the MTSO from Zaghouan, Bizerte, and Sousse as well as for nigella seed oil, data are also presented in Trolox equivalents: 1 mL of oil is equivalent to X moles (values shown in the table) of Trolox. Data shown are the mean of three independent experiments conducted in triplicate. ND: not detected.

3.3. Effects of Milk Thistle Seed Oil on 7-Ketocholesterol- and 24S-Hydroxycholesterol-Induced Mitochondrial Dysfunction and Cell Growth Inhibition, Assessed with the MTT and Crystal Violet Tests

To determine the impact of MTSO (0.1% *v/v*, final concentration) on the loss of mitochondrial activity and on cell growth inhibition triggered by 7KC and 24S (25 μM, 24 h), the MTT and crystal violet tests were used, respectively. With the MTT test, measurement of the enzymatic activity of succinate dehydrogenase (a mitochondrial enzyme of the Krebs cycle) showed lower MTT values following 7KC and 24S treatment, supporting a loss of $\Delta\Psi m$ and/or a reduced cell growth and/or a loss of cell adhesion [70–72] (Figure 1). The crystal violet test, which permits the evaluation of cell growth, also showed a significant decrease in 158N adherent cells and/or a loss of cell adhesion after treatment with 7KC and 24S for 24 h (Figure 1). In the presence of MTSO or α-tocopherol (400 μM), which was used as a positive control [34], the toxic effects of 7KC (lower MTT values, lower crystal violet values) were significantly reduced, whereas no cytoprotective effects of nigella seed oil were found (Figure 1). No significant differences were observed between the controls, vehicle (ethanol)-treated cells, MTSO, and α-tocopherol for cell growth evaluated with the crystal violet test (Figure 1). However, lower MTT and crystal violet values, similar to those observed with 7KC and 24S, were observed with nigella seed oil, and no cytoprotective effects of nigella seed oil were found; nigella seed oil did not prevent 7KC- and 24S-induced mitochondrial dysfunction and cell growth inhibition.

3.4. *Effects of Milk Thistle Seed Oil on 7-Ketocholesterol and 24S-Hydroxycholesterol-Induced Overproduction of Reactive Oxygen Species*

As 7KC induces oxidative stress, which can contribute to oxiapoptophagy, in numerous cell types (murine microglial BV-2 cells [35], human SK-N-BE neuroblastoma cells [72], human U937 monocytic cells [73], and murine oligodendrocyte 158N cells [39,74]), the ability of MTSO to prevent oxidative stress was studied. The effects of MTSO (0.1% *v*/*v*, final concentration) and α-tocopherol (400 μM) on reactive oxygen species (ROS) overproduction under treatment with 7KC and 24S (25 μM, 24 h) were evaluated by flow cytometry after staining with dihydroethidium (DHE). Under treatment with 7KC and 24S, an overproduction of ROS (compared to vehicle-treated cells) was observed. Thus, after treatment with 7KC and 24S, the percentage of DHE-positive cells significantly increased. Treatment with MTSO or α-tocopherol alone had no effect on the production of ROS. When MTSO and α-tocopherol were added with 7KC and 24S, the overproduction of ROS was greatly and significantly attenuated compared to the condition with 7KC and 24S alone (Figure 2). No significant differences were observed between untreated cells, vehicle (ethanol)-treated cells, and MTSO- or α-tocopherol-treated cells (Figure 2). However, an enhancement of ROS overproduction (similar to with 7KC and 24S) was observed with nigella seed oil, and no cytoprotective effects of nigella seed oil were found; nigella seed oil did not prevent 7KC- and 24S-induced ROS overproduction.

3.5. *Effects of Milk Thistle Seed Oil from Different Areas of Tunisia on Plasma Membrane Permeability under Treatment with 7-Ketocholesterol and 24S-Hydroxycholesterol*

The effects of milk thistle oils (0.1% *v*/*v*, final concentration) and α-tocopherol (400 μM) on the plasma membrane alterations induced by 7KC and 24S (25 μM, 24 h) were evaluated by flow cytometry with propidium iodide (PI). In 158N cells, 7KC and 24S induce an increase in plasma membrane permeability (evaluated by the percentage of PI-positive cells). Compared to control cells and vehicle (ethanol)-treated cells, the percentage of PI-positive cells under treatment with 7KC and 24S significantly increased. When MTSO and α-tocopherol were added with 7KC and 24S, the increase in plasma membrane permeability was strongly attenuated (Figure 3). Treatment with MTSO or α-tocopherol had no effect on the plasma membrane permeability. No significant differences between control, vehicle (ethanol), MTSO, and α-tocopherol were observed. (Figure 3). However, an enhancement of plasma membrane permeability (similar than with 7KC and 24S) was observed with nigella seed oil, and no cytoprotective effects of nigella seed oil were found with oxysterol-induced enhancement of membrane permeability.

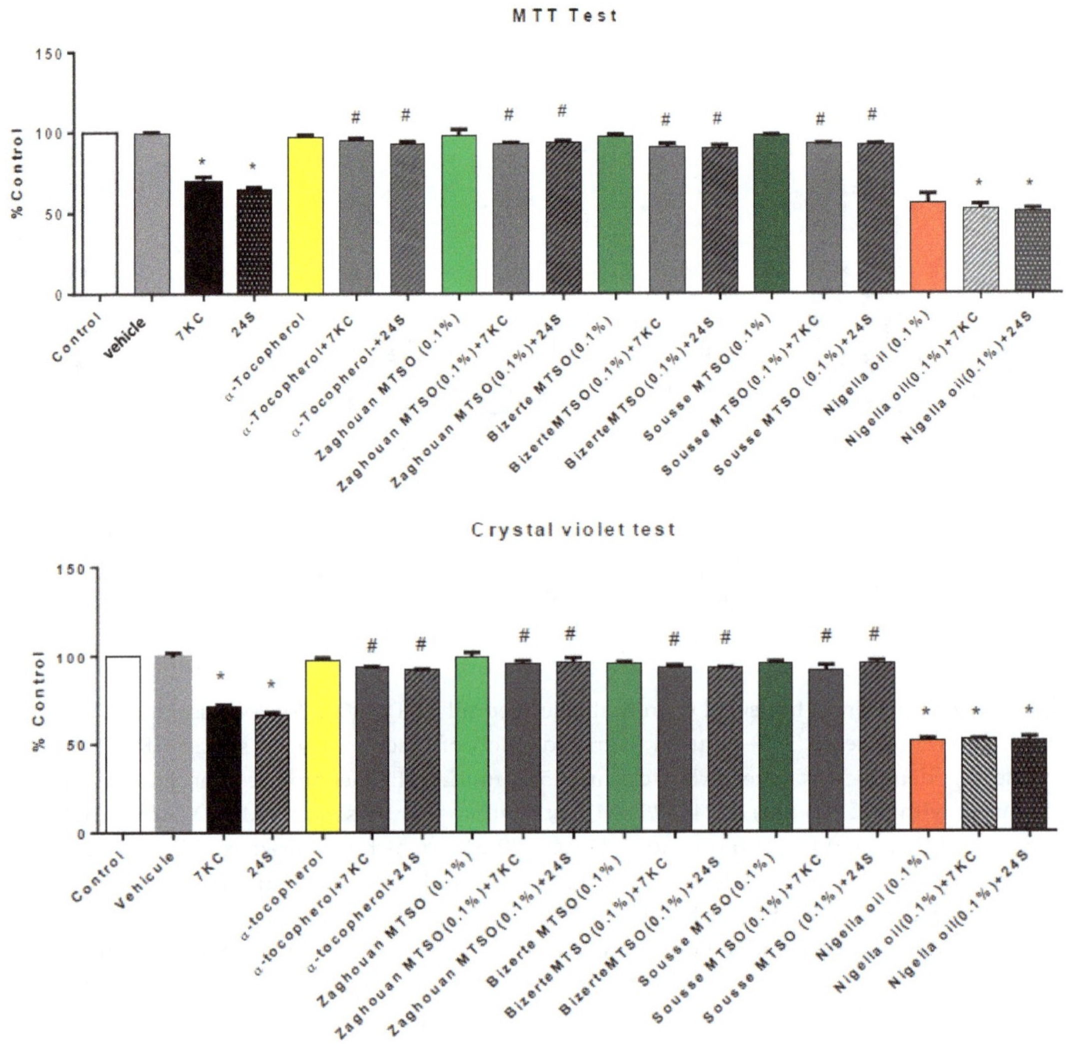

Figure 1. Evaluation of the effects of milk thistle seed oil (MTSO) on 7-ketocholesterol (7KC)- and 24S-hydroxycholesterol (24S)-induced mitochondrial dysfunction and cell growth inhibition in 158N murine oligodendrocytes with the MTT (Methylthiazolyldiphenyl-tetrazolium bromide) and crystal violet tests. After 24 h of culture, 158N murine oligodendrocytes were cultured for 24 h without or with 7KC or 24S (25 μM) in the absence or presence of milk thistle seed oils (MTSO; area: Zaghouan, Bizerte, and Sousse; 0.1% v/v) or α-tocopherol (400 μM), which was used as a positive control. MTSO and nigella seed oil (0.1% v/v), and α-tocopherol were added to the culture medium 2 h before 7KC and 24S. The cytoprotective effects of MTSO on 7KC- and 24S-induced mitochondrial dysfunction (decreased activity of succinate dehydrogenase, a mitochondrial enzyme belonging to the Krebs cycle) and inhibition of cell growth were evaluated with the MTT and crystal violet tests, respectively. Data are the means ± standard deviations (SDs) of two independent experiments carried out in triplicate. The significance of the difference between vehicle and cells treated with 7KC, 24S, MTSO and nigella seed oil or α-tocopherol was calculated with ANOVA tests (Sidak's multiple comparisons); * $p \leq 0.05$. The significance of the difference between cells treated with 7KC alone, 7KC or 24S with MTSO, or 7KC and 24S with α-tocopherol was calculated by ANOVA tests (Sidak's multiple comparisons); # $p \leq 0.05$. No significant differences were found between control and vehicle-treated cells (ethanol).

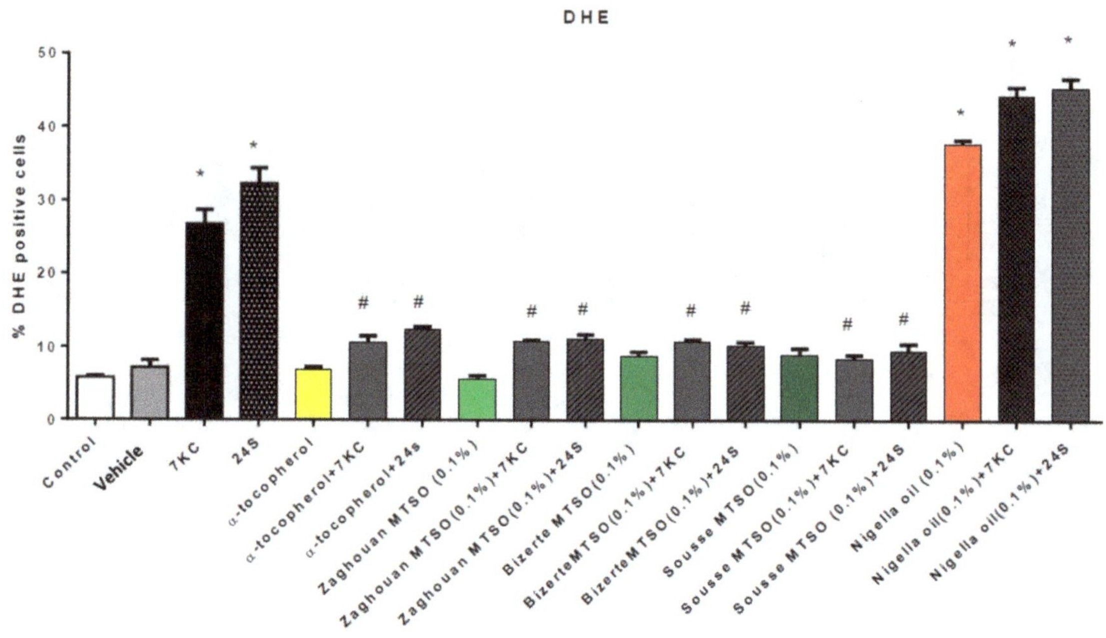

Figure 2. Evaluation of the effect of milk thistle seed oil (MTSO) on 7-ketocholesterol- (7KC) and 24S-hydroxycholesterol (24S)-induced overproduction of reactive oxygen species (ROS) in 158N murine oligodendrocytes. After 24 h of culture, 158N murine oligodendrocytes were cultured for 24 h without or with 7KC (25 μM) or 24S (25 μM) in the absence or presence of MTSO (Area: Zaghouan, Bizerte, and Sousse; 0.1% v/v) or α-tocopherol (400 μM), which was used as the positive control. MTSO, nigella seed oil, and α-tocopherol were added to the culture medium 2 h before 7KC and 24S. The cytoprotective effect of MTSO on 7KC- and 24S-induced ROS overproduction, mainly superoxide anions, was evaluated by flow cytometry after staining with dihydroethidine (DHE). ROS overproduction was determined by the percentage of dihydroethidine (DHE)-positive cells. Data are means ± SDs of two independent experiments carried out in triplicate. The significance of the differences between vehicle and cells treated with 7KC, MTSO, nigella seed oil, or α-tocopherol was calculated by ANOVA tests (Sidak's multiple comparisons); * $p \leq 0.05$. The significance of the differences between cells treated with 7KC or 24S, 7KC or 24S with MTSO, and 7KC or 24S with α-tocopherol was calculated by ANOVA tests (Sidak's multiple comparisons); # $p \leq 0.05$. No significant differences between control, vehicle (ethanol), MTSO, and α-tocopherol were observed.

3.6. Effects of Milk Thistle Seed Oil on 7-Ketocholesterol- and 24S-Hydroxycholesterol-Induced Apoptosis and Autophagy

The effects of MTSO (0.1% v/v) and α-tocopherol (400 μM) on 7KC- and 24S- (25 and/or 50 μM, 24 h) induced apoptosis and autophagy were evaluated by nuclear staining with Hoechst 33342, allowing the identification of cells with apoptotic nuclei (Supplementary Figure S1) by the activation of caspase-3 for apoptosis and by conversion of LC3-I in LC3-II leading to an increase in [LC3-II/LC3-I] for autophagy [74]. The MTSO from Zaghouan was chosen to determine the impact on caspase-3 activation and on the conversion of LC3-I in LC3-II, based on this oil having the highest content of α-tocopherol. As shown by staining with Hoechst 33342, in the presence of 7KC and 24S (25 and/or 50 μM; 24 h), both MTSO (0.1% v/v) and α-tocopherol (400 μM) were able to reduce apoptosis (Figure 4).

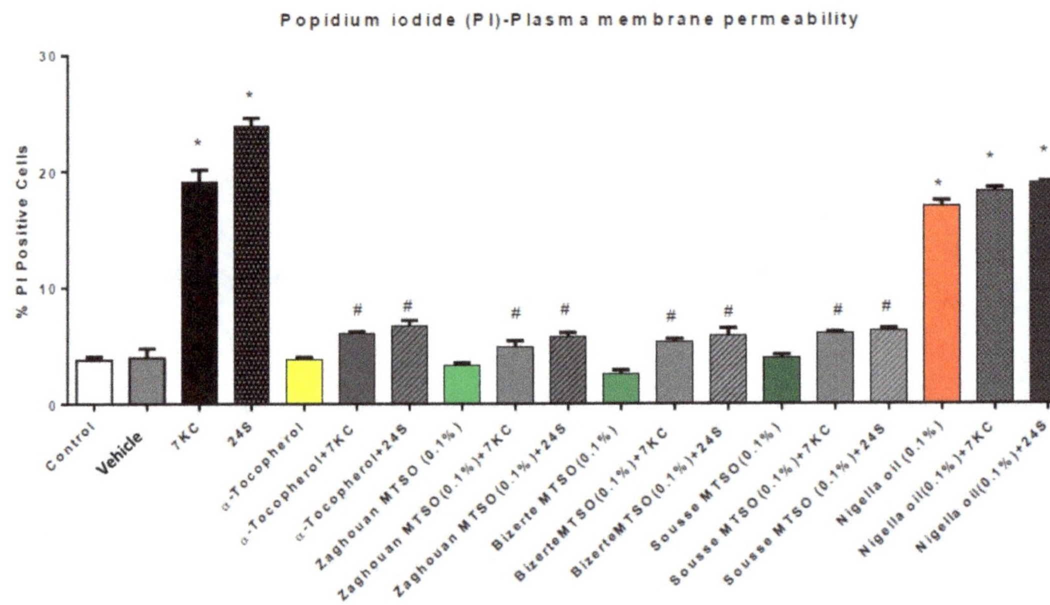

Figure 3. Effect of milk thistle seed oil (MTSO) on 7-ketocholesterol (7KC)- and 24S-hydroxycholesterol (24S)-induced plasma membrane permeability in 158N murine oligodendrocytes. After 24 h of culture, 158N murine oligodendrocytes were cultured for 24 h without or with 7KC or 24S (25 μM) in the absence or presence of MTSO (Area: Zaghouane, Bizerte, and Sousse; 0.1% v/v) or α-tocopherol (400 μM), which was used as a positive control. MTSO, nigella seed oil, and α-tocopherol were added to the culture medium 2 h before 7KC. The cytoprotective effects of MTSO and nigella seed oil on 7KC and 24S-induced plasma membrane permeability were evaluated by flow cytometry after staining with propidium iodide (PI). Plasma membrane permeability was determined by the percentage of PI positive cells. Data are means ± SDs of two independent experiments carried out in triplicate. The significance of the differences between the vehicle and cells treated with 7KC, MTSO, nigella seed oil, or α-tocopherol was calculated by ANOVA tests (Sidak's multiple comparisons); * $p \leq 0.05$. The significance of the differences between the cells treated with 7KC or 24S, 7KC or 24S with MTSO, and 7KC or 24S with α-tocopherol was calculated by ANOVA tests (Sidak's multiple comparisons); # $p \leq 0.05$. No significant difference between the control, vehicle (ethanol), MTSO, and α-tocopherol were observed.

As shown by Western blotting, in the presence of 7KC (25–50 μM; 24 h), both MTSO (0.1% v/v) and α-tocopherol (400 μM) were able to prevent (i) apoptosis, revealed by the presence of cleaved caspase-3, and (ii) autophagy, revealed by activation of LC3-I in LC3-II. In the presence of 7KC (25–50 μM, 24 h), caspase-3 was cleaved in a concentration dependent manner (Figure 5); similarly, the [LC3-II/LC3-I] ratio was increased in a concentration dependent manner (Figure 5). The cleavage of caspase-3 and the activation of LC3-I in LC3-II (revealed by an increase in the LC3-II/LC3-I ratio) were attenuated by MTSO from Zaghouan (Figure 5). When the 158N cells were treated with the vehicle (ethanol), MTSO from Zaghouan (0.1% v/v) or α-tocopherol (400 μM), no caspase-3 cleavage and no increase of the ratio [LC3-II/LC3-I] were observed (Figure 5).

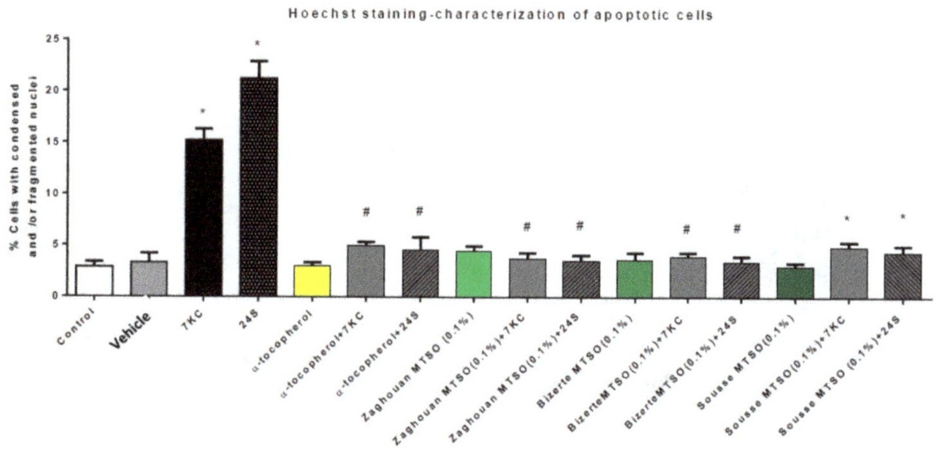

Figure 4. Effects of milk thistle seed oil (MTSO) on 7-ketocholesterol (7KC)- and 24S-hydroxycholesterol (24S)-induced apoptosis evaluated by condensation and/or fragmentation of the nuclei. After 24 h of culture, 158N murine oligodendrocytes were cultured for 24 h with or without 7KC (25 µM) in the absence or presence of MTSO (Area: Zaghouan, Bizerte, and Sousse; 0.1% v/v) or α-tocopherol (400 µM), which was used as the positive control. MTSO and α-tocopherol were added to the culture medium 2 h before 7KC and 24S. Apoptosis was evaluated by the percentage of apoptotic cells characterized by condensed and/or fragmented nuclei, whereas control cells (untreated cells) had round and regular nuclei. Data are the means ± SDs of two independent experiments carried out in triplicate. The significance of the differences between the vehicle and cells treated with 7KC, MTSO, nigella seed oil, or α-tocopherol was calculated by ANOVA tests (Sidak's multiple comparisons); * $p \leq 0.05$. The significance of the differences between cells treated with 7KC or 24S, 7KC or 24S with MTSO, 7KC or 24S with α-tocopherol was calculated by ANOVA tests (Sidak's multiple comparisons); # $p \leq 0.05$. No significant differences between the control, vehicle (ethanol), MTSO, and α-tocopherol were observed.

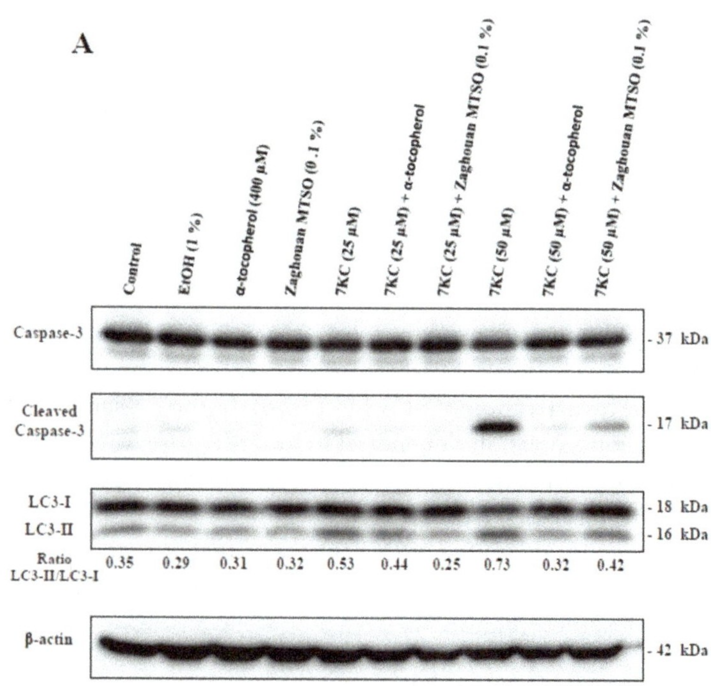

Figure 5. *Cont.*

B

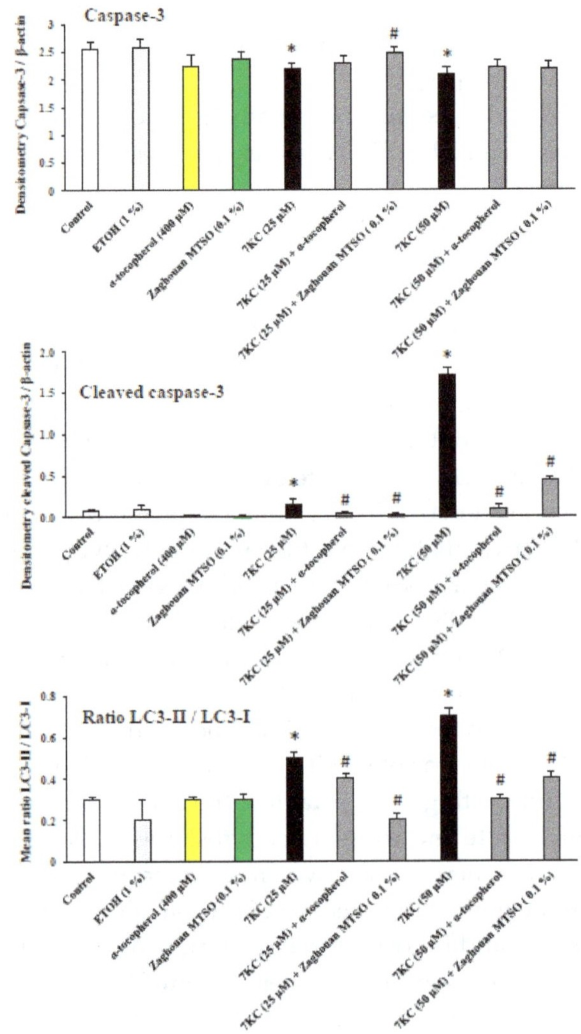

Figure 5. Effects of milk thistle seed oil (MTSO from Zaghouan area, Tunisia) on 7-ketocholesterol (7KC)-induced caspase-3 cleavage and activation of LC3-I in LC3-II. (**A**) After 24 h of culture, 158N murine oligodendrocytes were cultured for 24 h without or with 7KC (25 µM or 50 µM) in the absence or presence of MTSO (Zaghouan; 0.1% v/v) or α-tocopherol (400 µM), which was used as positive control. MTSO and α-tocopherol were added to the culture medium 2 h before 7KC. Apoptosis was evaluated by caspase-3 activation (cleaved caspase-3) and autophagy by conversion of LC3-I to LC3-II (increased LC3-II/LC3-I ratio). (**B**) The means ± SDs of the densitometric values of 3 independent experiments are shown. The ethanol (EtOH) value corresponds to the highest final EtOH concentration present in the culture medium with 7KC (50 µM) associated with MTSO. The significance of the differences between vehicle and cells treated with 7KC, MTSO or α-tocopherol was calculated by ANOVA tests (Sidak's multiple comparisons); * $p \leq 0.05$. The significance of the differences between the cells treated with 7KC, 7KC with MTSO, and 7KC with α-tocopherol was calculated by ANOVA tests (Sidak's multiple comparisons); # $p \leq 0.05$. No significant differences between control, vehicle (ethanol)-treated cells, MTSO, and α-tocopherol were observed. No differences were observed between the control, vehicle (ethanol), MTSO, and α-tocopherol.

3.7. Discussion

The prevalence of some diseases or syndromes increase with age, such as atherosclerosis, Alzheimer's disease, age-related macular degeneration, cataract, and osteoporosis. All of these diseases involve oxidative stress, inflammation, and/or cell death processes [11].

Oxysterols could play an important role in these different age-related pathologies, in particular, in the pathophysiology of the brain. Indeed, several oxysterols can induce several side effects contributing to neurodegeneration [11].

The most widely-considered oxysterols potentially involved in the pathogenesis of the processes of neurodegenerative diseases are 24S [75], which is of enzymatic origin, and 7KC resulting from cholesterol auto-oxidation [8,76].

In 158N murine oligodendrocytes, 7KC and 24S trigger a complex mode of cell death defined as oxiapoptophagy (OXIdation + APOPTOsis + autoPHAGY), simultaneously involving oxidative stress, apoptosis, and autophagy [73,74]. 7KC and 24S induce a decrease in cell proliferation, assessed by crystal violet; an alteration of mitochondrial activity, quantified with the MTT test; increased permeability of plasma membrane, revealed with propidium iodide; overproduction of reactive oxygen species, revealed by dihydroethidium staining; caspase-3 cleavage; and activation of LC3-I into LC3-II that are typical of oxiapoptophagy. In agreement with previous studies, this complex type of cell death induced by 7KC and 24S is attenuated by α-tocopherol [36,38,39,74].

Natural products are considered effective sources for the discovery of powerful and novel therapeutic agents, particularly dietary phytochemicals (polyphenols, terpenes, carotenoids, and others). As some of them are known to protect against oxidative stress, they could be effective in preventing 7KC- and 24S-induced side effects and in preventing and/or treating 7KC- and 24S-associated diseases. At the moment, various phytochemicals (fatty acids, polyphenols, phytosterols, and tocopherols) are able to counter the side effects of oxysterols in different age-related pathologies [68]. Some of these phytochemicals, either food extracts or pure compounds, are present in Mediterranean diet products, such as olive oil, fruits, and vegetables.

In this context, it was interesting (i) to establish the chemical profile of MTSO from different areas of Tunisia (Zaghouan, Bizerte and Sousse) in phytosterols, tocopherols, and polyphenols, since these compounds are potentially neuroprotective, (ii) to determine their antioxidant characteristics, and (iii) to precisely determine their cytoprotective effects on nerve cells.

Currently, oxidative stress and mitochondrial dysfunction are considered key events in several degenerative diseases [77]. Interestingly, the chemical profile of MTSO reveals the presence of numerous compounds that can prevent oxidative stress and mitochondrial dysfunction. Thus, MTSO contains high levels of antioxidant molecules (tocopherols, polyphenols) capable of reducing the overproduction of reactive oxygen species (ROS: ROO•, RO•) [78], which can induce lipid peroxidation leading to protein carbonylation and several types of cellular dysfunction that may contribute to neurodegeneration [79,80]. The presence of these compounds is consistent with the antioxidant properties of MTSO determined with the KRL, DPPH, and FRAP tests. In addition, MTSO is also rich in oleic acid (C18:1 n-9). Although (C18:1 n-9) is not an antioxidant [47], it has been shown in 7KC-treated murine microglia BV-2 cells that this fatty acid is able to attenuate the overproduction of ROS [43,48]. In addition, oleic acid as well as α- and γ-tocopherol have been shown to prevent mitochondrial, lysosomal, and peroxisomal dysfunction in different types of nerve cells [33,34,43,48]. As these compounds, which have been shown to inhibit 7KC- and 24S-induced neurotoxicity are present at low levels in MTSO (the final concentrations of oleic acid, and α- and γ-tocopherol were more than one hundred-fold lower than those in the culture medium when these compounds were used alone), it is possible that some of them may act in synergy to exert cytoprotective effects and/or that several other compounds of MTSO (polyphenolic compounds, sylimarine, etc.), could be involved in the beneficial effects. We must also consider that the different compounds present in MTSO could activate and suppress several signaling pathways contributing to cytoprotection.

It should be noted that when 7KC was used at 25 and 50 μM, two concentrations capable of inducing oxidative stress and favoring oxiapoptophagy [38,80,81], MTSO was able to attenuate the toxicity induced by 7KC (25–50 μM). As observed with α- and γ-tocopherol [47], docosahexahenoic acid [38], acid oleic [46] and dimethylfumarate [72], and argan oil [47], MTSO (0.1% v/v) was able to counteract the inhibition of cell growth associated with 7KC-induced loss of cell adhesion.

These results were highlighted by the crystal violet and the MTT assays. As observed with α- and γ-tocopherol [46,47], docosahexahenoic acid [39], oleic acid [46], polyphenols [82], and dimethylfumarate [72], MTSO also significantly reduced the oxidative stress revealed by DHE staining as well as the percentage of cells permeable to PI. This increased the values of PI positive cells either indicates an increase of dead cells and/or an increase of cells with damaged plasma membranes resulting from lipid peroxidation which could be the consequence of ROS overproduction [4,43]. These cytoprotective effects of MTSO on the plasma membrane evocate those observed with argan oil which protects against the cytotoxic effects induced by 7KC [47]. In addition, 7KC- and 24S-induced mitochondrial dysfunctions were attenuated by MTSO—the mitochondrial dysfunction revealed by the MTT test was attenuated. In addition, MTSO was able to prevent 7KC-induced LC3-I activation in LC3-II and the cleavage of caspase-3, which are the criteria for autophagy and apoptosis, respectively. Currently, the autophagic process associated with 7KC-induced cell death is considered rather beneficial [83,84]. Since some compounds present in MTSO can normalize autophagy and attenuate apoptosis, which are two events involved in neurodegeneration, this is an important argument in favor of the potentially neuroprotective activity of MTSO.

So, it can be considered that MTSO is a mixture of compounds (fatty acids, polyphenols, tocopherols, and phytosterols) that can act synergistically. Polyphenols are mainly hydrophilic molecules present at very low levels in oil; their cytoprotective activity on 7KC-induced oxiapoptophagy can be excluded. On the other hand, fatty acids (especially oleic acid) and tocopherols (mainly α- and γ-tocopherol) are present at high concentrations, and it has already been proved that they prevent 7KC-induced oxiapoptophagy [34,48,72]. It is, therefore, supposed that these compounds probably contribute to the cytoprotective effects of MTSO. Since several data are available on the signaling pathways activated by 7KC [85] and on the cellular targets of tocopherols and oleic acid involved in the attenuation of 7KC-induced side effects [43,86], it will be easy to determine whether this assumption is realistic.

It is noteworthy that in the presence of nigella seed oil, considered potentially toxic, major differences compared to MTSO are observed. Whereas MTSO is cytoprotective, nigella seed oil is not; it is cytotoxic and does not prevent 7KC- and 24S-induced side effects. In vivo, toxic effects of nigella seed oil have also been reported by Zaoui et al. [87], who showed that certain blood parameters were modified, especially the platelet count. Other more recent in vivo studies by Zaghloul et al. [88] confirmed the toxic effect of nigella seed oil on the renal cortex and, to a lesser degree, on hepatic cells. In addition, whereas the content of fatty acids is almost similar in MTSO and nigella seed oil, there are major differences in their sterol contents. It is suggested that, the cytotoxicity of nigella seed oil could be explained, at least in part, by the high content of cycloartenol and methylene cycloartenol which are not found in MTSO. Thymoquinone, which is a polyphenol known for its anti-inflammatory, antioxidant, and anti-proliferative properties, is also only found in MTSO, but its concentration is probably too low to induce side effects [89].

Altogether our data support that our in vitro assay on 158N cells, which is rapid and easy to standardize, could be used as a screening test in order to distinguish and identify oils with different biological activities.

In addition, the present study provides new data that reinforce the interest in the use of MTSO for the prevention of neurodegenerative diseases. The chemical profile of MTSO was quite similar in the three areas of Tunisia studied (Bizerte, Zaghouan, and Sousse), and revealed the presence of fatty acids, polyphenols, phytosterols, and tocopherols capable of attenuating the side effects associated with neurodegeneration (oxidative stress, mitochondrial dysfunction, and apoptosis/autophagy). These chemical characteristics reinforce the interest in the potential of MTSO to prevent age-related diseases including neurodegenerative diseases, since several of its compounds are theoretically capable of crossing the blood–brain barrier and have been shown to have neurotrophic (cytoprotective + differentiating) properties on nerve cells, mainly oleic acid and polyphenols [90,91]. In addition, MTSO has antioxidant properties and is also capable of counteracting 7KC- and 24S-induced oxiapoptophagy in 158N murine oligodendrocytes. Since 7KC and 24S can be increased in patients with neurodegenerative diseases, the cytoprotective effects of MTSO against the toxic effects of 7KC and 24S suggest that MTSO may have beneficial effects related to preventing or slowing down the development of 7KC- and 24S- associated neurodegenerative diseases. In addition, the results obtained on the cytoprotective effects of milk thistle seed oil on 158N cells encourage us to develop more elaborate cell models that take into account the selective passage of certain oil compounds through the blood–brain barrier. Models mimicking the blood–brain barrier by combining endothelial cells, pericytes, and nerve cells [92–94] should provide a more accurate evaluation of the activity of MTSO on brain cells under normal and pathologic conditions induced by mechanical, physical and/or chemical agents.

4. Conclusions

Based on the biochemical and antioxidant characteristics of MTSO, this oil may be beneficial for age-related diseases, including neurodegenerative diseases, and may be associated with diet as functional foods. Indeed, these oils contain numerous molecules (fatty acids, polyphenols, phytosterols, and tocopherols) that are theoretically capable of crossing the blood–brain barrier [92–94] and attenuating numerous neurodegenerative side effects: oxidative stress, mitochondrial dysfunctions, and cell death [36,37,39,46]. In addition, the various compounds present in the MTSO could act in synergy to counter the toxic effects of 7KC of 24S identified at increased levels in patients with neurodegenerative diseases. The data shown in this study also validate the development of a cellular model (158N cells treated with oxysterols) to apprehend the biological activities of oils on brain cells.

Author Contributions: Investigation, W.M., A.Z. and T.N.; Methodology, A.Z., T.N., M.P., L.B., L.R. and M.M.; Validation, W.M., A.Z., M.P., L.B. and T.N.; Writing-Original Draft Preparation, W.M., L.R., A.V. and G.L.; Funding acquisition, M.M. and G.L.; Project administration, M.M. and G.L.; Conceptualization, G.L.; Supervision, G.L.

Funding: This work was supported by grants from the University of Bourgogne (Dijon, France); the University of Carthage (Tunis, Tunisia), and the Faculty of Sciences Bizerte (Bizerte, Tunisia).

Acknowledgments: The authors acknowledge Stéphane Grégoire and Lucy Martine (Inra, Dijon, France) for fatty acids and tocopherols analyses, Emmanuelle Camus-Prost (Laboratoire Spiral, Couternon, France) for polyphenols analysis, and Philippe Durand (Laboratoire Spiral, Couternon, France) for the KRL test.

Conflicts of Interest: The authors declare no conflict of interest.

References

1. Harman, D. The free radical theory of aging. *Antioxid. Redox Signal.* **2003**, *5*, 557–561. [CrossRef] [PubMed]
2. Tosato, M.; Zamboni, V.; Ferrini, A.; Cesari, M. The aging process and potential interventions to extend life expectancy. *Clin. Interv. Aging* **2007**, *2*, 401–412. [PubMed]
3. Lordan, S.; Mackrill, J.J.; O'Brien, N.M. Oxysterols and mechanisms of apoptotic signaling: Implications in the pathology of degenerative diseases. *J. Nutr. Biochem.* **2009**, *20*, 321–336. [CrossRef] [PubMed]
4. Vejux, A.; Lizard, G. Cytotoxic effects of oxysterols associated with human diseases: Induction of cell death (apoptosis and/or oncosis), oxidative and inflammatory activities, and phospholipidosis. *Mol. Asp. Med.* **2009**, *30*, 153–170. [CrossRef] [PubMed]
5. Leoni, V.; Caccia, C. Oxysterols as biomarkers in neurodegenerative diseases. *Chem. Phys. Lipids* **2011**, *164*, 515–524. [CrossRef] [PubMed]
6. Poli, G.; Biasi, F.; Leonarduzzi, G. Oxysterols in the pathogenesis of major chronic diseases. *Redox Biol.* **2013**, *1*, 125–130. [CrossRef] [PubMed]
7. Schroepfer, G.J., Jr. Oxysterols: Modulators of cholesterol metabolism and other processes. *Physiol. Rev.* **2000**, *80*, 361–554. [CrossRef] [PubMed]
8. Iuliano, L. Pathways of cholesterol oxidation via non-enzymatic mechanisms. *Chem. Phys. Lipids* **2011**, *164*, 457–468. [CrossRef] [PubMed]

9. Vejux, A.; Samadi, M.; Lizard, G. Contribution of cholesterol and oxysterols in the physiopathology of cataract: Implication for the development of pharmacological treatments. *J. Ophthalmol.* **2011**, *2011*, 471947. [CrossRef] [PubMed]
10. Rodriguez, I.R.; Clark, M.E.; Lee, J.W.; Curcio, C.A. 7-ketocholesterol accumulates in ocular tissues as a consequence of aging and is present in high levels in drusen. *Exp. Eye Res.* **2014**, *128*, 151–155. [CrossRef] [PubMed]
11. Zarrouk, A.; Vejux, A.; Mackrill, J.; O'Callaghan, Y.; Hammami, M.; O'Brien, N.; Lizard, G. Involvement of oxysterols in age-related diseases and ageing processes. *Ageing Res. Rev.* **2014**, *18*, 148–162. [CrossRef] [PubMed]
12. El-Sayyad, H.; Bakr, E.; El-Ghawet, H.; El-Desoky, T. Overview of congenital, senile and metabolic cataract. *J. Ocular Biol.* **2015**, *3*, 12.
13. Testa, G.; Staurenghi, E.; Zerbinati, C.; Gargiulo, S.; Iuliano, L.; Giaccone, G.; Fantò, F.; Poli, G.; Leonarduzzi, G.; Gamba, P. Changes in brain oxysterols at different stages of Alzheimer's disease: Their involvement in neuroinflammation. *Redox Biol.* **2016**, *10*, 24–33. [CrossRef] [PubMed]
14. Balandrin, M.F.; Klocke, J.A.; Wurtele, E.S.; Bollinger, W.H. Natural plant chemicals: Sources of industrial and medicinal materials. *Science* **1985**, *228*, 1154–1160. [CrossRef] [PubMed]
15. Seifaddinipour, M.; Farghadani, R.; Namvar, F.; Mohamad, J.; Abdul Kadir, H. Cytotoxic Effects and Anti-Angiogenesis Potential of Pistachio (*Pistacia vera* L.) Hulls against MCF-7 Human Breast Cancer Cells. *Molecules* **2018**, *23*, 110. [CrossRef] [PubMed]
16. Parry, J.H.Z.; Luther, M.; Su, L.; Zhou, K.; Yu, L. Characterization of cold-pressed onion, parsley, cardamom, mullein, roasted pumpkin, and milk thistle seed oils. *J. Am. Oil Chem. Soc.* **2006**, *83*, 847–854. [CrossRef]
17. Rahal, N.B.; Barba, F.J.; Barth, D.; Chevalot, I. Supercritical CO_2 extraction of oil, fatty acids and flavonolignans from milk thistle seeds: Evaluation of their antioxidant and cytotoxic activities in Caco-2 cells. *Food Chem. Toxicol.* **2015**, *83*, 275–282. [CrossRef] [PubMed]
18. Parry, J.; Yu, L. Fatty acid content and antioxidant properties of cold-pressed black raspberry seed oil and meal. *J. Food Sci.* **2004**, *69*. [CrossRef]
19. Connor, W.E. Importance of n−3 fatty acids in health and disease. *Am. J. Clin. Nutr.* **2000**, *71*, 171S–175S. [CrossRef] [PubMed]
20. Tapiero, H.; Ba, G.N.; Couvreur, P.; Tew, K. Polyunsaturated fatty acids (PUFA) and eicosanoids in human health and pathologies. *Biomed. Pharmacother.* **2002**, *56*, 215–222. [CrossRef]
21. Singh, R.P.; Dhanalakshmi, S.; Tyagi, A.K.; Chan, D.C.; Agarwal, C.; Agarwal, R. Dietary feeding of silibinin inhibits advance human prostate carcinoma growth in athymic nude mice and increases plasma insulin-like growth factor-binding protein-3 levels. *Cancer Res.* **2002**, *62*, 3063–3069. [PubMed]
22. Zi, X.; Feyes, D.K.; Agarwal, R. Anticarcinogenic effect of a flavonoid antioxidant, silymarin, in human breast cancer cells MDA-MB 468: Induction of G1 arrest through an increase in Cip1/p21 concomitant with a decrease in kinase activity of cyclin-dependent kinases and associated cyclins. *Clin. Cancer Res.* **1998**, *4*, 1055–1064. [PubMed]
23. Deep, G.; Singh, R.; Agarwal, C.; Kroll, D.; Agarwal, R. Silymarin and silibinin cause G1 and G2–M cell cycle arrest via distinct circuitries in human prostate cancer PC3 cells: A comparison of flavanone silibinin with flavanolignan mixture silymarin. *Oncogene* **2006**, *25*, 1053–1069. [CrossRef] [PubMed]
24. Vinh, P.Q.; Sugie, S.; Tanaka, T.; Hara, A.; Yamada, Y.; Katayama, M.; Deguchi, T.; Mori, H. Chemopreventive Effects of a Flavonoid Antioxidant Silymarin on N-Butyl-N-(4-hydroxybutyl) nitrosamine-induced Urinary Bladder Carcinogenesis in Male ICR Mice. *Cancer Sci.* **2002**, *93*, 42–49. [CrossRef]
25. Tyagi, A.; Agarwal, C.; Harrison, G.; Glode, L.M.; Agarwal, R. Silibinin causes cell cycle arrest and apoptosis in human bladder transitional cell carcinoma cells by regulating CDKI–CDK–cyclin cascade, and caspase 3 and PARP cleavages. *Carcinogenesis* **2004**, *25*, 1711–1720. [CrossRef] [PubMed]
26. Kohno, H.; Tanaka, T.; Kawabata, K.; Hirose, Y.; Sugie, S.; Tsuda, H.; Mori, H. Silymarin, a naturally occurring polyphenolic antioxidant flavonoid, inhibits azoxymethane-induced colon carcinogenesis in male F344 rats. *Int. J. Cancer* **2002**, *101*, 461–468. [CrossRef] [PubMed]
27. Yang, S.-H.; Lin, J.-K.; Chen, W.-S.; Chiu, J.-H. Anti-angiogenic effect of silymarin on colon cancer lovo cell line. *J. Surg. Res.* **2003**, *113*, 133–138. [CrossRef]
28. Sharma, O.P.; Bhat, T.K. DPPH antioxidant assay revisited. *Food Chem.* **2009**, *113*, 1202–1205. [CrossRef]

29. Malewicz, B.; Wang, Z.; Jiang, C.; Guo, J.; Cleary, M.P.; Grande, J.P.; Lü, J. Enhancement of mammary carcinogenesis in two rodent models by silymarin dietary supplements. *Carcinogenesis* **2006**, *27*, 1739–1747. [CrossRef] [PubMed]
30. Vejux, A.; Aires, V.; Delmas, D. *Functional Foods and Cancer: Bioactive Compounds and Cancer Volume 4*, 1st ed.; Martirosyan, D.M., Zhou, J.-K., Eds.; CreateSpace Independent Publishing Platform: Lavergne, TN, USA, 2017; p. 204.
31. Kittur, S.; Wilasrusmee, S.; Pedersen, W.A.; Mattson, M.P.; Straube-West, K.; Wilasrusmee, C.; Jubelt, B.; Kittur, D.S. Neurotrophic and neuroprotective effects of milk thistle (Silybum marianum) on neurons in culture. *J. Mol. Neurosci.* **2002**, *18*, 265–269. [CrossRef]
32. Teerapattarakan, N.; Benya-aphikul, H.; Tansawat, R.; Wanakhachornkrai, O.; Tantisira, M.H.; Rodsiri, R. Neuroprotective effect of a standardized extract of Centella asiatica ECa233 in rotenone-induced parkinsonism rats. *Phytomedicine* **2018**, *44*, 65–73. [CrossRef] [PubMed]
33. Baarine, M.; Ragot, K.; Genin, E.C.; El Hajj, H.; Trompier, D.; Andreoletti, P.; Ghandour, M.S.; Menetrier, F.; Cherkaoui-Malki, M.; Savary, S. Peroxisomal and mitochondrial status of two murine oligodendrocytic cell lines (158N, 158JP): Potential models for the study of peroxisomal disorders associated with dysmyelination processes. *J. Neurochem.* **2009**, *111*, 119–131. [CrossRef] [PubMed]
34. Ragot, K.; Mackrill, J.J.; Zarrouk, A.; Nury, T.; Aires, V.; Jacquin, A.; Athias, A.; de Barros, J.-P.P.; Véjux, A.; Riedinger, J.-M. Absence of correlation between oxysterol accumulation in lipid raft microdomains, calcium increase, and apoptosis induction on 158N murine oligodendrocytes. *Biochem. Pharmacol.* **2013**, *86*, 67–79. [CrossRef] [PubMed]
35. Nury, T.; Zarrouk, A.; Ragot, K.; Debbabi, M.; Riedinger, J.-M.; Vejux, A.; Aubourg, P.; Lizard, G. 7-Ketocholesterol is increased in the plasma of X-ALD patients and induces peroxisomal modifications in microglial cells: Potential roles of 7-ketocholesterol in the pathophysiology of X-ALD. *J. Steroid Biochem. Mol. Biol.* **2017**, *169*, 123–136. [CrossRef] [PubMed]
36. Ragot, K.; Delmas, D.; Athias, A.; Nury, T.; Baarine, M.; Lizard, G. α-Tocopherol impairs 7-ketocholesterol-induced caspase-3-dependent apoptosis involving GSK-3 activation and Mcl-1 degradation on 158N murine oligodendrocytes. *Chem. Phys. Lipids* **2011**, *164*, 469–478. [CrossRef] [PubMed]
37. Leoni, V.; Nury, T.; Vejux, A.; Zarrouk, A.; Caccia, C.; Debbabi, M.; Fromont, A.; Sghaier, R.; Moreau, T.; Lizard, G. Mitochondrial dysfunctions in 7-ketocholesterol-treated 158N oligodendrocytes without or with α-tocopherol: Impacts on the cellular profil of tricarboxylic cycle-associated organic acids, long chain saturated and unsaturated fatty acids, oxysterols, cholesterol and cholesterol precursors. *J. Steroid Biochem. Mol. Biol.* **2017**, *169*, 96–110. [PubMed]
38. Zarrouk, A.; Nury, T.; Samadi, M.; O'Callaghan, Y.; Hammami, M.; O'Brien, N.M.; Lizard, G.; Mackrill, J.J. Effects of cholesterol oxides on cell death induction and calcium increase in human neuronal cells (SK-N-BE) and evaluation of the protective effects of docosahexaenoic acid (DHA; C22: 6 n-3). *Steroids* **2015**, *99*, 238–247. [CrossRef] [PubMed]
39. Nury, T.; Zarrouk, A.; Mackrill, J.J.; Samadi, M.; Durand, P.; Riedinger, J.-M.; Doria, M.; Vejux, A.; Limagne, E.; Delmas, D. Induction of oxiapoptophagy on 158N murine oligodendrocytes treated by 7-ketocholesterol-, 7β-hydroxycholesterol-, or 24 (S)-hydroxycholesterol: Protective effects of α-tocopherol and docosahexaenoic acid (DHA; C22: 6 n-3). *Steroids* **2015**, *99*, 194–203. [CrossRef] [PubMed]
40. Miguet, C.; Monier, S.; Bettaieb, A.; Athias, A.; Bessede, G.; Laubriet, A.; Lemaire, S.; Neel, D.; Gambert, P.; Lizard, G. Ceramide generation occurring during 7β-hydroxycholesterol-and 7-ketocholesterol-induced apoptosis is caspase independent and is not required to trigger cell death. *Cell Death Differ.* **2001**, *8*, 83–99. [CrossRef] [PubMed]
41. Kahn, E.; Ménétrier, F.; Vejux, A.; Montange, T.; Dumas, D.; Riedinger, J.-M.; Frouin, F.; Tourneur, Y.; Brau, F.; Stoltz, J.-F. Flow cytometry and spectral imaging multiphoton microscopy analysis of CD36 expression with quantum dots 605 of untreated and 7-ketocholesterol-treated human monocytic cells. *Anal. Quant. Cytol. Histol.* **2006**, *28*, 316–330. [PubMed]
42. Vurusaner, B.; Gamba, P.; Testa, G.; Gargiulo, S.; Biasi, F.; Zerbinati, C.; Iuliano, L.; Leonarduzzi, G.; Basaga, H.; Poli, G. Survival signaling elicited by 27-hydroxycholesterol through the combined modulation of cellular redox state and ERK/Akt phosphorylation. *Free Radic Biol. Med.* **2014**, *77*, 376–385. [CrossRef] [PubMed]

43. Debbabi, M.; Zarrouk, A.; Bezine, M.; Meddeb, W.; Nury, T.; Badreddine, A.; Sghaier, R.; Bretillon, L.; Guyot, S.; Samadi, M. Comparison of the effects of major fatty acids present in the Mediterranean diet (oleic acid, docosahexaenoic acid) and in hydrogenated oils (elaidic acid) on 7-ketocholesterol-induced oxiapoptophagy in microglial BV-2 cells. *Chem. Phys. Lipids* **2017**, *207*, 151–170. [CrossRef] [PubMed]
44. Moilanen, T.; Nikkari, T. The effect of storage on the fatty acid composition of human serum. *Clin. Chim. Acta* **1981**, *114*, 111–116. [CrossRef]
45. Morrison, W.R.; Smith, L.M. Preparation of fatty acid methyl esters and dimethylacetals from lipids with boron fluoride–methanol. *J. Lipid Res.* **1964**, *5*, 600–608. [PubMed]
46. Debbabi, M.; Nury, T.; Zarrouk, A.; Mekahli, N.; Bezine, M.; Sghaier, R.; Grégoire, S.; Martine, L.; Durand, P.; Camus, E. Protective effects of α-tocopherol, γ-tocopherol and oleic acid, three compounds of olive oils, and no effect of trolox, on 7-ketocholesterol-induced mitochondrial and peroxisomal dysfunction in microglial BV-2 cells. *Int. J. Mol. Sci.* **2016**, *17*, 1973. [CrossRef] [PubMed]
47. Badreddine, A.; Zarrouk, A.; Karym, E.M.; Debbabi, M.; Nury, T.; Meddeb, W.; Sghaier, R.; Bezine, M.; Vejux, A.; Martine, L. Argan Oil-Mediated Attenuation of Organelle Dysfunction, Oxidative Stress and Cell Death Induced by 7-Ketocholesterol in Murine Oligodendrocytes 158N. *Int. J. Mol. Sci.* **2017**, *18*, 2220. [CrossRef] [PubMed]
48. Mounts, T.; Abidi, S.; Rennick, K. Effect of genetic modification on the content and composition of bioactive constituents in soybean oil. *J. Am. Oil Chem. Soc.* **1996**, *73*, 581–586. [CrossRef]
49. Park, S.W.; Addis, P. HPLC determination of C-7 oxidized cholesterol derivatives in foods. *J. Food Sci.* **1985**, *50*, 1437–1441. [CrossRef]
50. Rossi, R.; Pastorelli, G.; Corino, C. Application of KRL test to assess total antioxidant activity in pigs: Sensitivity to dietary antioxidants. *Res. Vet. Sci.* **2013**, *94*, 372–377. [CrossRef] [PubMed]
51. Oyaizu, M. Studies on products of browning reaction. *Jpn. J. Nutr. Diet.* **1986**, *44*, 307–315. [CrossRef]
52. Benzie, I.F.; Strain, J.J. The ferric reducing ability of plasma (FRAP) as a measure of "antioxidant power": The FRAP assay. *Anal. Biochem.* **1996**, *239*, 70–76. [CrossRef] [PubMed]
53. Singleton, V.L.; Rossi, J.A. Colorimetry of total phenolics with phosphomolybdic-phosphotungstic acid reagents. *Am. J. Enol. Vitic.* **1965**, *16*, 144–158.
54. Colin, D.; Limagne, E.; Jeanningros, S.; Jacquel, A.; Lizard, G.; Athias, A.; Gambert, P.; Hichami, A.; Latruffe, N.; Solary, E. Endocytosis of resveratrol via lipid rafts and activation of downstream signaling pathways in cancer cells. *Cancer Prev. Res.* **2011**, *4*, 1095–1106. [CrossRef] [PubMed]
55. Lizard, G.; Gueldry, S.; Deckert, V.; Gambert, P.; Lagrost, L. Evaluation of the cytotoxic effects of some oxysterols and of cholesterol on endothelial cell growth: Methodological aspects. *Pathol. Biol.* **1997**, *45*, 281–290. [PubMed]
56. Mosmann, T. Rapid colorimetric assay for cellular growth and survival: Application to proliferation and cytotoxicity assays. *J. Immunol. Methods* **1983**, *65*, 55–63. [CrossRef]
57. Zarrouk, A.; Vejux, A.; Nury, T.; El Hajj, H.I.; Haddad, M.; Cherkaoui-Malki, M.; Riedinger, J.-M.; Hammami, M.; Lizard, G. Induction of mitochondrial changes associated with oxidative stress on very long chain fatty acids (C22: 0, C24: 0, or C26: 0)-treated human neuronal cells (SK-NB-E). *Oxid. Med. Cell. Longev.* **2012**, *2012*, 623257. [CrossRef] [PubMed]
58. Rothe, G.; Valet, G. Flow cytometric analysis of respiratory burst activity in phagocytes with hydroethidine and 2′,7′-dichlorofluorescin. *J. Leukoc. Biol.* **1990**, *47*, 440–448. [CrossRef] [PubMed]
59. Lizard, G.; Fournel, S.; Genestier, L.; Dhedin, N.; Chaput, C.; Flacher, M.; Mutin, M.; Panaye, G.; Revillard, J.P. Kinetics of plasma membrane and mitochondrial alterations in cells undergoing apoptosis. *Cytom. Part A* **1995**, *21*, 275–283. [CrossRef] [PubMed]
60. El-Mallah, H.M.; El-Shami, S.M.; Hassanein, M.M. Detailed studies on some lipids of *Silybum marianum* (L.) seed oil. *Grasas y Aceites* **2003**, *54*, 397–402.
61. Fathi-Achachlouei, B.; Azadmard-Damirchi, S. Milk thistle seed oil constituents from different varieties grown in Iran. *J. Am. Oil Chem. Soc.* **2009**, *86*, 643–649. [CrossRef]
62. Dabbour, I.; Al-Ismail, K.; Takruri, H.; Azzeh, F. Chemical characteristics and antioxidant content properties of cold pressed seed oil of wild milk thistle plant grown in Jordan. *Pak. J. Nutr.* **2014**, *13*, 67–78. [CrossRef]
63. Hasanlou, T.; Bahmani, M.; Sepehrifar, R.; Kalantari, F. Determination of tocopherols and fatty acids in seeds of *Silybum marianum* (L.) gaerth. *J. Med. Plants* **2008**, *7*, 69–76.

64. O'Brian, R.D. *Fats and Oils: Formulating and Processing for Applications*; Taylor & Francis Group, CRC Press: Boca Raton, FL, USA, 2009.
65. Benveniste, P. Biosynthesis and accumulation of sterols. *Annu. Rev. Plant Biol.* **2004**, *55*, 429–457. [CrossRef] [PubMed]
66. Behrman, E.; Gopalan, V. Cholesterol and plants. *J. Chem. Educ.* **2005**, *82*, 1791. [CrossRef]
67. Traber, M.G.; Stevens, J.F. Vitamins C and E: Beneficial effects from a mechanistic perspective. *Free Radic. Biol. Med.* **2011**, *51*, 1000–1013. [CrossRef] [PubMed]
68. Cilla, A.; Alegría, A.; Attanzio, A.; Garcia-Llatas, G.; Tesoriere, L.; Livrea, M.A. Dietary phytochemicals in the protection against oxysterol-induced damage. *Chem. Phys. Lipids* **2017**, *207*, 192–205. [CrossRef] [PubMed]
69. Otaegui-Arrazola, A.; Menéndez-Carreño, M.; Ansorena, D.; Astiasarán, I. Oxysterols: A world to explore. *Food Chem. Toxicol.* **2010**, *48*, 3289–3303. [CrossRef] [PubMed]
70. Lizard, G.; Deckert, V.; Dubrez, L.; Moisant, M.; Gambert, P.; Lagrost, L. Induction of apoptosis in endothelial cells treated with cholesterol oxides. *Am. J. Pathol.* **1996**, *148*, 1625–1638. [PubMed]
71. Zahm, J.M.; Baconnais, S.; Monier, S.; Bonnet, N.; Bessede, G.; Gambert, P.; Puchelle, E.; Lizard, G. Chronology of cellular alterations during 7-ketocholesterol–induced cell death on A7R5 rat smooth muscle cells: Analysis by time lapse-video microscopy and conventional fluorescence microscopy. *Cytom. Part A* **2003**, *52*, 57–69. [CrossRef] [PubMed]
72. Zarrouk, A.; Nury, T.; Karym, E.-M.; Vejux, A.; Sghaier, R.; Gondcaille, C.; Andreoletti, P.; Trompier, D.; Savary, S.; Cherkaoui-Malki, M. Attenuation of 7-ketocholesterol-induced overproduction of reactive oxygen species, apoptosis, and autophagy by dimethyl fumarate on 158 N murine oligodendrocytes. *J. Steroid Biochem. Mol. Biol.* **2017**, *169*, 29–38. [CrossRef] [PubMed]
73. Monier, S.; Samadi, M.; Prunet, C.; Denance, M.; Laubriet, A.; Athias, A.; Berthier, A.; Steinmetz, E.; Jürgens, G.; Nègre-Salvayre, A. Impairment of the cytotoxic and oxidative activities of 7β-hydroxycholesterol and 7-ketocholesterol by esterification with oleate. *Biochem. Biophys. Res. Commun.* **2003**, *303*, 814–824. [CrossRef]
74. Nury, T.; Zarrouk, A.; Vejux, A.; Doria, M.; Riedinger, J.M.; Delage-Mourroux, R.; Lizard, G. Induction of oxiapoptophagy, a mixed mode of cell death associated with oxidative stress, apoptosis and autophagy, on 7-ketocholesterol-treated 158N murine oligodendrocytes: Impairment by α-tocopherol. *Biochem. Biophys. Res. Commun.* **2014**, *446*, 714–719. [CrossRef] [PubMed]
75. Lütjohann, D.; Breuer, O.; Ahlborg, G.; Nennesmo, I.; Siden, A.; Diczfalusy, U.; Björkhem, I. Cholesterol homeostasis in human brain: Evidence for an age-dependent flux of 24S-hydroxycholesterol from the brain into the circulation. *Proc. Natl. Acad. Sci. USA* **1996**, *93*, 9799–9804. [CrossRef] [PubMed]
76. Sottero, B.; Gamba, P.; Gargiulo, S.; Leonarduzzi, G.; Poli, G. Cholesterol oxidation products and disease: An emerging topic of interest in medicinal chemistry. *Curr. Med. Chem.* **2009**, *16*, 685–705. [CrossRef] [PubMed]
77. Tritschler, H.-J.; Packer, L.; Medori, R. Oxidative stress and mitochondrial dysfunction in neurodegeneration. *Biochem. Mol. Biol. Int.* **1994**, *34*, 169–181. [PubMed]
78. Rimbach, G.; Minihane, A.M.; Majewicz, J.; Fischer, A.; Pallauf, J.; Virgli, F.; Weinberg, P.D. Regulation of cell signalling by vitamin E. *Proc. Nutr. Soc.* **2002**, *61*, 415–425. [CrossRef] [PubMed]
79. Grimsrud, P.A.; Xie, H.; Griffin, T.J.; Bernlohr, D.A. Oxidative stress and covalent modification of protein with bioactive aldehydes. *J. Biol. Chem.* **2008**, *283*, 21837–21841. [CrossRef] [PubMed]
80. Klionsky, D.J.; Abdelmohsen, K.; Abe, A.; Abedin, M.J.; Abeliovich, H.; Acevedo Arozena, A.; Adachi, H.; Adams, C.M.; Adams, P.D.; Adeli, K. Guidelines for the use and interpretation of assays for monitoring autophagy. *Autophagy* **2016**, *12*, 1–222. [CrossRef] [PubMed]
81. Guina, T.; Biasi, F.; Calfapietra, S.; Nano, M.; Poli, G. Inflammatory and redox reactions in colorectal carcinogenesis. *Ann. N. Y. Acad. Sci.* **2015**, *1340*, 95–103. [CrossRef] [PubMed]
82. Dugas, B.; Charbonnier, S.; Baarine, M.; Ragot, K.; Delmas, D.; Ménétrier, F.; Lherminier, J.; Malvitte, L.; Khalfaoui, T.; Bron, A. Effects of oxysterols on cell viability, inflammatory cytokines, VEGF, and reactive oxygen species production on human retinal cells: Cytoprotective effects and prevention of VEGF secretion by resveratrol. *Eur. J. Nutr.* **2010**, *49*, 435–446. [CrossRef] [PubMed]
83. He, C.; Zhu, H.; Zhang, W.; Okon, I.; Wang, Q.; Li, H.; Le, Y.-Z.; Xie, Z. 7-Ketocholesterol induces autophagy in vascular smooth muscle cells through Nox4 and Atg4B. *Am. J. Pathol.* **2013**, *183*, 626–637. [CrossRef] [PubMed]

84. Levine, B.; Kroemer, G. Autophagy in the pathogenesis of disease. *Cell* **2008**, *132*, 27–42. [CrossRef] [PubMed]
85. Vejux, A.; Malvitte, L.; Lizard, G. Side effects of oxysterols: Cytotoxicity, oxidation, inflammation, and phospholipidosis. *Braz. J. Med. Biol. Res.* **2008**, *41*, 545–556. [CrossRef] [PubMed]
86. Vejux, A.; Guyot, S.; Montange, T.; Riedinger, J.-M.; Kahn, E.; Lizard, G. Phospholipidosis and down-regulation of the PI3-K/PDK-1/Akt signalling pathway are vitamin E inhibitable events associated with 7-ketocholesterol-induced apoptosis. *J. Nutr. Biochem.* **2009**, *20*, 45–61. [CrossRef] [PubMed]
87. Zaoui, A.; Cherrah, Y.; Mahassini, N.; Alaoui, K.; Amarouch, H.; Hassar, M. Acute and chronic toxicity of Nigella sativa fixed oil. *Phytomedicine* **2002**, *9*, 69–74. [CrossRef] [PubMed]
88. Zaghlol, D.A.A.; Kamel, E.S.; Mohammed, D.S.; Abbas, N.H. The possible toxic effect of different doses of Nigella sativa oil on the histological structure of the liver and renal cortex of adult male albino rats. *Egypt. J. Histol.* **2012**, *35*, 127–136. [CrossRef]
89. Al-Ali, A.; Alkhawajah, A.A.; Randhawa, M.A.; Shaikh, N.A. Oral and intraperitoneal LD50 of thymoquinone, an active principle of Nigella sativa, in mice and rats. *J. Ayub Med. Coll. Abbottabad* **2008**, *20*, 25–27. [PubMed]
90. Giacoppo, S.; Galuppo, M.; Lombardo, G.E.; Ulaszewska, M.M.; Mattivi, F.; Bramanti, P.; Mazzon, E.; Navarra, M. Neuroprotective effects of a polyphenolic white grape juice extract in a mouse model of experimental autoimmune encephalomyelitis. *Fitoterapia* **2015**, *103*, 171–186. [CrossRef] [PubMed]
91. Gundimeda, U.; McNeill, T.H.; Schiffman, J.E.; Hinton, D.R.; Gopalakrishna, R. Green tea polyphenols potentiate the action of nerve growth factor to induce neuritogenesis: Possible role of reactive oxygen species. *J. Neurosci. Res.* **2010**, *88*, 3644–3655. [CrossRef] [PubMed]
92. Vandenhaute, E.; Dehouck, L.; Boucau, M.-C.; Sevin, E.; Uzbekov, R.; Tardivel, M.; Gosselet, F.; Fenart, L.; Cecchelli, R.; Dehouck, M.-P. Modelling the neurovascular unit and the blood-brain barrier with the unique function of pericytes. *Curr. Neurovasc. Res.* **2011**, *8*, 258–269. [CrossRef] [PubMed]
93. Figueira, I.; Tavares, L.; Jardim, C.; Costa, I.; Terrasso, A.P.; Almeida, A.F.; Govers, C.; Mes, J.J.; Gardner, R.; Becker, J.D.; et al. Blood-brain barrier transport and neuroprotective potential of blackberry-digested polyphenols: An in vitro study. *Eur. J. Nutr.* **2017**. [CrossRef] [PubMed]
94. Gosselet, F. Modelling of the blood-brain barrier. *Med. Sci.* **2017**, *33*, 423–431.

3

Betalains in Some Species of the Amaranthaceae Family

Maria Graça Miguel

Faculdade de Ciências e Tecnologia, MeditBio, Universidade do Algarve, Campus de Gambelas, 8005-139 Faro, Portugal; mgmiguel@ualg.pt

Abstract: Natural pigments are largely distributed in the plant kingdom. They belong to diverse groups, with distinct biochemical pathways. Betalains with colours that range from yellow to red-violet can de divided into two main subgroups: betaxanthins and betacyanins. These types of pigments are confined into 13 families of the order Caryophyllales and in some genera of higher fungi (*Amanita muscaria*, *Hygrocybe* and *Hygrophorus*). The Amaranthaceae family includes diverse genera in which betalains are present: *Alternanthera*, *Amaranthus*, *Beta*, *Chenopodium*, *Celosia* and *Gomphrena*. The biosynthesis of betalains and their general biological properties were reviwed in the present work. In addition, the types of betalains present in some species of the aforementioned genera, their stability and production, as well as biological attributes, were reviewed.

Keywords: betalains; alternanthera; amaranthus; beta; chenopodium; celosia; gomphrena

1. Introduction

The colour of flowers, fruits, vegetables and grains result from the presence of chlorophylls, carotenoids, flavonoids and of the water-soluble anthocyanins and betalains [1,2]. Anthocyanins and betalains have never been detected jointly in plant tissues. Anthocyanin pigments (orange, red, purple, blue) occur in all members of the Angiospermae, whereas betalains occur only in 13 families of the order Caryophyllales [3,4].

Betalains are water-soluble pigments classified into betacyanins (red colour) and betaxanthins (yellow colour). They are dissolved inside the vacuoles as *bis*-anions. Betalains can be found in edible fruits and roots, flowers, stems and bracts of species belonging to the families of Caryophyllales, except for Caryophyllaceae and Molluginaceae [5]. These pigments have also been detected in some genera of higher fungi (*Amanita muscaria*, *Hygrocybe* and *Hygrophorus*) [6].

The present work aims to make a review of the betalains present in some species of the genera *Alternanthera*, *Amaranthus*, *Beta*, *Chenopodium*, *Celosia* and *Gomphrena*, which belong to the *Amaranthaceae* family.

2. Betalains

2.1. General Chemical Aspects of Betalains

Betalains are immonium derivatives of betalamic acid [4-(2-oxoethylidene)-1,2,3,4-tetrahydropyridine-2,6-dicarboxylic acid]. The condensation of this structure with amines and/or their derivatives generates yellow betaxanthins (dLatin: beta = beet; Greek: xanthos = yellow), whereas the condensation of betalamic acid with *cyclo*-dopa [*cyclo*-3-(3,4-dihydroxyphenylalanine)] or its glucosyl derivatives gives rise to violet betacyanins (Latin: beta = beet; Greek: kyaneos = blue) (Figure 1) [7,8]. The resulting glycosides of betacyanins can be linked to acylation groups, leading to several structures [9].

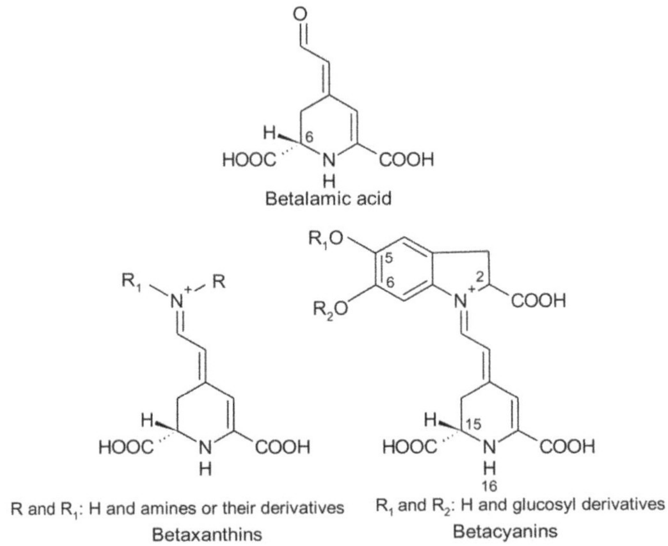

Figure 1. Structures of betalamic acid, betaxanthins and betalains.

Four structural types of betacyanins have been reported: betanin, gomphrenin, amaranthin and bougainvillein [6]. These structures differ by the attachment of glucosyl groups to the oxygen atoms in the *o*-position on the *cyclo*-dopa moiety [6]. Betanin-type group has a hydroxyl attached to the C_6 carbon and a glucosyl or derivative on the C_5 carbon (Figure 2), whereas gomphrenin-type group possesses a hydroxyl attached to the C_5 carbon and a glucosyl or derivative on the C_6 carbon (Figure 2). Amaranthin-type group has the glucuronylglucosyl moiety or derivative linked to the C_5 carbon. Bougainvillein-type group may possess a diglucosyl moiety or derivative linked to the C_5 carbon or to the C_6 carbon of carboxylated or decarboxylated betacyanins [6]. Betaxanthins are divided into two groups: amino acid-derived conjugate group and amine-derived conjugate group. In both cases, they are linked to the conjugated moiety of betalamic acid [10].

The 1,7-diazaheptamethinium resonance system with conjugated double bonds of betalamic acid (Figure 1) is responsible for its lemon-yellow colour [7]. The conjugation of a substituted aromatic nucleus to this chromophore shifts the absorbance maximum from 480 nm in yellow betaxanthins to 540 nm in red purple betacyanins [1]. In addition, betacyanins display other absorption maxima: 270–280 nm due to the *cyclo*-dopa structure. Acylation with hydroxycinnamic acids generates a third maximum at about 300–330 nm. The addition of aliphatic acid derivatives did not affect the absorption. Decarboxylation at C-2 produces a slight hypsochromic shift of about 5 nm [7].

The absorption maximum of the betacyanins is influenced by the introduction of substituents in the backbone of the molecule. For example, glycosylation of betanidin (violet-red) at C_5 gives rise to betanin (magenta). Generally, the introduction of a glucosyl group at C_5 comes along with a hypsochromic shift of about 6 nm of the resulting betacyanin. The introduction of the same group at C_6 brings about a greater bathochromic shift than 5-glycosylation. A second sugar moiety attached to the first apparently did not affect the spectroscopic properties [2,7]. Acylation with aromatic acids leads to a bathochromic shift up to 12 nm, whereas esterification with aliphatic acyl moieties only slightly or did not alter the maximum absorption of betacyanins [2,7].

As for betacyanins, in betaxanthins, structural modifications in the backbone may produce hypso- or bathochromic shifts. For instance, amine conjugates exhibit a lower absorption maximum than their respective amino acid counterparts [11].

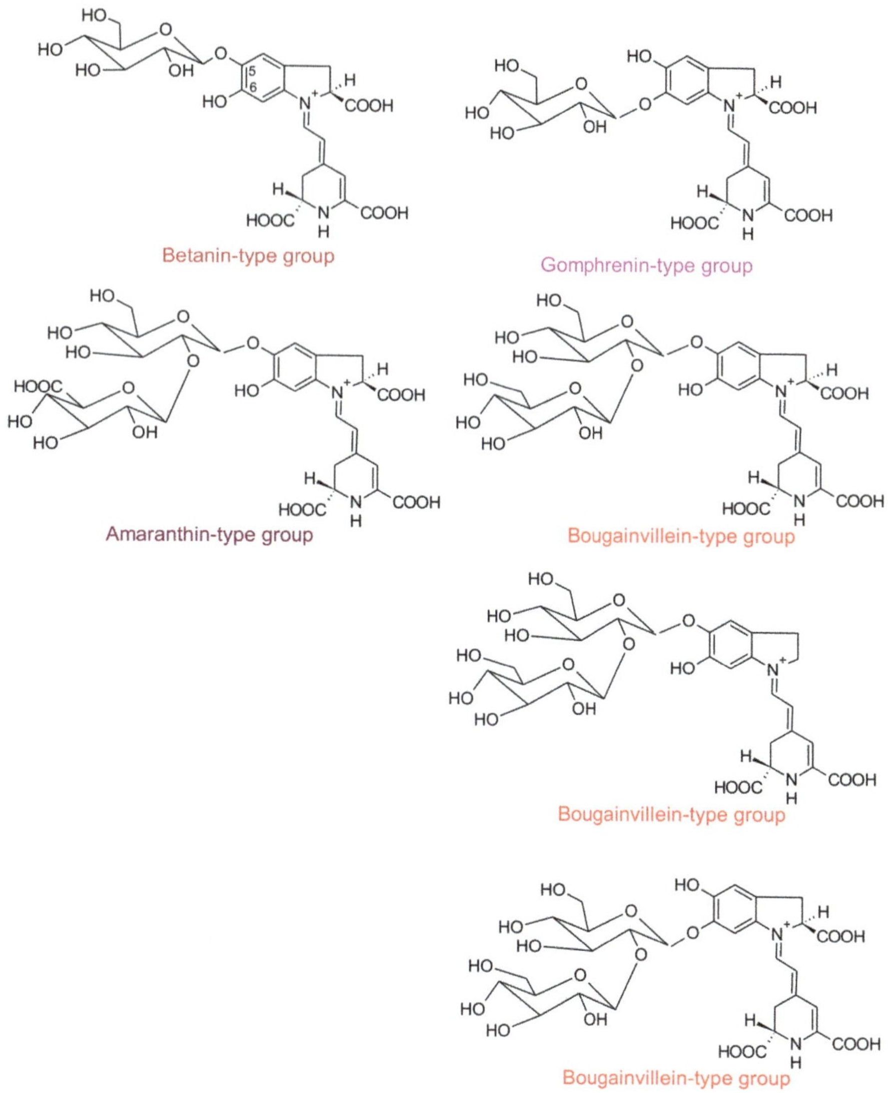

Figure 2. Example of structures of the different types of betacyanins.

Betaxanthins are fluorescent pigments which present maximum excitation wavelengths between 320 and 475 nm that correspond to blue light and emission maxima between 506 and 660 nm that correspond to green light. The fluorescence of betacyanins is weaker than that of betaxanthins but the intensity is enhanced by carboxyl groups or reduced by aromatic ring and hydroxyl groups [6,12].

2.2. *Stability of Betalains*

Despite betalains pigments are considered more stable than anthocyanins [13] there are several factors that negatively affect their stability: pH < 3 or pH > 7; high a_w (water activity); metal cations (Fe^{3+}, Fe^{2+}, Cu^{2+}, Cu^{+}, Sn^{2+}, Al^{3+}, Hg^{2+}, Cr^{3+}); high temperature; light; O_2; H_2O_2, low pigment content; among other factors [7]. For these reasons, betalains have had little application in food industry as colourants, unless if they can be used in frozen foods, low temperature dairy products or short-shelf life foods [14].

Heat mostly induces dehydrogenation in the presence of oxygen (oxidation), aldimine bond hydrolysis and decarboxylation of batalains, which induce a colour change to orange-yellow. At pH values < 3, the betalain structure is converted from anionic form (red) to cationic form (violet), generating a visible colour change from red to blue-violet shade. At pH values > 7, there is the aldimine bond hydrolysis of betalain, giving rise to betalamic acid and *cyclo*-dopa-5-*O*-glucoside and the colour change to yellow-brown. Metal ions can accelerate oxidation of betalains with the consequent loss of colours [15]. Epimerization is another process that can occur [16]. Figure 3 represents the possible chemical processes that can occur in betanin when exposed to acid or basic conditions or when submitted to heating, according to that previously reported by Gonçalves et al. [16].

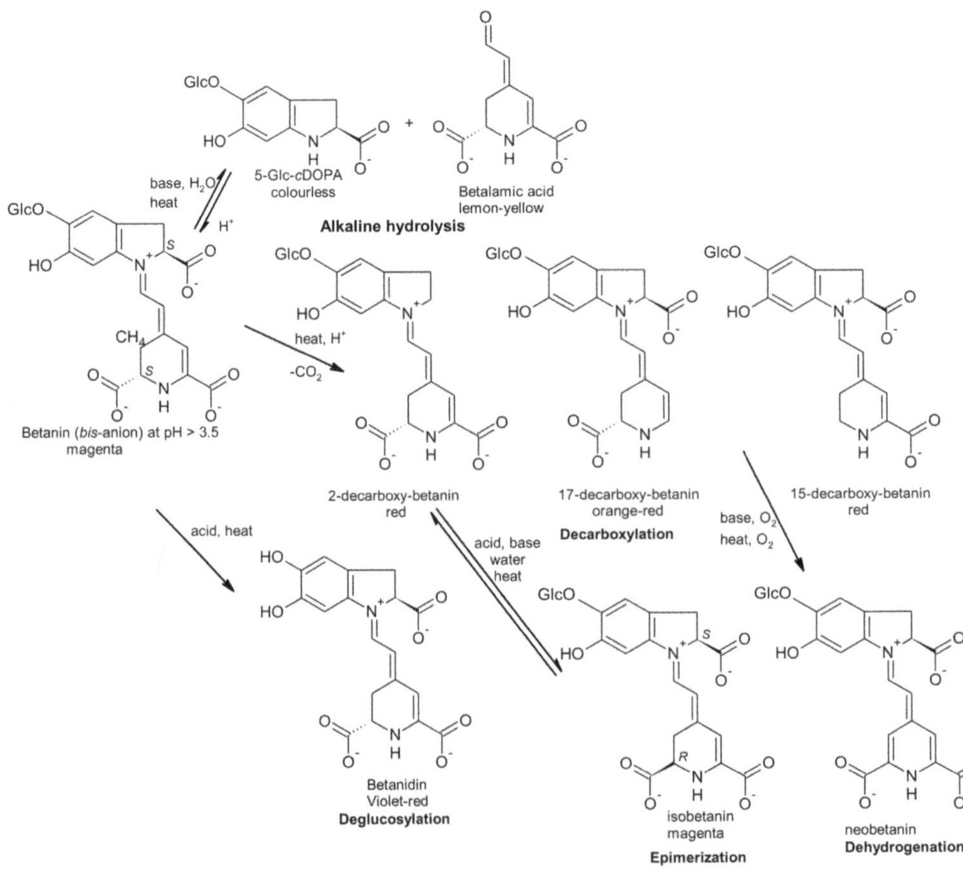

Figure 3. Betanin degradation products and some degradation pathways (adapted from [16]).

2.3. *Extraction, Separation, Identification and Quantification of Betalains*

Betalains are generally extracted from ground plant material by maceration extraction with water, cold, or at room temperature or Soxhlet extraction. For a complete extraction, it is preferable to use methanol or ethanol solutions (20–50%, *v*/*v*). Before extraction, a short heat treatment (70 °C, 20 min) can be made for inactivating degradative enzymes, despite the possible destruction of some pigments. A slight acidification with HCl or citric acid or acidified ethanol (0.4 to 1% HCl) can be used for the precipitation of betacyanins. The addition of aqueous ethanol (95%) will give betaxanthins [1]. However, other techniques have been assayed to extract betalains, particularly from red beet, in order to enhance the yields in a shorter time period, to increase the cell membrane permeabilisation and to be more environmentally friendly—diffusion extraction, ultrafiltration and reverse osmosis and loose reverse osmosis (LRO), cryogenic freezing, aqueous two-phase extraction, pulsed electric fields and gamma irradiation, microwave and ultrasound-assisted extractions [11,17–19].

Purification and isolation of betalains is needed before their qualitative and quantitative analysis for eliminating possible interfering compounds. Chromatographic and electrophoretic procedures have been used to separate and/or purify betalains. For the separation of these pigments, ion chromatography on cation exchange resins followed by adsorption chromatography on polyamide column or a sequential chromatography on a series of Sephadex ion exchangers can be used [20]. Separation, identification and quantification of betalains have been carried through high performance liquid chromatography (HPLC) coupled to ultraviolet-visible (UV-Vis), photodiode array (PDA) mass spectrometry (MS) and nuclear magnetic resonance detection (NMR) by using reversed phase columns and binary gradient dilutions (acidified water with formic acid 2–5%, *v*/*v*) and acetonitrile or methanol. As betaxanthins are fluorescent pigments, the detection of these pigments may be done using fluorescence methods [20].

2.4. Biosynthesis of Betalains

The biosynthesis of betalains will be described according to the review by Gandía-Herrero and García-Carmona [21]. The pathways are schematised in Figure 4.

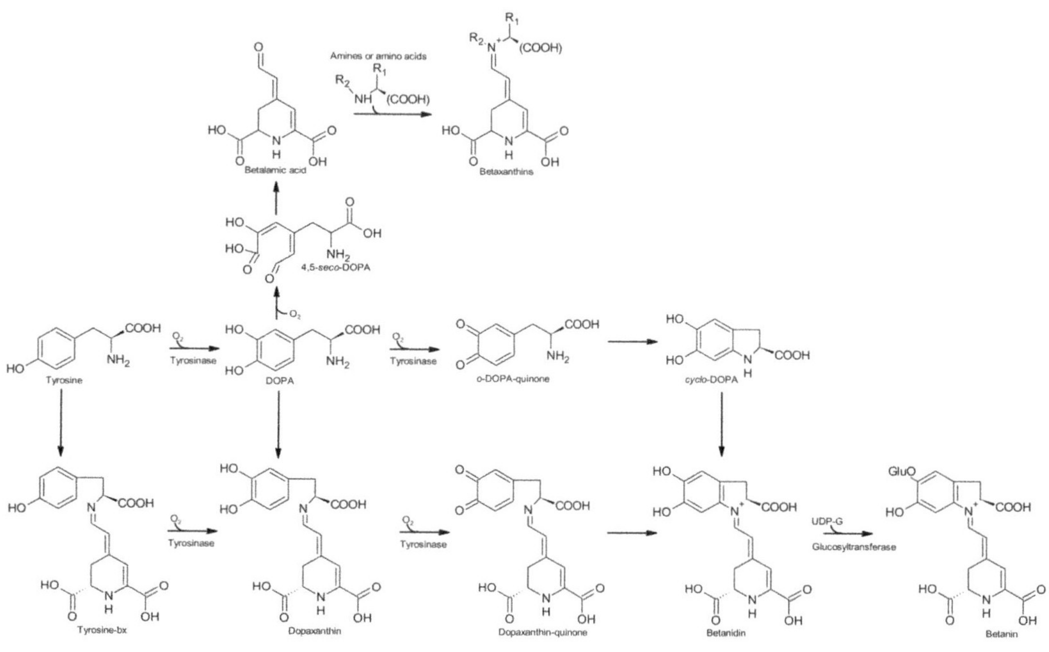

Figure 4. Simple scheme for the biosynthetic pathway of betalains (adapted from [21]).

Betalains are secondary metabolites derived from the amino acid L-tyrosine. The amino acid undergoes hydroxylation and L-dopa is formed—the reaction is catalysed by the enzyme tyrosinase (or polyphenoloxidase). A second enzyme (4,5-dopa extradiol dioxygenase) catalyses the cleavage of dopa to form the intermediate 4,5-*seco*-dopa. A spontaneous intramolecular condensation occurs between the amine group and the aldehyde group of 4,5-*seco*-dopa, giving rise to betalamic acid (Figure 4).

Betalamic acid, a structure that holds the chromogenic electron resonance, may accept spontaneously amines or amino acids, which leads, by the reaction between the amine group of the amine and the aldehyde group of betalamic acid, to the formation of yellow betaxanthins.

For the formation of betacyanins two pathways could be considered:

Pathway 1. Formation of betanidin through the condensation with free L-dopa derivatives

L-Dopa, in the absence of a reducing agent (ascorbic acid or an analogous reducing agent), is transformed by tyrosinase to *o*-dopa-quinone in the presence of molecular oxygen. Then, a spontaneous cyclization takes place involving the amine group of the *o*-quinone that, through an intramolecular nucleophilic attack on the ring, forms the molecule *leuko*-dopa-chrome, also known as *cyclo*-dopa. This compound may react with betalamic acid to generate the pigment betanidin. This pigment is an intermediate in the formation of betacyanins. In the absence of a reducing agent, *cyclo*-dopa (unstable) undergoes a spontaneous oxidation with the formation of dopa-chrome with the simultaneous reduction of a molecule of dopa-quinone back to L-dopa. This mechanism was reported by Schliemann et al. [22], nevertheless is considered improbable to occur at a biological level [21].

Pathway 2. Formation of betanidin through tyrosine-betaxanthin (tyrosine-bx) and dopa-bx (dopaxanthin)

The reaction starts with the condensation of L-tyrosine with betalamic acid originating the pigment tyrosine-bx. This pigment is the substrate for tyrosinase that converts it in dopa-bx. This pigment is also substrate for tyrosinase that transforms it in dopaxanthin-quinone. In the absence of a reducing agent, this quinone undergoes an intramolecular nucleophilic attack with a consequent cyclization and formation of betanidin. Another possibility is the condensation of betalamic acid with L-dopa to form dopaxanthin [21].

Betanidin can incorporate a glucose residue in position 5, reaction catalysed by the enzyme betanidin-5-*O*-glucosyltransferase and betanin is formed. Other reactions of glycosylation and acylations may occur that lead to a wide variety of known betacyanins [21].

2.5. *Role of Betalains in Plants*

The function of betalains in plants is diverse: for plant propagation through pollen transfer or the dispersion of indigestible seeds by animals that are attracted by the colour of flowers and fruits; as a repelling signal to deter herbivores; to screen tissue against damaging ultraviolet (UV) radiation; for increasing pathogen resistance and improving viral defence; for providing higher tolerance to heat stress; as osmoregulators by modelling the amino acid pool from betaxanthins, among other functions [2,23–25].

2.6. *Importance of Betalains for Consumers*

Some species are edible sources of betalains: red beet roots (*Beta vulgaris* subsp. *vulgaris* convar. *vulgaris* var. *vulgaris*; Conditiva Group); fruits of cacti, particularly *Opuntia ficus-indica*; the dragon fruits from *Hylocereus polyrhizus*; Swiss chard (*Beta vulgaris* subsp. *vulgaris* convar. *cicla*. var. *flavescens*; Flavescens Group). For instance, the extracts of beetroot containing betalains are pink or violet pigments used as food additive under the E-162 code (betanin), in the European Union, or 73.40 of the Food and Drug Administration (FDA) [5]. E-162 is mainly applied for colouring fruit yogurts, ice-creams, jams, chewing gums, sauces and soups. The same pigment has also been used in cosmetics and pharmaceuticals [26].

Beyond the application of betalains as colourants in food industry, these secondary metabolites also possess biological properties beneficial for human health: anti-inflammatory, antioxidant, inhibitory effect towards skin and lung cancer in mice and chemo-preventive properties (positive effects on metabolic, cardiovascular and gastrointestinal health in humans), with the advantage to be devoid of toxicity, mutagenic action or allergic reactions [2,5,27–34].

The colouring properties of betalains along with their biological properties have led to the development of in vitro strategies for producing these secondary metabolites, however this has been without success. Georgiev et al. [35] reviewed progress in plant in vitro systems for producing betalains. At the same time, the authors cited the factors that could be manipulated for improving the betalain yields as well as the bioreactor systems that could be used.

2.7. *Production of Betalains*

Owing to the importance of betalains as natural pigments, there has been research with the aim to obtain them by synthetic procedures. Generally, it starts with the production of betalamic acid or even better, with extraction in ethyl acetate from natural sources and then condensation with amines or amino acids. Nevertheless, this procedure gives rise to very low yields. Another way to produce betalains is based on a combined procedure of betanin degradation and betalains synthesis. This methodology requires an immediate purification to avoid reverse reactions [36,37].

New methods have been developed and one of them consists of betalamic acid derivatized by a support generated from a primary amine polymer. This material is stable for months. The imine bond between polymer surface and betalamic acid may be broken at mild conditions through the addition of amines in water over a pH range at room temperature. Betalains (betaxanthins and betalains) originate from the displacement of betalamic acid from the surface polymer and its reaction with amines or amino acids. This procedure is optimized for the formation of betalains derived from tyramine, dopamine, pyrrolidine and indoline [38].

Plant cell and tissue cultures have also been used to produce betalains because such production is independent on the climate or soil properties, pest and diseases; it also allows continuous supplies with uniform quality and yield. However, the yield production is generally low and almost always needing bioreactor systems for improving large scale production [35]. Some examples include the production of betalains by hairy root cultures, cell suspension and callus culture of beetroot [39–46]. Generally, in these works, the authors used methods and studied factors that could improve the production or recovery of betalains by cell cultures of *Beta vulgaris* (radiation, light, utilization of adsorbents, changes in the composition of the culture medium, alterations of the bioreactors, among other factors). Other approaches include improving betalain yield in beet through the improvement of the utilization of tyrosine or enhancement of its production, depending on the beet genotype [47] or developing new betalains sources (microbes and/or plants) by metabolic engineering [48].

2.8. Biological Properties of Betalains

The antioxidant activity of betalains is well documented in several works and using diverse methodologies, e.g., scavenging of the 2,2′-azino-bis-(3-ethyl-benzthiazoline-6-sulfonic acid) ($ABTS^{\bullet +}$) and 1,1-diphenyl-2-picrylhydrazyl (DPPH) free radicals [49]. The relationship between the chemical structure of betalains and the activity was also investigated and different pigments exhibited diverse capacity for scavenging free radicals. The tested betalains decreased its scavenging capacity in the following order: simple gomphrenins > acylated gomphrenins > dopaminebetaxanthin > (*S*)-tryptophan-betaxanthin > 3-methoxytyraminebetaxanthin > betanin/isobetanin > celosianins > iresinins > amaranthine/isoamaranthine. Betalains, particularly red-violet gomphrenin type betacyanins and yellow betaxanthins, had strong antioxidant activity when compared to the traditional standards (ascorbic acid, rutin and catechin). There is an impact of the chemical structure of betalains on the antioxidant activity: the capacity for scavenging free radicals increased with the number of hydroxyl groups and imino groups and decreased with more glycosylation of aglycones in the molecule. The capacity for scavenging other free radicals, such as peroxyl (ROO•) free radicals or nitric oxide (NO•), by some betacyanins was also dependent on the number of hydroxyls. For example, betanin was less effective than betanidin [50,51]. Additive effects were observed when betanin or betanidin were blended with α-tocopherol and incorporated in liposomes [51]. However, and according to some authors [52], the antioxidant activity of betalains, particularly betaxanthins, is not linked to the presence of hydroxyl groups or aromaticity of the pigment structure. According to the same authors there is an 'intrinsic activity' of betaxanthins which might be associated with the common resonance system supported by the two nitrogen atoms of the betaxanthin. Nevertheless, the presence of hydroxyl groups in betaxanthins increase their ABTS free radicals scavenging activity [52].

The capacity for scavenging $ABTS^{\bullet +}$ of betalamic acid was better when compared to that of trolox. The same pigment was also able to reduce Fe^{3+} to Fe^{2+}. These activities were attributed to the extended conjugated system of betalamic acid, nevertheless dependent on the pH of the environment: pH values above 5.5 increased the activity of betalamic acid [53]. The importance of the pH on the activity was also reported for betanin, the main pigment of red beet [28] and other betalains [12].

The oxidation mechanisms of betanin and some of its derivatives (2-decarboxybetanin, 17-decarboxybetanin, 2,17-bidecarboxybetanin and neobetanin) in the presence of ABTS and the intermediates that are generated during the reactions, was studied by Wybraniec et al. [54].

Betanin and betanidin were able to prevent lipid peroxidation in microemulsions, membranes and low-density lipoprotein (LDL) catalysed by cytochrome c, H_2O_2-activated metmyoglobin, iron redox cycle and lipoxygenase [55]. Betanin could also inhibit 71% lipid peroxidation in a liposome system [56]. The protection of LDL oxidation in vivo by betalains was attributed to the transactivation of paraoxonase 1 (PON1), an antioxidant enzyme produced in the liver [57].

Beta vulgaris extract was able to inhibit protein oxidation induced by hypochlorous acid released from active neutrophils. This property is beneficial on pain associated with osteoarthritis [58].

Lipoxygenase (LOX) and cyclooxygenase (COX) are enzymes that are involved in the conversion of arachidonic acid to inflammatory mediators leukotrienes and prostaglandins, which are inflammatory mediators. Betanidin and betanin were able to inhibit soybean LOX, being this activity higher than catechin (control) [55]. Betanin was able to inhibit COX-1 and COX-2 [56]. Betaxanthins had also capacity for inhibiting COX, phenethylamine-bx was a potent inhibitor of this enzyme by interaction with Tyr-385 and Ser-530 residues close to the active site of COX [34]. The anti-inflammatory activity of betalains may also be due to their action against cellular mediators of inflammation, such as intercellular cell adhesion molecule-1 (ICAM-1) significantly repressed by betanin [59].

In different studies, betanin and betalain-rich red beet extract induced phase II enzyme quinine reductase [60,61]. This activity is related to the hepatoprotective effect of these pigments: Feeding rats with betalain-rich red beet juice diminished the action of the hepatotoxic compounds *N*-nitrosodiethylamine, carbon tetrachloride and 7,12-dimethylbenz(a)anthracene, due to the improved antioxidant status and increased expression of quinine reductase [62,63]. Moreover, administration of *Amaranthum tricolor* extracts containing betalains to diabetic rats significantly reduced blood cholesterol, triglycerides and LDL (low density lipoproteins) level and increased the high-density lipoproteins level (HDL), having thus the potential to prevent cardiovascular disorders [64,65]. Betalains from red beet juice and chips inhibited neutrophil oxidative metabolism in obese individuals [66], suggesting that betalains may have an interesting role in the management of hyperlipidaemia [64]. The antimalarial activity of betanin/amaranthin-rich extract of *Amaranthus spinosus* in mice was due to the capacity of these pigments for chelating the inner cations Ca^{2+}, Fe^{2+} and Mg^{2+} and for blocking the choline intracellular transport of parasites [30].

Beet root pomace and betalains were able to reduce the growth of several Gram-positive and Gram-negative microorganisms, nevertheless the mechanisms involved in the microbial inhibition is scarce [64]. Other attributes have been found in vitro and in vivo for betalains such as anti-diabetic, anti-tumoural, regulator of metabolic dysfunctions, among other properties that are compiled in three recent reviews [5,14,64].

3. Amaranthaceae

Amaranthaceae family is characterised by its diversity in secondary metabolites: essential oils, sesquiterpenes, diterpenes, triterpenes, phenolic acids, flavonoids and betalains [67]. This family includes diverse genera in which betalains have been reported: *Alternanthera*, *Amaranthus*, *Beta*, *Chenopodium*, *Celosia* and *Gomphrena* [27,29,68–70].

Several properties have been attributed to some of these genera: antioxidant, positive effects on metabolic, cardiovascular and gastrointestinal health in humans; antimalarial, inhibitors of LOX and COX [27–30,33,34,49,70].

3.1. Gomphrena globosa L.

Gomphrena globosa L. (globe amaranth) is native to Panama and Guatemala and presents some resistance to drought and high adaption ability to poor soils or colder lands [71]. It is an ornamental plant largely cultivated in mild climatic regions [72]. Leaves and inflorescences' decoctions and other parts of globe amaranth are used in folk medicine in the treatment of some inflammatory respiratory diseases, such as bronchial asthma, acute and chronic bronchitis or whooping cough;

jaundice; hypertension; some kidney problems such as gall stones; prostate problems; diabetes; and to stop local haemorrhage [71,73–75].

G. globosa inflorescences can have purple-, red- and orange colour [76]. According to the variety, the levels of betacyanins and betaxanthins changed. Purple inflorescences had the highest amounts of betacyanins (556.8 mg/kg, fresh weight) and only traces of betaxanthins. The lowest concentrations of betacyanins were found in orange varieties (30.6 mg/kg, fresh weight), whereas the red variety had the highest concentrations of betaxanthins (75.0 mg/kg, fresh weight) [76]. For the first time, betaxanthins histidine-bx (muscaarin VII), arginine-bx, glutamine-bx (vulgaxanthin I), lysine-bx, isoleucine-bx and tryptophan-bx (Figure 5) were reported in the red petals of globe amaranth [76]. The betacyanins identified in the red and purple petals of globe amaranth were amaranthin, betanin, gomphrenin I, gomphrenin II, gomphrenin III, isogomphrenin I, isogomphrenin II, isogomphrenin III, isoamaranthin, isobetanin, betanidin, isobetanidin, celosianin II and isocelosianin II [76,77]. In addition, six more betacyanins were tentatively identified [76]: 17-decarboxy-amaranthin, sinapoyl-amaranthin, *cis*-isomer of gomphrenin III, *cis*-isomer of gomphrenin II, sinapoyl-gomphrenin I and sinapoyl-isogomphrenin I (Figure 6).

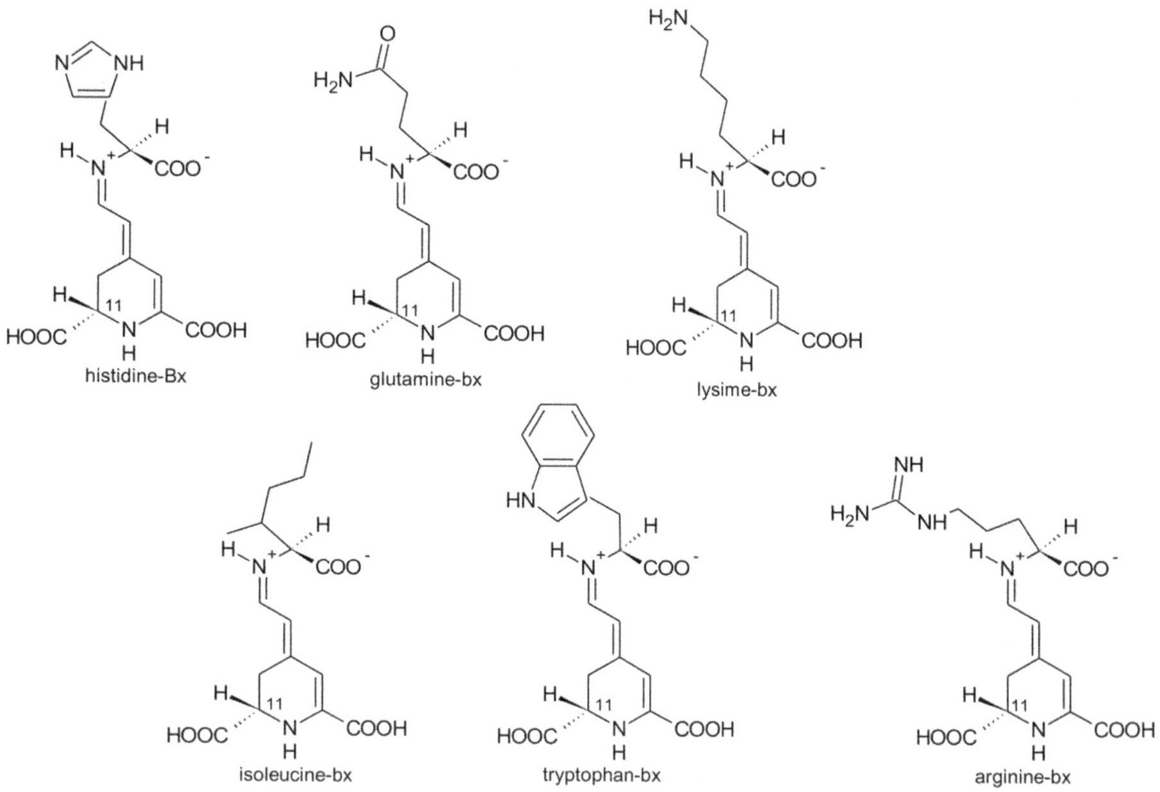

Figure 5. Betaxanthins found in red inflorescences of *G. globosa* L.

17-Decarboxy-amaranthin, 17-decarboxy-isoamaranthine, sinapoyl-gomphrenin I, amaranthin, isoamaranthin, betanin, isobetanin, gomphrenin I, gomphrenin II, gomphrenin III, isogomphrenin II, isogomphrenin III, isogomphrenin I, celosianin II and isocelosianin II were found in extracts of red inflorescences of *G. globosa* [49,72,78–83].

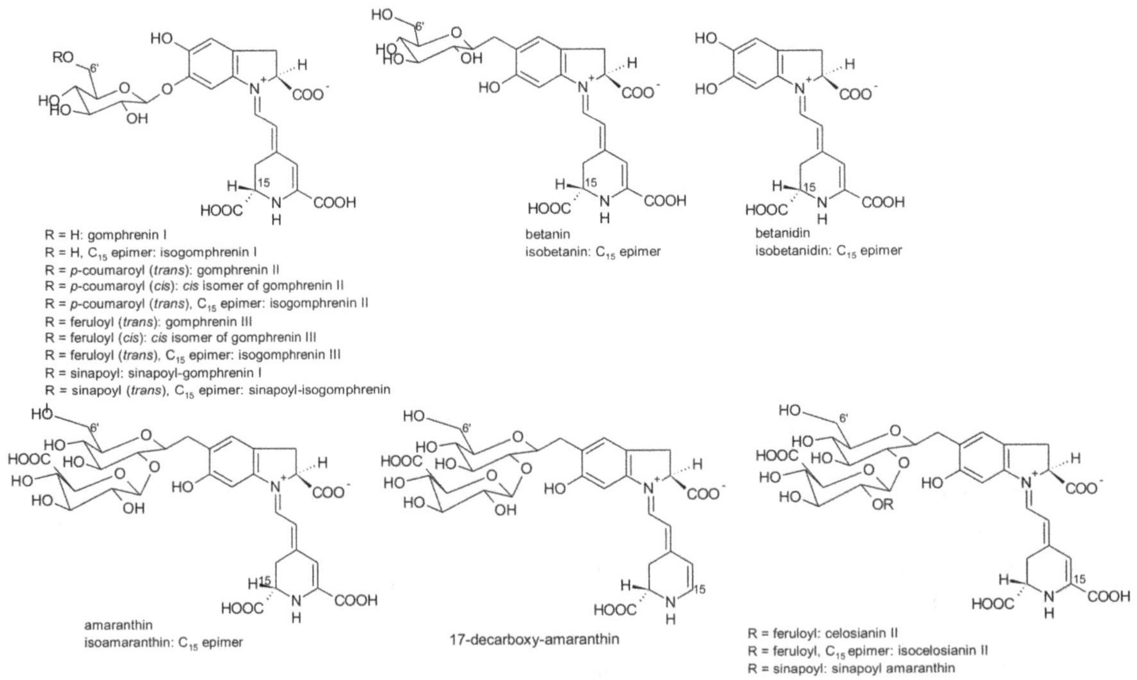

Figure 6. Betacyanins found in *G. globosa* L. inflorescences and *Amaranthus*.

The type of extraction and extraction solvent used for obtaining betacyanins from *G. globosa* inflorescences gave rise to quantitative differences in the betacyanins identified by Silva et al. [71]. Maceration of inflorescences with methanol for 30 min, at room temperature, with agitation (400 rpm) revealed to be the most effective extraction, capable to extract higher amounts of betacyanins (gomphrenin I, gomphrenin II, gomphrenin III, isogomphrenin I, isogomphrenin II, isogomphrenin III, sinapoyl-gomphrenin I and isosinapoyl-gomphrenin I), being isogomphrenin III the most abundant (1.25 mg/g) [71]. The same components have been already reported by Ferreres et al. [80] in aqueous extracts of *G. globosa* inflorescences obtained by maceration for 30 min at room temperature, in obscurity and with agitation (400 rpm).

In order to obtain the maximal amount of betacyanins, Roriz et al. [81] used the response surface methodology (RSM), with which it is possible to optimize the maceration conditions simultaneously (time, temperature, ethanol-water proportion and solid-liquid ratio). The betacyanins identified were gomphrenin and isogomphrenin II and III and the best conditions of extraction for obtaining the highest pigment content (~45 mg/g) were: 165 min, 25 °C, 0% ethanol and 5 g/L of solid-liquid ratio. The best extraction method of gomphrenin and isogomphrenin II and III from flowers, bract and bracteoles of *G. globosa* was ultrasound assisted extraction in the following conditions: time = 22 min; power = 500%; Ethanol = 0%; and ratio solid/liquid = 5 g/L [82].

Matrix-assisted laser desorption/ionization quadrupole ion trap time-of-flight mass spectrometry (MALDI-QIT-TOF-MS) was a method of identification betacyanins of crude extracts from *G. globosa* without any previous purification [72]. The identification by this method revealed to be rapid without any previous purification of extracts but presented some limitations, including the difficulty to distinguish the isomers of the betacyanins, which needs an additional analysis by HPLC or LC-MS [72].

Extracts of *G. globosa* had antioxidant activity, through the capacity for scavenging diverse free radicals (DPPH, superoxide, nitric oxide) and anti-inflammatory activity since they were able to decrease the nitric oxide content in the supernatant of the lipopolysaccharide (LPS)-stimulated RAW 264.7 macrophages culture [71]. However, the authors were unable to attribute these activities only to the betalains present in the extracts. Other components had also a role on the activities detected.

Roriz et al. [79] studied the antioxidant activity of three extracts (*Pterospartum tridentatum* (L.) Willk. *Gomphrena globosa* L. and *Cymbopogon citratus* (DC) Stapf.), using four methods (DPPH scavenging activity, reducing power and inhibition of lipid peroxidation by β-carotene bleaching inhibition and TBARS assays). They found that *G. globosa* extract, the sole possessing betalains together with the lowest amounts of phenols, had the worst activity. Therefore and according to the authors, the antioxidant activity found in samples was highly dependent on the profile in phenolic compounds and their amounts.

3.2. *Alternanthera*

The *Alternanthera* genus includes 80 species. Many species of *Alternanthera* have been used in folk medicine for the treatment of infections, genital inflammation and fever [84–86]. *Alternanthera brasiliana* (L.) Kuntze and *Alternanthera tenella* Colla are native to tropical and sub-tropical regions of Australia and South America [69].

In Brazil, the leaves of *A. brasiliana* (Brazilian joyweed) have been used in folk medicine as galactogogue, cholagogue and a diuretic for the treatment of indigestion and abortifacient [87,88]. In Peru, whole plant is used to treat bronchitis and asthma. Laboratorial studies have demonstrated that the extracts of *A. brasiliana* possess modest antioxidant activity; anti-inflammatory; wound healing; analgesic, antiviral and antitumor activities [88–93]. These findings were generally attributed to the phenols, terpenes and sterols present in the leaves and not to their pigments or betalains. Such does not mean the absence of activity of these secondary metabolites, only very few works can be found that aimed to study the betalains of leaves from *A. brasiliana* [69]. The antimicrobial activity of *A. brasiliana* extracts on several microorganisms (*Staphylococcus aureus, S. epidermidis, Escherichia coli, Bacillus subtilis, Micrococcus luteus, Candida albicans* and *Saccharomyces cerevisiae*) was weak [94,95].

Alternanthera tenella Colla (joyweed) is a weed that occurs in crops and uncultivated areas in northwest Brazil but also in other regions, like the state of São Paulo [85,96,97]. *A. tenella* has been used in popular medicine to treat the infections, fevers, bruises and itches [98,99]. The plant has been also used as diuretic [100,101]. Laboratorial experiments have revealed that *A. tenella* extracts have immunomodulatory, antioxidant, anti-hyperalgesic, antimicrobial and antiparasitic properties [85,96,101–104]. As reported for *A. brasiliana*, these activities have been generally attributed to the phenols, particularly flavonoids. However, the possible role of betalains in such activities was not evaluated by the authors. In some locations of India there are diverse tribes that use the leaves of *A. brasiliana* and *A. tenella* as vegetables that can be consumed fresh or cooked or even fried in diverse ways, along with rice [69,105,106].

A. brasiliana and *A. tenella* leaves and stems are strongly coloured. Betalains from these parts of both species were extracted by Deladino et al. [69]. In both species, leaves had higher amounts of total betalains than the respective stems. The highest amounts of betalains were found in the leaf extracts of *A. brasiliana* (89.40 μg/g, dry weight), while the leaf extracts of *A. tenella* only had 17.29 μg/g (dry weight) [69]. Amaranthin, isoamaranthin, betanin and isobetanin (Figure 6) were quantified in the leaf and stems extracts of *A. brasiliana* and *A. tenella*. In all samples, amaranthin predominated. Dopamine-bx and 3-methoxytyramine-bx (Figure 7) were the sole betaxanthins tentatively identified in the same extracts but in very small amounts [69].

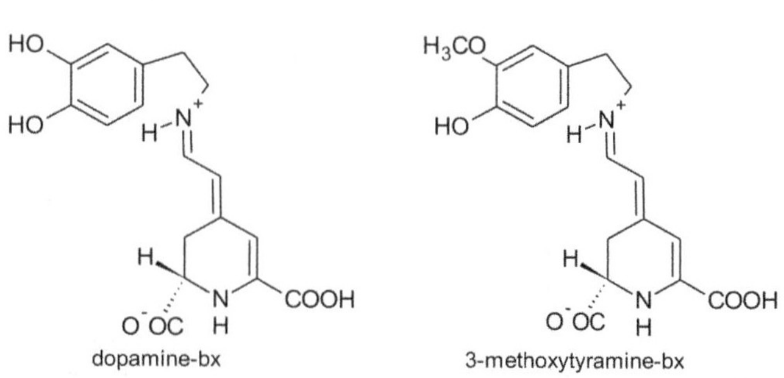

Figure 7. Betaxanthins found in Alternanthera brasiliana and *Alternanthera tenella*.

The antioxidant activity, measured trough the ferric reducing antioxidant power, was evaluated in leaf and stems' extracts of *A. brasiliana* and *A. tenella*. Leaf extracts of *A. tenella* possessed the highest antioxidant activity, being coincident with the highest amounts of flavones found in this extract, particularly vitexin and its C-glycosides derivatives. The authors concluded that this activity could only be attributed to these flavones and not to betalains [69]. These results disagree with those reported by Rodrigues-Brandão [103], since the antioxidant activity was related to the betacyanins accumulated by *A. tenella* growing in vitro. Both increased with the addition of salicylic acid to the culture medium. In order to enhance the production of betalains, some authors assayed the action of tyrosine added to the in vitro cultures of *A. tenella* [98]. The authors reported a negative effect on in vitro growth of this species, affecting the formation of shoot and roots, nevertheless increased the biosynthesis of betacyanins, measured as total amaranthin. Higher production of betaxanthins and betacyanins was observed when *A. brasiliana* plants were submitted to blue and white light, whereas *A. tenella* plants did not show any significant differences in the amounts of these pigments accumulated when submitted to the same light types [102].

3.3. *Amaranthus*

The word *Amaranthus is* derived from the Greek word "Anthos" (Flower) which means everlasting, immortal [107,108]. *Amaranthus* known as amaranth is a genus of herbs that includes 60–70 species. Most of the species are annual weeds. Species of this genus can be a source of pseudo-cereals, vegetable and ornamentals. In Europe and America, *Amaranthus* are used as pseudo-cereals, whereas in Africa they are planted as vegetables [109,110].

Amaranth species were classified in vegetable *Amaranthus* (*A. tricolor* L.); grain *Amaranthus* (*A. hypochondriacus*, *A. caudatus*, *A. cruentus*); weed *Amaranthus* (*A. spinosus*, *A. viridis*, *A. retroflexus*, *A. graecizans*, *A. dubius* and *A. hybridus*) [109,110]. Vegetable *Amaranthus* possess inflorescences formed by mostly or exclusively axillary glomerules or with short spikes; whereas grain *Amaranthus* possesses an apical large to moderately large complex inflorescence with aggregates of cymes. Some weed species may present morphological similarity with leafy vegetable form and others with grain form of *Amaranthus* [109,110].

Despite that classification, some species may be used either as vegetable or grain. For example, leaves of the young *A. cruentus* plants may be used in salads and soups and the grains are utilized into breads, cakes, cookies, confectionary and soups [111]. Leaves of the young *A. tricolor* plants are used in salads and soups and the applications of *A. caudatus* grains are the same of those reported for *A. cruentus*. *Amaranthus spinosus* is not considered safe for consumption either by humans or livestock [111].

Grains of amaranth have been considered as possessing high nutritional value owing to their protein content, levels of essential amino acids (lysine and methionine) when compared to other grains. Amaranth grain is also considered a good source of insoluble fibre. Amaranth is also a rich source of soluble fibre, vitamins (riboflavin, niacin, ascorbic acid) and mineral contents (calcium and magnesium) [111]. Beyond these components, there are also secondary metabolites such as phenols and pigments (betacyanins) in the leaves of the vegetable amaranth *A. tricolor* as well as in the grain amaranth *A. cruentus* and *A. caudatus* [112]. Some genotypes of grain amaranth have much higher betacyanins over a longer growth period than vegetable amaranth species [113,114].

Amaranthus tricolor L. (Chinese spinach, tampala, Joseph's coat), the main type of vegetable amaranth, is native to south or south-east Asia and then was dispersed all over the tropical and temperate regions [115]. This species adapts well to adverse growing conditions, is resistant to heat and drought, with the advantage to be rich in carotenoids, proteins, vitamins and dietary fibre [116]. This has made *A. tricolor* as an alternative source of nutrition for people living in developing countries with little access to protein-rich food [116,117]. This species has diverse leaf colours (red, purple) owing to the accumulation of various pigments, such as betacyanins [118].

A. tricolor was used as sudorific, febrifuge, emollient, blood purifier, on the treatment of menstrual disorders, eruptive fevers, pain, colic, anaemia, dysentery, skin diseases, dropsy, toothache, sore throat, cough, bronchitis, bilious disorder and diabetes [119,120]. Extracts of *A. tricolor* have been reported as antioxidant; hepatoprotetive; antimicrobial; antiproliferative on human AGS (gastric), CNS (central nervous system, SF-268), HCT-116 (colon), NCl-H460 (lung) and MCF-7 (breast) cancer cell lines; anti-inflammatory by inhibiting both cyclooxygenases isoenzymes (COX-1 and COX-2) and also by downregulating proinflammatory cytokine gene expression (TNF-α (tumour necrosis factor-α, IL-1(interleukin-1) and IL-6) in advanced glycation end products-induced cells; among other properties [120–125]. Generally, the authors related these activities with phenolic compounds including flavonoids.

Amaranthin and isoamarathin were extracted from seedlings and leaves of three genotypes of *A. tricolor* (Figure 6) [83,113]. Amaranthin was at higher concentrations. The authors found a relationship between betacyanins and proteins quantified in the samples [113]. Later on, [72] using MALDI-QIT-TOF-MS also identified amaranthin and isoamaranthin in the extracts of *A. tricolor* seedlings without previous purification.

As aforementioned, amaranthin (betanidin 5-*O*-β-glucuronosylglucoside) is the main betacyanin pigment of the vegetable amaranth. Betanidin glucosyltransferase is the enzyme that catalyses the transfer reaction of glucose molecule from UDP-glucose (uridine diphosphate-glucose) to betanidin. Betanidin glucosyltransferase has been isolated from several sources, for the first time from the leaves of *A. tricolor* by Das et al. [119]. In this work, the authors reported that this enzyme was able to catalyse the transfer of glucose to betanidin as well as to the flavonoids kaempferol and quercetin.

Total betaxanthins and betacyanins were quantified in the leaves of four cultivars of vegetable amaranth (Rocto alta, Rocto ranga, Alto pati, Baromashi), from Bangladesh [115]. Betaxanthins were in higher concentration than betacyanins in Alto pati, Baromashi cultivars. The amounts of both groups of pigments as well as the antioxidant activity were highly dependent on the cultivars [115]. The antioxidant property was related with the phenols and not with the betalains [115,126]. Differences in the amounts of betacyanins among cultivars were also previously reported by some authors [113,127,128]. Factors that may influence the accumulation of these pigments in the leaves of the vegetable amaranth include the growth stage (older plants had higher amounts of betacyanins); the position of the leaves within the shoot canopy (the apical leaves accumulated higher betacyanins than those of middle and basal leaves) [128]; photoperiod (12 h photoperiod revealed to be the best for the accumulation of betacyanins), which were coincident with the highest antioxidant activity found by the authors [129]; and food processing factors (low temperature, darkness and absence of oxidants maintained the stability of betalains of vegetable amaranth) [128].

The betacyanin accumulation in leaves of vegetable amaranth in response to natural climatic conditions (temperature, humidity and sunlight) was dependent on the cultivar [127]. This study permitted to separate the cultivars in different groups, according to the response to the natural climatic changes and may facilitate the selection and development of appropriate cultivars with desired traits in relation to the influence of climate [127].

Betacyanins' accumulation by red amaranth cultivar Rocto alta can be affected by different coloured shade polyethylene, the highest betacyanins' content occurred under blue colour polyethylene shade followed by yellow and white polyethylene shade, whereas green polyethylene shaded leaves exhibited the lowest amounts of betacyanins [118].

The biotechnological production of secondary metabolites is independent on the climate variations and soil properties, pests and diseases. In addition, such approach is also appropriate for studying the metabolic pathways. Biswas et al. [130] were able to obtain stable *callus* line of *A. tricolor* with enhanced production of betacyanins. Beyond the red-violet amaranthin and its C_{15}-epimer isoamaranthin, the authors reported the production of new pigments belonging to the betaxanthins' group: methyl derivative of arginine-bx and an unidentified betaxanthin. The production of betacyanins by seedlings obtained from *callus* cell line of *A. tricolor* was also reported and positively influenced by light and cytokinins [131]. The expression of five betalains' biosynthesis genes was modulated by phytohormones but there are presumably also other factors that influence betalain production [132].

3.4. *Beta vulgaris* L.

There are four agriculturally groups within the subspecies *vulgaris* (cultivated beets): sugar beet (*B. vulgaris* ssp. *vulgaris* convar. *vulgaris* var. *altissima*), garden beet, table or red beet (*B. vulgaris* ssp. *vulgaris* convar. *vulgaris* var. *vulgaris*), fodder beet (*B. vulgaris* ssp. *vulgaris* convar. *vulgaris* var. *crassa*) and leaf beet, mangold, chard or silver beet (*B. vulgaris* ssp. *vulgaris* convar. *cicla*) [133].

The red beet is a traditional and popular vegetable in many parts of the world and has been also used to produce red juice and natural pigment in dairy products, beverages, candies and beef [134,135]. The red beetroot is the major commercially exploited betalain crop is red beetroot, being among the top ten vegetables known with the strongest antioxidant activity [11,136].

Over 80% of the total pigments of red beetroot are constituted by betacyanins, particularly betanin and its C_{15} isomer, isobetanin, whereas vulgaxanthin I is the predominant betaxanthin (yellow) [135,137].

Lee et al. [135] reported four main betalains in 9 cultivars of red beetroot, whose concentrations and proportions were cultivar dependent: betanin and isobetanin (betacyanins) and vulgaxantin I and miraxanthin V. Betacyanin:betaxanthin content ratio in red beetroot generally ranges about 1:3, depending on the cultivar and technology for obtaining juices [138].

Slatnar et al. [138] identified and quantified 15 betacyanins and 7 betaxanthins in red and yellow coloured cultivars grown in the field and at the same time compared the content of the analysed compounds in beetroot flesh, peel and petiole. The betacyanins identified included: 2′-*O*-glucosyl-betanin, betanin, 2′-*O*-glucosyl-isobetanin, isobetanin, isoprebetanin, betanidin, 2,17-bidecarboxy-neobetanin, 17-decarboxy-neobetanin, 2-decarboxy-neobetanin, neobetanin, 2,17-bidecarboxy-2,3-dehydro-neobetanin, 6′-*O*-feruloyl-2′-*O*-glucosyl-betanin, 6′-*O*-feruloyl-2′-*O*-glucosyl-isobetanin, 2-decarboxy-2,3-dehydro-neobetanin, 6′-*O*-feruloyl-betanin/isobetanin. The betaxanthins identified were: glutamine-bx (vulgaxanthin I), proline-isobx (isoindicaxanthin), proline-bx (indicaxanthin), valine-isobx, isoleucine-isobx, isoleucine-bx/leucine-isobx (isovulgaxanthin IV) and phenylalanine-isobx.

Not all identified compounds were present in all parts of the plant [138]. For example, betanin and 2-decarboxy-neobetanin were only detected in the peel. Others were absent in flesh: 2,17-bidecarboxy-2,3-dehydro-neobetanin, 6′-*O*-feruloyl-2′-*O*-glucosyl-betanin, 6′-*O*-feruloyl-2′-*O*-glucosyl-isobetanin and 6′-*O*-feruloyl-betanin/isobetanin. In red beetroot, only vulgaxanthin, isoleucine-isobx, isoleucine-bx/leucine-isobx (isovulgaxanthin IV) were present and only in flesh and peel.

More recently, Sawicki et al. [136] reported eighteen betacyanins and twelve betaxanthins in thirteen varieties and in the root parts of red beet, dominating betanin and isobetanin (betacyanins) and vulgaxanthin I (betaxanthins) as previously described [135,137]. The root peel had the highest betalain concentration.

According to Sawicki et al. [136], the betacyanins identified were: prebetanin, betanin, isoprebetanin, betanidin, isobetanin, 17-decarboxy-neobetanin, 17-decarboxy-betanidin/isobetanidin, neobetanin, 15-decarboxy-betanidin/isobetanidin, 17-decarboxy-betanin, 17-decarboxy-isobetanin, 2-decarboxy-neobetanin, 2,17-bidecarboxy-betanin/isobetanin, 2,17-bidecarboxy-neobetanin, 6′-*O*-feruloyl betanin, 6′-*O*-feruloyl-isobetanin, 2-decarboxy-isobetanin, 2-decarboxy-betanin (Figure 8). The betaxanthins identified were: glutamine-bx (vulgaxanthin I), valine-bx, leucine-bx (vulgaxanthin IV), asparagine-bx (vulgaxanthin III), phenylalanine-isobx, tryptophan-bx, tyramine-bx (miraxanthin III), 3-methoxytyramine-bx, phenylalanine-bx, threonine-bx, aspartic acid-bx (miraxanthin II) and γ-aminobutyric acid-bx.

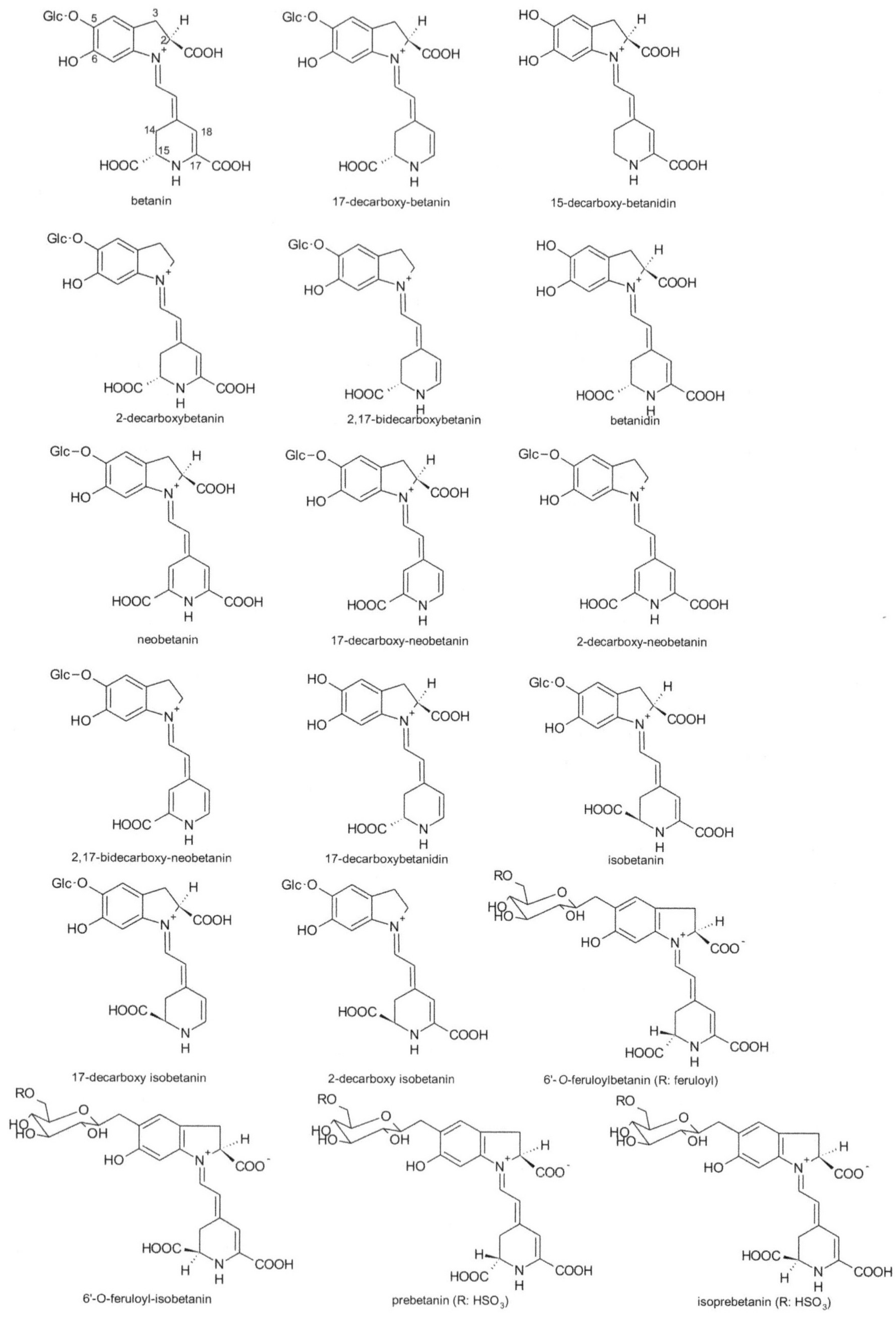

Figure 8. Betacyanins identified in the root parts of red beet.

Several factors have been evaluated (some constituents of culture media, light, pH, type and inoculum cultures, utilization of adsorbents) in order to enhance the production of betalains by Beta tissue cultures [40,44], particularly hairy roots [39,41–43,45,139–142].

Several factors may influence the amounts of betalain pigments in the red beetroot such as water stress, growth of plants in the greenhouse or field, different radiation sources either in the nature or in cell cultures, thermal treatment either in industrial or home processing [46,134,135,142–147]. In some cases, the biological activities were affected by these factors. For example, the capacity for scavenging free radicals (DPPH, ABTS) and the reductive power are strongly affected by beet root processing [144]. The gamma ray radiation at 30 kGy also influenced the antioxidant activity of betalain extracts, decreasing it. The capacity for inhibiting tyrosinase activity presented a similar behaviour of that reported for the capacity for scavenging DPPH free radicals [134].

Antioxidant activity of betalains from red beet is largely reported, using diverse methodologies for its evaluation. Generally, betacyanins have higher antioxidant activity than betaxanthins. Glycosylation of betalains reduces their ability for scavenging free radicals and consequently decrease their antioxidant activity. The position of glycosylation also affects the radical scavenging property (6-*O*-glycosylated betacyanins exhibit higher free radical scavenging activity than 5-*O*-glycosylated counterparts). The antioxidant activity of betaxanthins is function of the number of hydroxyl and imino residues. Betaxanthins without phenolic hydroxyl groups present only moderate radical scavenging ability [6,26,60,148].

The pH is also an important factor influencing the capacity of betalains for scavenging free radicals. At higher values of pH, the antioxidant activity of betalains generally increases, in contrast to their stability that decreases [7,14]. The encapsulation of some betalains has been made for improving the stability, not affecting their capacity for scavenging free radicals [14,149].

For preventing losses of betalains and respective antioxidant activity, due to thermal treatment of juices, Slavov et al. [150] treated the pressed red beet juice with microwave irradiation. This procedure was able to improve its capacity for scavenging peroxyl radicals. In this case, the amounts of betacyanins decreased in contrast to those of betaxanthins and polyphenols. According to the authors, the best extraction of polyphenols using microwave irradiation may partly explain the best activity found. In addition, the highest amounts of betaxanthins could be result of the synthesis of these pigments during the microwave pre-treatment [150].

Beyond the capacity for scavenging DPPH, ABTS, peroxyl radicals, some authors [151,152] also showed that beet root pomace extracts were able to scavenge other free radicals, such as hydroxyl and superoxide anion radical, being the activities found dose-dependent. A correlation was found between the activities and all phytochemical components (phenols, such as ferulic acid, betacyanins and betaxanthins) detected in the extracts [151,152].

Synergistic antioxidant activity between phenolic compounds and betalains in *B. vulgaris* root extracts was reported [31]. Even in the same organ (root), different antioxidant activities (outer layer had higher activity than the inner part) were found [136]. The harvesting season has also influenced the capacity of red beet root to scavenge the DPPH free radicals. Fresh spring red beet had higher amounts of betalains and antioxidant activity than those samples collected in autumn [153].

A powder derived from beetroot juice, obtained by spray drying, showed stability and antioxidant activity but dependent on the water activity at which they are stored. The greatest stability of the powder was verified for storage atmospheres of a_w (water activity) lower than 0.521, whereas the best antioxidant activity was observed for a_w values higher than 0.748. However, the powder cannot be stored at this atmosphere a_w because rapidly the powder would dissolve [154]. For this reason, the antioxidant activity must be sacrificed in detriment of the stability of the powder.

Beyond the importance of this species for obtaining natural dyes, many properties have been attributed to the beet root betalains, which can prevent some degenerative illnesses, coronary diseases and cancer if consumed in a balanced diet [68].

3.5. Celosia argentea L.

The genus *Celosia* consists of about 60 species worldwide and is native in subtropical and temperate zones of Africa, South America and South East Asia [155]. There has been a great controversy in the designations of *Celosia argentea*, *Celosia argentea* var. *cristata* and *Celosia cristata*. Some consider *Celosia cristata* as a synonymous of *Celosia argentea*, others as a variety of *Celosia argentea* (var. *cristata* (L.) Kuntze), or a separate species [156]. However, several biometric, cytological and molecular studies have revealed that *Celosia cristata* and *Celosia argentea* can be considered as two species, being *C. argentea* the direct progenitor of *Celosia cristata* [157–163].

C. argentea is considered a wild form, whereas *C. cristata* and *C. plumosa* are considered cultivars. Such designation is based on the flower head form. *C. argentea* has cylindrical pink or rose flower heads with longer bloom stalk; *C. cristata* has crested tightly grouped flowers that form into a wide cockscomb, being these flowers known as brain celosia, wool-flowers or cockscombs; and *C. plumosa* that has feathery plume like flower heads [164–166]. In the present work, *C. cristata* and *C. plumosa* are considered species.

The name *Celosia* is derived from the Greek word "kelos"—which means "burned, burning"—owing to the colour of the inflorescences (yellow, red and orange), particularly for *C. plumosa*, which resembles flames erupting from the stems [165,166].

Celosia plumosa and *C. cristata* are largely used as ornamental plants but the seedlings, young leaves and inflorescences are also utilised as vegetables in Asia, Africa and South America. Green leaves possess a characteristic sweet taste appreciated in soups [167–170]. In folk medicine, dried leaves, inflorescences and seeds (semem celosiae) of *C. argentea* are used as disinfectant and ailments for eyes (to improve eyesight) and the liver, in the treatment of dysentery, dysuria, blood and gynaecologic diseases, hypertension, sarcoptidosis, among other disorders [167,171–174].

Beyond those attributes and applications, *C. argentea* is also considered a weed that may affect the growth of many crops since it inhibits germination and seedling growth of associated crops, such as *Sorghum bicolor*, *Phaseolus aureus*, *Arachis hypogaea*, *Dolichos lablab* and *Vigna unguiculata* [175]. Perveen et al. [176] reported on the possibility of *C. argentea* to be a substitute of herbicides to control some weeds, such as *Lepidium sativum*, that attack crops, due to the results obtained with phenolic-rich extracts of *C. argentea* that were able to control the growth of *L. sativum*.

Laboratorial research has demonstrated diverse biological properties of extracts either in vitro or in vivo conditions: antimicrobial [177,178], anti-inflammatory [179], immunomodulatory [180–183], antidiabetic [184], antimetastatic [182], anticancer [172,185], healing effects on burn wounds [186,187], inhibitor of α-amylase and α-glucosidase [188]; inhibitor of acetylcholinesterase and tyrosinase [189]; hepatoprotective [174,180,181,190] and antioxidant [168,169,191]. However, there are also reports of the pro-oxidant activity of aqueous and methanolic extracts of *C. argentea*, due to the possible interaction between the molecules with other antioxidants (vitamin C) and minerals (copper, iron) also present in the extract, generating cuprous and ferrous ions that are potent pro-oxidants [192,193]. The biological properties found were generally attributed to phenols [172,183,185] including flavonoids [179], polysaccharides [180,181], saponins [174,190] and bicyclic peptides [194].

The seeds of *C. argentea* (Semen celosiae) are a Chinese herbal medicine for eye and hepatic diseases [195]. The dried ripe seeds are known in China as "Qing Xiang Zi" and are used for the treatment of some diseases such as hepatitis, hypertension, sarcoptidosis and to improve eyesight [173,196]. Saponins (celosins), phenol glycosides and flavonoids may explain some of those properties [67,190,196]. In the seeds, there are also the bicyclic peptides (celogentins and moroidin) that exhibit a huge tubulin polymerization inhibition, with the exception of celogentin K [194,195,197–200].

The colour of *Celosia* inflorescences may vary from yellow to various shades of red and violet, particularly for the garden *Celosia* (*cristata* and *plumosa*). The pigments involved in these colours are betalains [155]. Six pigments have been reported: amaranthin, isoamaranthin, betalamic acid, dopamine-bx, 3-methoxytyramine-bx and *S*-tryptophan-bx (Figures 4, 6, 7 and 9). However, the amounts of these pigments were different according to the colour of the inflorescences and species.

Thus, for the species *cristata*, in the yellow inflorescences predominated dopamine-bx; in the orange inflorescences, amaranthin/isoamaranthin and dopamine-bx were found in similar amounts; whereas in red inflorescences, amaranthin/isoamaranthin were the main pigments. In addition, the amounts of total betalains were also dependent on the colour of the inflorescences. By ascending order, the total amounts of betalains in the inflorescences of the species *cristata* were: yellow < orange < red [155]. In the cultivated *C. plumosa*, dopamine-bx predominated in the yellow inflorescences (Figure 9), such as in the species *cristata*, nevertheless 4 times higher than in this species. In orange-red inflorescences similar amounts of amaranthin/isoamaranthin and dopamine-bx were reported by the authors [155]. Shortly, the red inflorescences of *C. cristata* contained minor amounts of betaxanthins which were in higher amounts in the yellow and orange-red inflorescences. Such results may indicate that there is a gradual reversion of the pigments' biosynthesis: dopa-*cyclo*-dopa to amaranthin and dopa-dopamine to betaxanthins [155].

The yellow and orange-red inflorescences of the species *plumosa* had always higher amounts of betaxanthins than the yellow and orange inflorescences of the species *cristata* [155]. Cai et al. [167] also described a higher ratio of betaxanthins to betacyanins in the orange-red inflorescences of *C. plumosa* than in the correspondent inflorescences' colour of the *C. cristata*.

Schliemann et al. [155] did not find celosianins (Figure 9), amaranthin-type (substituted at C-5 of betanidin) betacyanins with acyl groups (*p*-coumaroyl and feruloyl groups) which were already reported by Piatelli and Minale [201] and, later, also reported by Cai et al. [202] for *C. cristata*. The remaining betacyanins and betaxanthins were also reported for the same species [155].

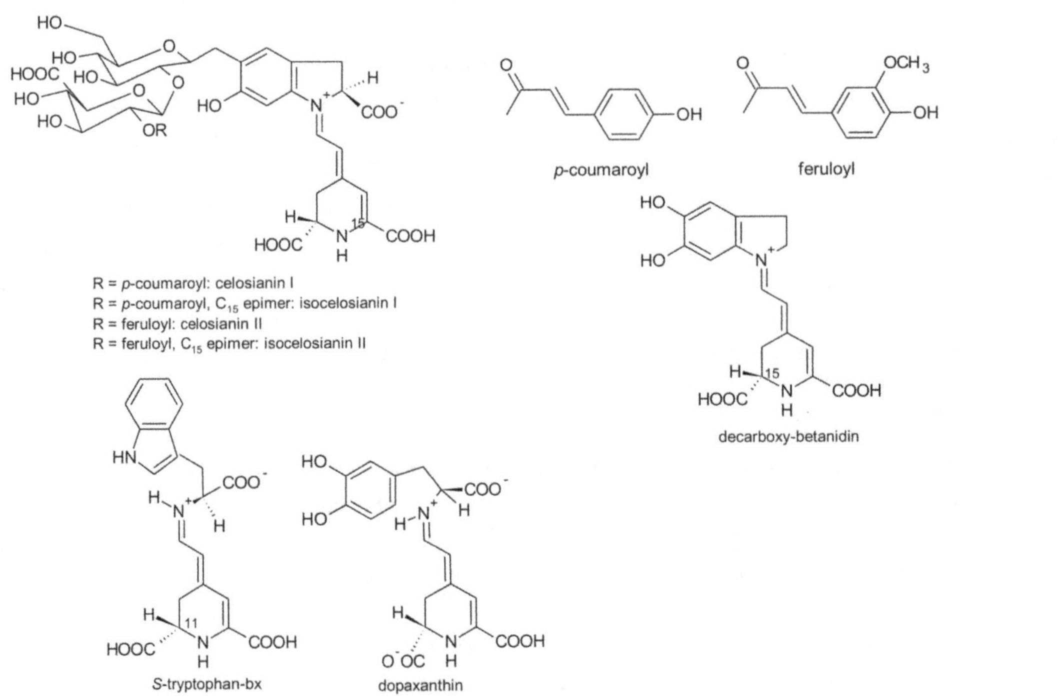

Figure 9. Celosianins, dihydroxylated betalains and *S*-tryptophan-bx from *Celosia*.

In the yellow inflorescences of *Celosia*, Schliemann et al. [155] found high levels of dopamine, thousand-fold higher than 3-methoxytyramine, thereby the authors warn the possible toxicological effect of these inflorescences when consumed as a vegetable or as an herb in traditional Chinese medicine.

Cai et al. [202] studied the chemical stability and colorant properties of the betaxanthins isolated from *C. argentea*. They found that these pigments were bright yellow in the pH range 2.2–7.0, being more stable at pH 5.5. In addition, the betaxanthins of *Celosia* were more stable than betacyanins at 40 °C but as unstable as red betacyanins (betanin and amaranthin) at temperatures higher than 40 °C.

Lyophilised betaxanthins had much higher storage stability than the corresponding aqueous solutions at 22 °C, although refrigeration increased the stability.

In cell culture of *Celosia plumosa*, established from hypocotyls, the new betalains dopaxanthin, betanidin and decarboxy-betanidin (Figure 9) were found beyond dopamine-bx [203]. Cell suspension cultures showed increased production of the dihydroxylated betalains dopaxanthin, betanidin and decarboxy-betanidin. There was also secretion of these pigments from the cells to the culture medium reaching maximal values after 8 days of culture. Along with betalains, the precursor molecules betalamic acid and dopamine were also obtained in the same cell cultures [203].

The effect of light and type of light on the biosynthesis of betalains of *Celosia* was studied [204]. The authors found that white and prolonged far-red irradiation induce the accumulation of betalains in that species. They suggested that the accumulation of these pigments induced by the prolonged far-red irradiation is controlled by the photosynthetic system.

Dopa feeding did not induce an accumulation of betaxanthins by *Celosia*. The same behaviour was observed for other species of the *Amarantaceae* family (particularly of the genera *Gomphrena* and *Iresine*), however for some species of *Portulacaceae*, *Chenopodiaceae* and *Aizoaceae*, when dopa had been added to the apical stem parts with single flower buds or inflorescences, a higher accumulation of betaxanthins were observed [205].

The action of phytohormones on the synthesis of betalains was also studied [206]. These authors reported that indolacetic acid, kinetin, abscisic acid and ethrel at lower concentrations stimulated the betacyanin synthesis and depressed the hypocotyl length of dark grown *Celosia cristata* seedlings. The authors concluded that those compounds, at specific concentrations, control de biosynthesis of betalains through ethylene production in plant tissues.

Bodhipadma et al. [207] investigated and compared the inflorescences of *Celosia cristata*, obtained either in vitro or in vivo. The authors detected that both inflorescences have the same shape but the floret size was smaller in those plants obtained in vitro, despite presenting the same number of bracts, tepals, stamens, ovaries and styles. Both in vitro and in vivo pollen had similar shape, size and germination percentage; however, the formation of seeds did not occur in vitro. The plant regeneration of *Celosia* using in vitro methodologies was also reported [171,208,209] and in vitro plants could be obtained from diverse explants (leaf, stem, shoot tips) and *callus*. Higher percentage of regeneration was possible in well-defined conditions and in vitro plants produced lower mean cell areas but higher nuclear areas when compared to in vivo plants. Somaclonal variation did not occur [208].

3.6. *Chenopodium quinoa* Willd

The term *Chenopodium* is derived from the Greek words "chenos", which means "goose", and "podos", which means "foot", because the leaves often resemble goose feet [210]. *Chenopodium quinoa* Willd (quinoa) is a dicotyledonous herbaceous plant and a seed-producing crop native to the Andean regions of Chile, Peru, Ecuador and Bolivia. The seeds are small, round and flat, are the main edible parts of the crop and their colours range from white and yellow to purple and black [211–214], although the main commercial varieties are white or black [215].

Quinoa was a staple food of the Incas until the Spanish conquest that introduced wheat and barley although the considerable production losses of these crops due to their poor adaptability to the environmental conditions of the Andean region. In contrast, *C. quinoa* is well adapted to the environmental conditions of that region: frequent drought, frost, hail and wind at an elevation of 3500–3900 m above sea level [211,213,216–218]. Quinoa is able to survive with salinity levels as high as those present in sea water (electrical conductivity 40 dS/m to 400 mM NaCl) [216,217,219].

Quinoa is a facultative halophyte that comprises wild relatives and domesticated populations. It exhibits great genetic variability which permits to the crop to grow since altitudes from sea level up to 3900 m above sea level, from extreme aridity (annual rainfall 80 mm) to 2000 mm; in soils with a great range of pH; different photoperiods (short-day and day-neutral cultivars); and withstand temperatures between −8 and 38 °C. Moreover, it has high potential to be cultivated outside its native range [214,218,220–222].

There has been an increase of the production of quinoa outside the Andean region, such as United States of America, Canada, India, Italy and China. The interest for the production of that crop is due to the high nutritional and functional properties of seeds. They have a high concentration of proteins (≤23%) providing all of the essential amino acids (lysine, threonine and methionine) nutritionally well balanced; lipids in which prevails linoleic and oleic acids; vitamins (vitamin E and folate); and minerals recommended in the human diet [220,223,224]. Quinoa, a pseudocereal, has been considered gluten-free because it contains very little or no prolamin, and therefore is adequate for celiac patients and for people allergic to wheat [212,225,226]. However, some few cultivars had celiactoxic epitopes, that is, such cultivars had been able to activate the adaptive and innate immune responses in some patients with celiac disease [227].

The traditional uses of quinoa in the Andean region includes whole seeds in soups, "quispiño" (cooked quinoa bread made from raw flour and animal fat), "tactte" (small cake made from quinoa flour fried in fat animal), "pesqhe" (salted porridge with sweet quinoa seeds), bread, noodles and biscuits [221]. The quinoa seeds can be fermented for beer or for a traditional alcoholic beverage called "chichi". The leaves are also used like spinach and the germinated quinoa seedlings can be incorporated in salads. The whole plant is also used to feed cattle, pigs and poultry [29]. More recently, the application of quinoa broadened and in other regions of the world it has been used in the production of bread (sourdough and non-sourdough), Chinese steamed bread, pasta (tagliatelle and spaghetti), snacks, cookies, edible films and food-grade Pickering emulsions [224].

The leaves, stems and grain have folk medicinal uses in cicatrization, inflammation, analgesia against toothache and as a disinfectant of the urinary tract. It is also used in the case of fractures and internal haemorrhaging and as an insect repellent [228].

Beyond the important nutritional properties of quinoa seeds, they also present antinutritional and bitter-tasting saponins, which must be removed by washing the grain or by mechanical abrasion. The amounts of saponins in seeds determine the "bitter" or "sweet" genotypes. "Bitter" variety contains >0.11% of free saponins, whereas or "sweet" variety contains <0.11% of free saponins [212,229,230]. The main structures of saponins include oleanolic acid, hederagenin and phytolaccagenic acid [231,232].

In one study [231], the authors reported that the amount of saponins in quinoa seeds decrease under saline and drought conditions, thereby a deficit of irrigation could be an interesting and sustainable way to reduce the saponin levels, nevertheless the authors did not describe the effect of the same abiotic factors (salt and drought) on the crop yield. According to the authors, the reduction of saponin content would avoid the necessity to eliminate the outer layers of the seeds where vitamins and minerals are distributed.

Other secondary metabolites can be found in quinoa seeds: phytosterols (β-sitosterol, campestrol, brassicasterol and stigmasterol); phytoecdysteroids [20-hydroxyecdysone, makisterone A, 24-*epi*-makisterone A and 24(28)-dehydromakisterone A]; phenolic acids (ferulic, vanillic and *p*-coumaric) and particularly flavonoids (quercetin, acacetin, apigenin, kampferol and respective glycosides) and betalains [29,214,231–233].

Only very few works report the presence of betalains in the coloured seeds of quinoa. Until a recent past, the pigments described for coloured seeds of quinoa were anthocyanins [234]. Only in a work of Tang et al. [214] that, for the first time, the authors identified betacyanins (betanin and isobetanin) in the red and black seeds of quinoa from Canada. Later, Escribano et al. [215] reported more betalains than betanin and isobetanin: amaranthin, dopaxanthin, dopamine-bx or miraxanthin V and proline-bx or indicaxanthin, after analysis of 29 extracts obtained from seeds of different colour (white-black) from Peru. Betacyanins predominated in the red-violet seeds, whereas in yellow ones, betaxanthins predominated. These results contrast with those previously reported [233]. The authors did not detect the presence of betacyanins in some Peruvian red seeds of quinoa. Nevertheless, Abderrahim et al. [235] detected and quantified total betalains (betacyanis and betaxanthins) in

Peruvian red seeds of quinoa. The presence of betalains was qualitatively confirmed by the change in the initial colour from red to yellow, after treatment with 2 M sodium hydroxide. According to the absorption spectra of the extracts, the authors [235] classified them in two groups, one presenting a similar spectrum to the beet root extract and the second one in which the peak related to the betaxanthins was absent.

Phenolic fractions of *C. quinoa* seeds revealed capacity for scavenging peroxyl and DPPH free radicals, as well as capacity for reducing Fe^{3+}. The authors [214] did not assay the betalain extracts in what concerns antioxidant activity. The capacity for scavenging peroxyl radicals and for reducing metal ions was attributed to the relative high levels of HMF (hydroxymethylfurfural) and not to the phenolic compounds. The presence of this sugar degradation product in the extracts is due to the acid hydrolysis method, at relatively high temperature, that the extracts were submitted without previous remotion of free sugars. Other authors [234,236,237] also reported antioxidant activity of seed extracts of quinoa through the capacity for scavenging free radicals (DPPH, ABTS) and reducing power, which activities were related with phenol content and not with betalains.

Escribano et al. [215] evaluated the antioxidant capacity of extracts obtained from diverse coloured seeds of quinoa (white-black) from Peru. The authors found a correlation between the activity, measured through diverse methods and the colour of seeds. The most active samples were those obtained from red-violet and yellow seeds, that is, in those that exhibited the highest amounts of betacyanins (red-violet) and betaxanthins (yellow).

A direct procedure without previous extraction of antioxidants was followed by Abderrahim et al. [235] for determining the antioxidant activity of diverse coloured seeds of quinoa from Peru, using Cu^{2+} oxidizing reagents. The results showed a positive correlation between the phenols/betalains (betacyanins and betaxanthins) content and antioxidant activity.

Other components, like saponins, which are considered to be anti-nutritionals, may possess some interesting biological properties. Yao et al. [238] showed that saponin-rich quinoa extracts were anti-inflammatory by decreasing the production of the inflammatory mediator nitric oxide and by inhibiting the release of the inflammatory cytokines tumour necrosis factor alpha (TNF-α) and interleukin 6 (IL-6) in LPS-stimulated RAW 264.7 macrophages.

In vivo studies demonstrated that quinoa intake may reduce the risk of developing cardiovascular disease and beneficially modulate metabolic parameters by decreasing the levels of triglycerides, cholesterol, LDL, preventing lipid peroxidation and increasing glutathione (GSH) [29,239–241].

The phytoecdysteroid 20-hydroxyecdysone was reported to show neuroprotective effects by modulation of $GABA_A$ (γ-aminobutyric acid) receptors as well as hypocholesterolemic activity through the increase of cholesterol transformation into bile acids [242]. The same phytoecdysteroid also had anti-obesity and antidiabetic activity detected in rats that were fed with a high fat diet. The authors linked such attributes to a reduction of absorption of lipids and increase of glucose oxidation, mitochondrial oxidative phosphorylation and energy expenditure [241,243,244].

4. Conclusions

Natural pigments, namely carotenoids, flavonoids, anthocyanins or betalains, have been used in food and pharmaceutical industries, replacing the synthetic pigments, since they are considered less deleterious for human health. However, particularly anthocyanins possess limitations: weak stability to processing and storage conditions. The weak stability of the pigments to pH or temperature is, however, less important for betalains since they are stable for broader pH range and are also able to regenerate after thermal treatment. Nevertheless, natural resources are not inexhaustible being also highly dependent on the climatic conditions. In addition, the possibility to obtain diverse hue colours with synthetic pigments is generally easier when compared to the natural ones, unless diverse pigments of different groups are mixed.

Therefore, several approaches need to be followed in order to obtain natural pigments in a sustainable way, cheaper and closer to the consumer requirements. Biotechnological production of betalains through plant cell culture from betalain producing species, so far showing weak yield, or microbes must be more deeply studied and even considered as alternatives to the traditional production of betalains. Studies regarding the encapsulation of natural pigments, such as betalains, for enhancing their colour stabilities, are possibilities to take into account. Nevertheless, the utilization of these natural products requires that they do not interfere on the final quality of the product where the pigments are applied.

Acknowledgments: The author wishes to acknowledge the financial support provided by the Portuguese National Funding Agency for Science, Research and Technology (Fundação para a Ciência e a Tecnologia—FCT; Portugal), under the projects UID/BIA/04325/2013-MeditBio.

Conflicts of Interest: The author declares no conflict of interest.

References

1. Delgado-Vargas, F.; Jiménez, A.R.; Paredes-López, O. Natural pigments: Carotenoids, anthocyanins and betalains—Characterisitcs, biosynthesis, processing and stability. *Crit. Rev. Food Sci. Nutr.* **2000**, *40*, 173–189. [CrossRef] [PubMed]
2. Stintzing, F.C.; Carle, R. Functional properties of anthocyanins and betalains in plants, food and in human nutrition. *Trends Food Sci. Technol.* **2004**, *15*, 19–38. [CrossRef]
3. Clement, J.S.; Mabry, T.J. Pigment evolution in the Caryophyllales: A systematic overview. *Bot. Acta* **1996**, *109*, 360–367. [CrossRef]
4. Stintzing, F.C.; Trichterborn, J.; Carle, R. Characterisation of anthocyanin–betalain mixtures for food colouring by chromatic and HPLC-DAD-MS analyses. *Food Chem.* **2006**, *94*, 296–309. [CrossRef]
5. Gandía-Herrero, F.; Escribano, J.; García-Carmona, F. Biological activities of plant pigments betalains. *Crit. Rev. Food Sci. Nutr.* **2016**, *56*, 937–945. [CrossRef] [PubMed]
6. Slimen, I.B.; Najar, T.; Abderrabba, M. Chemical and antioxidant properties of betalains. *J. Agric. Food Chem.* **2017**, *65*, 675–689. [CrossRef] [PubMed]
7. Herbach, K.M.; SDtintzing, F.C.; Carle, R. Betalain stability and degradation-structural and chromatic aspects. *J. Food Sci.* **2006**, *71*, R41–R50. [CrossRef]
8. Khan, M.I.; Giridhar, P. Plant betalains: Chemistry and biochemistry. *Phytochemistry* **2015**, *117*, 267–295. [CrossRef] [PubMed]
9. Sigurdson, G.T.; Tang, P.; Giusti, M.M. Natural colorants: Food colorants from natural sources. *Ann. Rev. Food Sci. Technol.* **2017**, *8*, 261–280. [CrossRef] [PubMed]
10. Strack, D.; Vogt, T.; Schliemann, W. Recent advances in betalain research. *Phytochemistry* **2003**, *62*, 247–269. [CrossRef]
11. Azeredo, H.M.C. Betalains: Properties, sources, applications and stability—A review. *Int. J. Food Sci. Technol.* **2009**, *44*, 2365–2376. [CrossRef]
12. Gandía-Herrero, F.; Escribano, J.; García-Carmona, F. Structural implications on color, fluorescence and antiradical activity in betalains. *Planta* **2010**, *232*, 449–460. [CrossRef] [PubMed]
13. Tanaka, Y.; Sasaki, N.; Ohmiya, A. Biosynthesis of plant pigments: Anthocyanins, betalains and carotenoids. *Plant J.* **2008**, *54*, 733–749. [CrossRef] [PubMed]
14. Khan, M.I. Plant betalains: Safety, antioxidant activity, clinical efficacy and bioavailability. *Compr. Rev. Food Sci. Food Saf.* **2016**, *15*, 316–330. [CrossRef]
15. Ngmwonglumlert, L.; Devahastin, S.; Chiewchan, N. Natural colorants: Pigment stability and extraction yield enhancement via utilization of appropriate pre-treatment and extraction methods. *Crit. Rev. Food Sci. Nutr.* **2017**, *57*, 3243–3259. [CrossRef] [PubMed]
16. Gonçalves, L.C.P.; di Genova, B.M.; Dörr, F.A.; Pinto, E.; Bastos, E.L. Effect of dielectric microwave heating on the color and antiradical capacity of betanin. *J. Food Eng.* **2013**, *118*, 49–55. [CrossRef]
17. Cardoso-Ugarte, G.A.; Sosa-Morales, M.E.; Ballard, T.; Liceaga, A.; San Martín-González, M.F. Microwave-assited extraction of betalains from red beet (*Beta vulgaris*). *LWT Food Sci. Technol.* **2014**, *59*, 276–282. [CrossRef]
18. Celli, G.B.; Brooks, M.S.-L. Impact of extraction and processing conditions on betalains and comparison of proerties with anthocyanins—A current review. *Food Res. Int.* **2017**, *100*, 501–509. [CrossRef] [PubMed]

19. Mereddy, R.; Chan, A.; Fanning, K.; Nirmal, N.; Sultanbawa, Y. Betalain rich functional extract with reduced salts and nitrate content from red beetroot (*Beta vulgaris* L.) using membrane separation technology. *Food Chem.* **2017**, *215*, 311–317. [CrossRef] [PubMed]
20. Mulinacci, N.; Innocenti, M. Anthocyanins and betalains. Chapter 22. In *Food Analysis by HPLC*, 3rd ed.; Nollet, M.L.L., Toldrà, F., Eds.; CRC Press: Boca Raton, FL, USA; Taylor & Francis Group: Didcot, UK, 2013; pp. 757–776.
21. Gandía-Herrero, F.; García-Carmona, F. Biosynthesis of betalains: Yellow and violet plant pigments. *Trends Plant Sci.* **2013**, *18*, 334–343. [CrossRef] [PubMed]
22. Schliemann, W.; Steiner, U.; Strack, D. Betanidin formation from dihydroxyphenylalanine in a model assay system. *Phytochemistry* **1998**, *49*, 1593–1598. [CrossRef]
23. Niveyro, S.L.; Mortensen, A.; Fomsgaerd, I.S.; Salvo, A. Differences among five amaranth varieties (*Amaranthus* spp.) regarding secondary metabolites and foliar herbivory by chewing insects in the field. *Arthropod Plant Interact.* **2013**, *7*, 235–245. [CrossRef]
24. Shao, L.; Chen, X.; Chen, Y.; Sun, B.; Chow, W.; Peng, C. Differential responses of photosystem II activity to photooxidation in red and green tissues of *Amaranthus tricolour* leaves. *Pak. J. Bot.* **2013**, *45*, 1905–1912.
25. Shu, Z.; Shao, L.; Huang, H.-Y.; Zeng, X.-Q.; Lin, Z.-F.; Chen, G.-Y.; Peng, C.-L. Comparison of thermostability of PSII between the chromatic and green leaf cultivars of *Amaranthus tricolour* L. *Phytosynthetica* **2009**, *47*, 548–558. [CrossRef]
26. Esatbeyoglu, T.; Wagner, A.E.; Schini-Kert, V.B.; Rimbach, G. Betanin—A food colorant with biological activity. *Mol. Nutr. Food Res.* **2015**, *59*, 36–47. [CrossRef] [PubMed]
27. Cai, Y.-Z.; Sun, M.; Corke, H. Characterization and application of betalain pigments from plants of the *Amaranthaceae*. *Trends Food Sci. Technol.* **2005**, *16*, 370–376. [CrossRef]
28. Gliszczyńska-Świgło, A.; Szymusiak, H.; Malinowska, P. Betanin, the main pigment of red beet: Molecular origin of its exceptionally high free radical-scavenging activity. *Food Addit. Contam.* **2006**, *23*, 1079–1087. [CrossRef] [PubMed]
29. Graf, B.L.; Rojas-Silva, P.; Rojo, L.E.; Delatorre-Herrera, J.; Baldeón, M.E.; Raskin, I. Innovations in health value and functional food development of quinoa (*Chenopodium quinoa* Willd.). *Compr. Rev. Food Sci. Food Saf.* **2015**, *14*, 431–445. [CrossRef] [PubMed]
30. Hilou, A.; Nacoulma, O.G.; Guiguemde, T.R. In vivo antimalarial activities of extracts from *Amaranthus spinosus* L. and *Boerhaavia erecta* L. in mice. *J. Ethnopharmacol.* **2006**, *103*, 236–240. [CrossRef] [PubMed]
31. Koubaier, H.B.H.; Snoussi, A.; Essaidi, I.; Chaabouni, M.M.; Thonart, P.; Bouzouita, N. Betalain and phenolic compositions, antioxidant of Tunisian red beet (*Beta vulgaris* L. *conditiva*) roots and stems extracts. *Int. J. Food Prop.* **2014**, *17*, 1934–1945. [CrossRef]
32. Lin, S.-M.; Lin, B.-H.; Hsieh, W.-M.; Ko, H.-J.; Liu, C.-D.; Chen, L.-G.; Chiou, R.Y.-Y. Structural identification and bioactivities of red-violet pigments present in *Basella alba* fruits. *J. Agric. Food Chem.* **2010**, *58*, 10364–10372. [CrossRef] [PubMed]
33. Pavlov, A.; Kovatcheva, P.; Tuneva, D.; Ilieva, M.; Bley, T. Radical scavenging activity and stability of betalains from *Beta vulgaris* hairy root culture in simulated conditions of human gastrointestinal tract. *Plant Food Hum. Nutr.* **2005**, *60*, 43–47. [CrossRef]
34. Vidal, P.J.; López-Nicolás, J.M.; Gandía-Herrero, F.; García-Carmona, F. Inactivation of lipoxygenase and cyclooxigenase by natural betalains and semi-synthetic analogues. *Food Chem.* **2014**, *154*, 246–254. [CrossRef] [PubMed]
35. Georgiev, V.; Ilieva, M.; Bley, T.; Pavlov, A. Betalain production in plant in vitro systems. *Acta Physiol. Plant.* **2008**, *30*, 581–593. [CrossRef]
36. Gandía-Herrero, F.; García-Carmona, F.; Escribano, J. Development of a protocol for the semi-synthesis and purification of betaxanthins. *Phytochem. Anal.* **2006**, *17*, 262–269. [CrossRef] [PubMed]
37. Schliemann, W.; Kobayashi, N.; Strack, D. The decisive step in betaxanthin biosynthesis is a spontaneous reaction. *Plant Physiol.* **1999**, *119*, 1217–1232. [CrossRef] [PubMed]
38. Cabanes, J.; Gandía-Herrero, F.; Escribano, J.; García-Carmona, F.; Jiménez-Atiénzar, M. One-step synthesis of betalains using a novel betalamic acid derivatized support. *J. Agric. Food Chem.* **2014**, *62*, 3776–3782. [CrossRef] [PubMed]
39. Pavlov, A.; Bley, T. Betalains biosynthesis by *Beta vulgaris* L. hairy root culture in a temporary immersion cultivation system. *Proc. Biochem.* **2006**, *41*, 848–852. [CrossRef]

40. Weller, T.A.; Lasure, L.L. Betalains in beet root tissue culture. *J. Food Sci.* **1981**, *47*, 162–163. [CrossRef]
41. Böhm, H.; Mäck, G. Betaxanthin formation and free amino acids in hairy roots of *Beta vulgaris* var. *lutea* depending on nutrient medium and glutamate or glutamine feeding. *Phytochemistry* **2004**, *65*, 1361–1368. [PubMed]
42. Neelwarne, B.; Thimmaraju, R. Bioreactor for cultivation of red beet hairy roots and in situ recovery of primary and secondary metabolites. *Eng. Life Sci.* **2009**, *9*, 227–238. [CrossRef]
43. Pavlov, A.; Kovatcheva, P.; Georgiev, V.; Koleva, I.; Ilieva, M. Biosynthesis and radical scavenging activity of betalains during the cultivation of red beet (*Beta vulgaris*) hairy root cultures. *Z. Naturforsch.* **2002**, *57*, 640–644. [CrossRef]
44. Križnic, B.; Pavoković, D. Enhancement of betanin yield in transformed cells of sugar beet (*Beta vulgaris* L.). *Acta Bot. Croat.* **2010**, *69*, 173–182.
45. Rudrappa, T.; Neelwarne, B.; Aswathanarayana, R.G. In situ and ex situ adsorption and recovery of betalains from hairy root cultures of *Beta vulgaris*. *Biotechnol. Prog.* **2004**, *20*, 777–785. [CrossRef] [PubMed]
46. Shin, K.S.; Murthy, H.N.; Heo, J.W.; Paek, K.Y. Unduction of betalain pigmetantion in hairy roots of red beet under different radiation sources. *Biol. Plant.* **2003**, *47*, 149–152. [CrossRef]
47. Wang, M.; Lopez-Nieves, S.; Goldman, I.L.; Maeda, H.A. Limited tyrosine utilization explains lower betalain contents in yellow than red table beet genotypes. *J. Agric. Food Chem.* **2017**, *65*, 4305–4313. [CrossRef]
48. Polturak, G.; Aharoni, A. "La vie en rose": Biosynthesis, sources and applications of betalain pigments. *Mol. Plant* **2018**, *11*, 7–22. [CrossRef] [PubMed]
49. Cai, Y.-Z.; Sun, M.; Corke, H. Antioxidant activity of betalains from plants of the *Amaranthaceae*. *J. Agric. Food Chem.* **2003**, *51*, 2288–2294. [CrossRef] [PubMed]
50. Taira, J.; Tsuchida, E.; Katoh, M.C.; Uehara, M.; Ogi, T. Antioxidant capacity of betacyanins as radical scavengers for peroxyl radical and nitric oxide. *Food Chem.* **2015**, *166*, 531–536. [CrossRef] [PubMed]
51. Tesoriere, L.; Allegra, M.; Gentile, C.; Livrea, M.A. Betacyanins as phenol antioxidants. Chemistry and mechanistic aspects of the lipoperoxyl radical-scavenging activity in solution and liposomes. *Free Radic. Res.* **2009**, *43*, 706–717. [CrossRef] [PubMed]
52. Gandía-Herrero, F.; Escribano, J.; García-Carmona, F. The role of phenolic hidroxi groups in the free radical scavenging activity of betalains. *J. Nat. Prod.* **2009**, *72*, 1142–1146. [CrossRef] [PubMed]
53. Gandía-Herrero, F.; Escribano, J.; García-Carmona, F. Purification and antiradical properties of the structural unit of betalains. *J. Nat. Prod.* **2012**, *75*, 1030–1036. [CrossRef] [PubMed]
54. Wybraniec, S.; Starzak, K.; Skopińska, A.; Nemzer, B.; Pietrzkowski, Z.; Michałowsli, T. Studies on nonenzymatic oxidation mechanisms in neobetanin, betanin and decarboxylated betanins. *J. Agric. Food Chem.* **2013**, *61*, 6465–6476. [CrossRef] [PubMed]
55. Kanner, J.; Harel, S.; Granit, R. Betalains—A new class of dietary cationized antioxidants. *J. Agric. Food Chem.* **2001**, *49*, 5178–5185. [CrossRef] [PubMed]
56. Reddy, M.K.; Alexander-Lindo, R.L.; Nair, M.G. Relative inhibition of lipid peroxidation, cyclooxygenase enzymes and human tumor cell proliferation by natural food colors. *J. Agric. Food Chem.* **2005**, *53*, 9268–9273. [CrossRef] [PubMed]
57. Esatbeyoglu, T.; Wagner, A.E.; Motafakkerazad, R.; Nakajima, Y.; Matsugo, S.; Rimbach, G. Free radical scavenging and antioxidant activity of betanin: Electron spin resonance spectroscopy studies and studies in cultured cells. *Food Chem. Toxcicol.* **2014**, *73*, 119–126. [CrossRef] [PubMed]
58. Pietrzkowski, Z.; Nemzer, B.; Spórna, A.; Stalica, P.; Tresher, W.; Keller, R.; Jiminez, R.; Michalowski, T.; Wybraniec, S. Influence of betalin-rich extracts on reduction of discomfort associated with osteoarthritis. *New Med.* **2010**, *1*, 12–17.
59. Gentile, C.; Tesoriere, L.; Allegra, M.; Livrea, M.A.; D'Alessio, P. Antioxidant betalains from cactus pear (*Opuntia ficus-indica*) inhibit endothelial ICAM-1 expression. *Ann. N. Y. Acad. Sci.* **2004**, *1028*, 481–486. [CrossRef] [PubMed]
60. Wettasinghe, M.; Bolling, B.; Plhak, L.; Xiao, H.; Parkin, K. Phase II enzyme-inducing and antioxidant activities of beetroot (*Beta vulgaris* L.) extracts from phenotypes of different pigmentation. *J. Agric. Food Chem.* **2002**, *50*, 6704–6709. [CrossRef] [PubMed]
61. Lee, C.-H.; Wettasinghe, M.; Bolling, B.W.; Ji, L.-L.; Parkin, K.L. Betalains, phase II enzyme-inducing components from red beetroot (*Beta vulgaris* L.) extracts. *Nutr. Cancer* **2005**, *53*, 91–103. [CrossRef] [PubMed]

62. Kujawska, M.; Ignatowicz, E.; Murias, M.; Ewertowsca, M.; Mikolajczyk, K.; Jodynis-Liebert, J. Protective effect of red beetroot against carbon tetrachloride- and *N*-nitrosodiethylamine-induced oxidative stress in rats. *J. Agric. Food Chem.* **2009**, *57*, 2570–2575. [CrossRef] [PubMed]
63. Szaefer, H.; Krajka-Kuźniak, V.; Ignatowicz, E.; Adamska, T.; Baer-Dubowska, W. Evaluation of the effect of beetroot juice on DMBA-induced damage in liver and mammary gland of female Sprague-Dawley rats. *Phytother. Res.* **2014**, *28*, 55–61. [CrossRef] [PubMed]
64. Gengatharan, A.; Dykes, G.A.; Choo, E.S. Betalains: Natural plant pigments with potential application in functional foods. *LWT Food Sci. Technol.* **2015**, *64*, 645–649. [CrossRef]
65. Clemente, A.C.; Desai, P.V. Evaluation of the haematological, hypoglycemic, hypolipidemic and antioxidant properties of *Amaranthus tricolor* leaf extract in rat. *Trop. J. Pharm. Res.* **2011**, *10*, 595–602.
66. Zielinbska-Przyjemska, M.; Olejnik, A.; Dobrowolska-Zachwieja, A.; Grajek, W. In vitro effects of beetroot juice and chips on oxidative metabolism and apoptosis neutrophils from obese individuals. *Phytother. Res.* **2009**, *23*, 49–55. [CrossRef] [PubMed]
67. Mroczek, A. Phytochemistry and bioactivity of triterpene saponins from *Amaranthaceae* family. *Phytochem. Rev.* **2015**, *14*, 577–605. [CrossRef]
68. Clifford, T.; Howatson, G.; West, D.J.; Stevenson, E.J. The potential benefits of red beetroot supplementation in health and disease. *Nutrients* **2015**, *7*, 2801–2822. [CrossRef] [PubMed]
69. Deladino, L.; Alvarez, I.; de Ancos, B.; Sánchez-Moreno, C.; Molina-García, A.D.; Teixeira, A.S. Betalains and phenolic compounds of leaves and stems of *Alternanthera brasiliana* and *Alternanthera tenella*. *Food Res. Int.* **2017**, *97*, 240–249. [CrossRef] [PubMed]
70. Tsai, P.-J.; Sheu, C.-H.; Wu, P.-H.; Sun, Y.-F. Thermal and pH stability of betacyanin pigment of djulis (*Chenopodium formosanum*) in Taiwan and their relation to antixodant activity. *J. Agric. Food Chem.* **2010**, *58*, 1020–1025. [CrossRef] [PubMed]
71. Silva, L.R.; Valentão, P.; Faria, J.; Ferreres, F.; Sousa, C.; Gil-Izquierdo, A.; Pinho, B.R.; Andrade, P.B. Phytochemical investigations and biological potential screening with cellular and non-cellular models of globe amaranth (*Gomphrena globosa* L.) inflorescences. *Food Chem.* **2012**, *135*, 756–763. [CrossRef] [PubMed]
72. Cai, Y.-Z.; Xing, J.; Sun, M.; Corke, H. Rapid identification of betacyanins from *Amaranthus tricolor*, *Gomphrena globosa* and *Hylocereus polyrhizus* by matrix-assisted laser desorption/ionization quadrupole ion trap time-of-flight mass spectrometry (MALDI-QIT-TOF-MS). *J. Agric. Food Chem.* **2006**, *54*, 6520–6526. [CrossRef] [PubMed]
73. Dinda, B.; Ghosh, B.; Achari, B.; Arima, S.; Sato, N.; Harigaya, Y. Chemical constituents of *Gomphrena globosa*. II. *Nat. Prod. Sci.* **2006**, *12*, 89–93.
74. Lans, C. Ethnomedicines used in Trinidad and Tobago for urinary problems and diabetes mellitus. *J. Ethnobiol. Ethnomed.* **2006**, *2*, 45. [CrossRef] [PubMed]
75. Lans, C. Ethnomedicines used in Trinidad and Tobago for reproductive problems. *J. Ethnobiol. Ethnomed.* **2007**, *3*, 13. [CrossRef] [PubMed]
76. Kugler, F.; Stintzing, F.C.; Carle, R. Characterisation of betalain patterns of differently coloured inflorescences from *Gomphrena globosa* L. and *Bougainvillea* sp. By HPLC-DAD-ESI-MSn. *Anal. Bioanal. Chem.* **2007**, *387*, 637–648. [CrossRef] [PubMed]
77. Heuer, S.; Wray, V.; Metzaer, J.W.; Strack, D. Betacyanins from flowers of *Gomphrena globosa*. *Phytochemistry* **1992**, *31*, 1801–1807. [CrossRef]
78. Spórna-Kucab, A.; Hołda, E.; Wybraniec, S. High-speed counter-current chromatography in separation of betacyanins from flowers of red *Gomphrena globosa* L. cultivars. *J. Chromatogr. B* **2016**, *1033–1034*, 421–427. [CrossRef] [PubMed]
79. Roriz, C.L.; Barros, L.; Carvalho, A.M.; Santos-Buelga, C.; Ferreira, I.C.F.R. *Pterospartum tridentatum*, *Gomphrena globosa* and *Cymbopogon citratus*. A phytochemical study focused on antioxidant compounds. *Food Res. Int.* **2014**, *62*, 684–693. [CrossRef]
80. Ferreres, F.; Gil-Izquierdo, A.; Valentão, P.; Andrade, P.B. Structural characterization of phenolics and betacyanins in *Gomphrena globosa* by high-performance liquid chromatography-diode array detection/electrospray ionization multi-stage masss pectrometry. *Rapid Commun. Mass Spectrom.* **2011**, *25*, 3441–3446. [CrossRef] [PubMed]

81. Roriz, C.L.; Barros, L.; Prieto, M.A.; Morales, P.; Ferreira, I.C.F.R. Floral parts of *Gomphrena globosa* L. as a novel alternative source of betacyanins: Optimization of the extraction using response surface methodology. *Food Chem.* **2017**, *229*, 223–234. [CrossRef] [PubMed]
82. Roriz, C.L.; Barros, L.; Prieto, M.A.; Barreiro, M.F.; Morales, P.; Ferreira, I.C.F.R. Modern extraction techniques optimized to extract betacyanins from *Gomphrena globosa* L. *Ind. Crops Prod.* **2017**, *105*, 29–40. [CrossRef]
83. Cai, Y.-Z.; Sun, M.; Corke, H. Identification and distribution of simple and acylated betacyanins in the *Amaranthaceae*. *J. Agric. Food Chem.* **2001**, *49*, 1971–1978. [CrossRef] [PubMed]
84. Aquino, D.F.; Piccinelli, C.; Soares, F.L.P.; Arena, A.C.; Salvador, M.J.; Kassuya, A.L. Anti-hyperalgesic and anti-inflammatory activity of *Alternanthera maritima* extract and 2″-*O*-α-L-rhamnopyranosylvitexin in mice. *Inflammation* **2015**, *38*, 2057–2066. [CrossRef] [PubMed]
85. Guerra, R.N.M.; Pereira, H.-A.W.; Silveira, L.M.S.; Olea, R.S.G. Immunomodulatory properties of *Alternathera tenella* Colla aqueous extracts in mice. *Braz. J. Med. Biol. Res.* **2003**, *36*, 1215–1219. [CrossRef] [PubMed]
86. Souza, J.G.; Tomei, R.R.; Kanashiro, A.; Kabeya, L.M.; Azzolini, A.E.C.S.; Dias, D.A.; Salvador, M.J.; Lucisano, Y. Ethanolic crude extract and flavonoids isolated from *Alternanthera maritima*: Neutrophil chemiluminescence inhibition and free radical scavenging activity. *Z. Naturforsch.* **2007**, *62*, 339–347. [CrossRef]
87. Kumar, S.; Singh, P.; Mishra, G.; Srivastav, S.; Jha, K.K.; Khosa, R.L. Phytopharmacological review of *Alternanthera brasiliana* (*Amaranthaceae*). *Asian J. Plant Sci. Res.* **2011**, *1*, 41–47.
88. Samudrala, P.K.; Augustine, B.B.; Kasala, E.R.; Bodduluru, L.N.; Barua, C.; Lahkar, M. Evaluation of antitumor activity and antioxidant status of *Alternanthera brasiliana* against Ehrlich ascites carcinoma in Swiss albino mice. *Pharmacogn. Res.* **2015**, *7*, 66–73. [CrossRef] [PubMed]
89. Barua, C.C.; Talukdar, A.; Begum, S.A.; Sarma, D.K.; Pathak, D.C.; Barua, A.G.; Bora, R.S. Wound healing activity of methanolic extract of leaves of *Alternanthera brasiliana* Kuntze using in vivo and in vitro model. *Indian J. Exp. Biol.* **2009**, *47*, 1001–1005. [PubMed]
90. Brochado, C.O.; Almeida, A.P.; Barreto, B.P.; Costa, L.P.; Ribeiro, L.S.; Pereira, R.L.C.; Koatz, V.L.G.; Costa, S.S. Flavonol robinobiosides and rutinosides from *Alternanthera brasiliana* (*Amaranthaceae*) and their effects on lymphocyte proliferation in vitro. *J. Braz. Chem. Soc.* **2003**, *14*, 449–451. [CrossRef]
91. Lagrota, M.H.C.; Wigg, M.D.; Santos, M.M.G.; Miranda, M.M.F.S.; Camara, F.P.; Couceiro, J.N.S.S.; Costa, S.S. Inhibitory activity of extracts of *Alternanthera brasiliana* (*Amaranthaceae*) against the *Herpes simplex* virus. *Phytother. Res.* **1994**, *8*, 358–361. [CrossRef]
92. Pereira, D.F.; Zanon, R.B.; Santos, M.; Boligon, A.A.; Athayde, M.L. Antioxidant activities and triterpenoids isolated from *Alternanthera brasiliana* (L.) Kuntze leaves. *Nat. Prod. Res.* **2013**, *27*, 1660–1663. [CrossRef] [PubMed]
93. Souza, M.M.; Kern, P.; Floriani, A.E.O.; Cechinel-Folho, V. Analgesic properties of a hydroalcoholic extract obtained from *Alternanthera brasiliana*. *Phytother. Res.* **1998**, *12*, 279–281. [CrossRef]
94. Souza, G.C.; Haas, A.P.S.; von Poser, G.L.; Schapoval, E.E.S.; Elisabetsky, E. Ethnopharmacological studies of antimicrobial remedies in the South of Brazil. *J. Ethnopharmacol.* **2004**, *90*, 135–143. [CrossRef] [PubMed]
95. Bussmann, R.W.; Glenn, A.; Sharon, D. Antibacterial activity of medicinal plants of Northern Peru—Can traditional applications provide leads for modern science? *Indian J. Tradit. Knowl.* **2010**, *9*, 742–753.
96. Biella, C.A.; Salvador, M.J.; Dias, D.A.; Dias-Baruffi, M.; Pereira-Crott, L.S. Evaluation of immunomodulatory and anti-inflammatory effects and phytochemical screening of *Alternanthera tenella* Colla (*Amaranthaceae*) aqueous extracts. *Mem. Inst. Pswaldo Cruz* **2008**, *103*, 569–577. [CrossRef]
97. Harthman, V.C.; Souza, L.A. Ontogenia do fruto em desenvolvimento de *Alternanthera tenella* Colla e *Amaranthus blitum* Linnaeus (*Amaranthaceae*). *Acta Bot. Bras.* **2012**, *26*, 642–650. [CrossRef]
98. Kleinowski, A.M.; Brandão, I.R.; Einhardt, A.M.; Ribeiro, M.V.; Peters, J.A.; Braga, E.J.B. Pigment production and growth of *Alternanthera* plants cultured in vitro in the presence of tyrosine. *Braz. Arch. Biol. Technol.* **2014**, *57*, 253–260. [CrossRef]
99. Vendruscolo, G.S.; Mentz, L.A. Levantamento etnobotânico das plantas utilizadas como medicinais por moradores do bairro Ponta Grossa, Porto Alegre do Sul, Brasil. *Iheringa Sér. Bot.* **2006**, *61*, 83–103.
100. Salvador, M.J.; Zucchi, O.L.A.D.; Candido, R.C.; Ito, I.Y.; Dias, D.A. In vitro antimicrobial activity of crude extracts and isolated constituents of *Alternanthera maritima* (*Amaranthaceae*). *Pharm. Biol.* **2004**, *42*, 138–148. [CrossRef]

101. Salvador, M.J.; Ferreira, E.O.; Mertens-Talcott, S.U.; Castro, V.; Butterweck, V.; Derendorf, H.; Dias, D.A. Isolation and HPLC quantitative analysis of antioxidant flavnoids from *Alternanthera tenella* Colla. *Z. Naturforsch.* **2006**, *61*, 19–25.
102. Reis, A.; Kleinowski, A.M.; Klein, F.R.S.; Telles, R.T.; Amarante, L.; Braga, E.J.B. Light quality on the in vitro growth and production of pigments in the genus *Alternanthera*. *J. Crop Sci. Biotechnol.* **2015**, *18*, 349–357. [CrossRef]
103. Rodrigues-Brandão, I.; Kneinowski, A.M.; Einhardt, A.M.; Lima, M.C.; Amarante, M.C.L.L.; Peters, J.A.; Braga, E.J.B. Salicylic acid on antioxidant activity and betacyanins in production from leaves of *Alternanthera tenella*. *Ciênc. Rural* **2014**, *44*, 1893–1898. [CrossRef]
104. Moraes, V.L.G.; Santos, L.F.M.; Castro, S.B.; Loureiro, L.H.; Lima, D.A.; Souza, M.L.M.; Yien, L.M.K.; Rossi-Bergmann, B.; Costa, S.S. Inhibition of lymphocyte activation by extracts and fractions of *Kalanchoe*, *Alternanthera*, *Paullinia* and *Mikania* species. *Phytomedicine* **1994**, *1*, 199–204. [CrossRef]
105. Narayanan, M.R.; Anilkumar, N.; Balakrishnan, V.; Sivadasan, M.; Alfarhan, H.A.; Alatar, A. Wild edible plants used by the Kattunaikka, Paniya and Kuruma tribes of Wayanad District, Kerala, India. *J. Med. Plant Res.* **2011**, *5*, 3520–3529.
106. Ramachandran, V. Wild edible plants of the Anamalais, Coimbatore district, Western Ghats, Tamil Nadu. *Indian J. Tradit. Knowl.* **2007**, *6*, 173–176.
107. Peter, K.; Gandhi, P. Rediscovering the therapeutic potential of *Amaranthus* species a review. *J. Basic Appl. Sci.* **2017**, *4*, 196–205. [CrossRef]
108. Rastogi, A.; Shukla, S. Amaranth: A new millennium crop of nutraceutical values. *Crit. Rev. Food Sci. Nutr.* **2013**, *53*, 109–125. [CrossRef] [PubMed]
109. Achigan-Dako, E.G.; Sogbohossou, O.E.D.; Maundu, P. Current knowledge on *Amaranthus* spp.: Research avenues for improved nutritional value and yield in leafy amaranths in sub-Saharan Africa. *Euphytica* **2014**, *197*, 303–317. [CrossRef]
110. Das, S. Systematics and taxonomic delimitation of vegetable, grain and weed amaranths: A morphological and biochemical approach. *Genet. Resour. Crop Evol.* **2012**, *59*, 289–303. [CrossRef]
111. Caselato-Sousa, V.M.; Amaya-Farfán, J. State of knowledge on amaranth grain: A comprehensive review. *J. Food Sci.* **2012**, *77*, R93–R104. [CrossRef] [PubMed]
112. Cai, Y.; Corke, H. *Amaranthus* betacyanin pigments applied in model food systems. *J. Food Sci.* **1999**, *64*, 869–873. [CrossRef]
113. Cai, Y.; Sun, M.; Wu, H.; Huang, R.; Corke, H. Characterization and quantification of betacyanin pigments from diverse *Amaranthus* species. *J. Agric. Food Chem.* **1998**, *46*, 2063–2070. [CrossRef]
114. Cai, Y.; Sun, M.; Corke, H. Colorant properties and stability of *Amaranthus* betacyanin pigments. *J. Agric. Food Chem.* **1998**, *46*, 4491–4495. [CrossRef]
115. Khanam, U.K.S.; Oba, S. Bioactive substances in leaves of two amaranth species, *Amaranthus tricolor* and *Amaranthus hypochondriacus*. *Can. J. Plant Sci.* **2013**, *93*, 47–58. [CrossRef]
116. Shukla, S.; Bhargava, A.; Chatterjee, A.; Srivastava, A.; Singh, S.P. Genotypic variability in vegetable amaranth (*Amaranthus tricolor* L.) for foliage and its contributing traits over successive cuttings and years. *Euphytica* **2006**, *151*, 103–110. [CrossRef]
117. Sarker, U.; Islam, M.T.; Rabbani, M.G.; Oba, S. Variability, heritability and genetic association in vegetable amaranth (*Amaranthus tricolor* L.). *Span. J. Agric. Res.* **2015**, *13*. [CrossRef]
118. Khandaker, L.; Akond Asmgm, A.S.M.G.; Ali Md, B.; Oba, S. Biomass yield and accumulations of bioactive compounds in red amaranth (*Amaranthus tricolor* L.) grown under colored shade polyethylene in spring season. *Sci. Hortic.* **2010**, *123*, 289–294. [CrossRef]
119. Das, S.S.; Gauri, S.S.; Misra, B.B.; Biswas, M.; Dey, S. Purification and characterization of a betanidin glucosyltransferase from *Amaranthus tricolor* L. catalyzing non-specific biotransformation of flavonoids. *Plant Sci.* **2013**, *211*, 61–69. [CrossRef] [PubMed]
120. Liu, S.Q.; Zhang, Y.; Wang, C.; Su, P.; Liao, X.L.; Bai, L.Y. Preliminary study on component analysis of *Amaranthus tricolor* leaf extracts against plant pathogenic bacteria. *Egypt. J. Biol. Pest Control* **2016**, *26*, 643–650.
121. Al-Dosari, M.S. The effectiveness of ethanolic extract of *Amaranthus tricolor* L.: A natural hepatoprotetive agent. *Am. J. Chin. Med.* **2010**, *38*, 1051–1064. [CrossRef] [PubMed]

122. Amornrit, W.; Santiyanont, R. Effect of *Amaranthus* on advanced glycation end-products induced cytotoxicity and proinflammatory cytokine gene expression in SH-SY5Y cells. *Molecules* **2015**, *20*, 17288–17308. [CrossRef] [PubMed]
123. Amornrit, W.; Santiyanont, R. Neuroprotective effect of *Amaranthus lividus* and *Amaranthus tricolor* and their effects on gene expression of RAGE during oxidative stress in SH-SY5Y cells. *Gen. Mol. Res.* **2016**, *15*, 15027562. [CrossRef] [PubMed]
124. Jayaprakasam, B.; Zhang, Y.; Nair, M.G. Tumor cell proliferation and cyclooxygenase enzyme inhibitory compounds in *Amaranthus tricolor*. *J. Agric. Food Chem.* **2004**, *52*, 6939–6943. [CrossRef] [PubMed]
125. Li, H.; Deng, Z.; Liu, R.; Zhu, H.; Draves, J.; Marcone, M.; Sun, Y.; Tsao, R. Characterization of phenolics, betacyanins and antioxidant activities of the seed, leaf, sprout, flower and stalk extracts of three *Amaranthus* species. *J. Food Compos. Anal.* **2015**, *37*, 75–81. [CrossRef]
126. Khandaker, L.; Ali, M.B.; Oba, S. Total polyphenol and antioxidant activity of red amaranth (*Amaranthus tricolor* L.) as affected by different sunlight level. *J. Jpn. Soc. Hortic. Sci.* **2008**, *77*, 395–401. [CrossRef]
127. Khanam, U.K.S.; Oba, S. Phenotypic plasticity of vegetable amaranth *Amaranthus tricolor* L. under a natural climate. *Plant Prod. Sci.* **2014**, *17*, 166–172. [CrossRef]
128. Khandaker, L.; Babar, A.M.; Shynia, O. Influence of cultivar and growth stage on pigments and processing factors on betacyanins in red amaranth (*Amaranthus tricolor* L.). *Food Sci. Technol. Int.* **2009**, *15*, 259–265. [CrossRef]
129. Ali, M.B.; Khandaker, L.; Oba, S. Comparative study on functional componenrs, antioxidant activity and color parameters of selected colored leafy vegetables as affected by photoperiods. *J. Food Agric. Environ.* **2009**, *7*, 392–398.
130. Biswas, M.; Das, S.S.; Dey, S. Establishment of a stable *Amaranthus tricolor callus* line for production of food colorant. *Food Sci. Biotechnol.* **2013**, *22*, 1–8. [CrossRef]
131. Bianco-Colomas, J.; Hugues, M. Establishment and characterization of a betacyanin producing cell line of *Amaranthus tricolor*: Inductive effects of light and cytokinins. *J. Plant Physiol.* **1990**, *136*, 734–739. [CrossRef]
132. Zheng, X.; Liu, S.; Cheng, C.; Guo, R.; Chen, Y.; Xie, L.; Mao, Y.; Lin, Y.; Zhang, Z.; Lai, Z. Cloning and expression analysis of betalain biosynthesis genes in *Amaranthus tricolor*. *Biotechnol. Lett.* **2016**, *38*, 723–729. [CrossRef] [PubMed]
133. Pin, P.A. Life Cycle and Flowering Time Control in Beet. Ph.D. Thesis, Swedish University of Agricultural Sciences, Umeå, Sweden, 2012.
134. Lee, S.S.; Le, E.M.; Hong, S.H.; Bai, H.-W.; Lee, I.C.; Chung, B.Y. Gamma rays as an effective tool for removing undesirable color without adverse changes in biological activities of red beet extracts. *Radiat. Phys. Chem.* **2012**, *81*, 1147–1151. [CrossRef]
135. Lee, E.J.; An, D.; Nguyen, C.T.T.; Patil, B.S.; Kim, J.; Yoo, K.S. Betalain and betaine composition of greenhouse- or field-produced beetroot (*Beta vulgaris* L.) and inhibition of HepG2 cell proliferation. *J. Agric. Food Chem.* **2014**, *62*, 1324–1331. [CrossRef] [PubMed]
136. Sawicki, T.; Baczek, N.; Wiczkowski, W. Betalain profile, content and antuioxidant capacity of red beetroot dependent on the genotype and root part. *J. Funct. Food* **2016**, *27*, 249–261. [CrossRef]
137. Stintzing, F.C.; Schieber, A.; Carle, R. Identification of betalains from yellow beet (*Beta vulgaris* L.) and cactus pear [*Opuntia ficus-indica* (L.) Mill.] by high-performance liquid chromatography-electrospray ionization mass spectrometry. *J. Agric. Food Chem.* **2002**, *50*, 2302–2307. [CrossRef] [PubMed]
138. Slatnar, A.; Stampar, F.; Vebaric, R.; Jakopic, J. HPLC-MS^n identification of betalains profile of different beetroot (*Beta vulgaris* L. ssp. *vulgaris*) parts and cultivars. *J. Food Sci.* **2015**, *80*, 1952–1958. [CrossRef] [PubMed]
139. Mukundan, U.; Bhide, V.; Singh, G.; Curtis, W.R. pH-mediated release of betalains from transformed root cultures of *Beta vulgaris* L. *Appl. Microbiol. Biotechnol.* **1998**, *50*, 241–245. [CrossRef]
140. Pavlov, A.; Georgiev, V.; Ilieva, M. Betalain biosynthesis by red beet (*Beta vulgaris* L.) hairy root culture. *Proc. Biochem.* **2005**, *40*, 1531–1533. [CrossRef]
141. Pavlov, A.; Georgiev, M.; Bley, T. Batch and fed-batch production of betalains by red beet (*Beta vulgaris*) hairy roots in a bubble column reactor. *Z. Naturforsch.* **2007**, *62*, 439–446. [CrossRef]
142. Pavoković, D.; Rusak, G.; Besendorfer, V.; Krsnik-Rasol, M. Light-dependent betanin production by transformed cells of sugar beet. *Food Technol. Biotechnol.* **2009**, *47*, 153–158.

143. Liu, X.; Gao, Y.; Xu, H.; Wang, Q.; Yang, B. Imapct of high-pressure carbon dioxide combined with thermal treatment on degradation of red beet (*Beta vulgaris* L.) pigments. *J. Agric. Food Chem.* **2008**, *56*, 6480–6487. [CrossRef] [PubMed]
144. Guldiken, B.; Toydemir, G.; Memis, K.N.; Okur, S.; Boyacioglu, D.; Capanoglu, E. Home-processed red beetroot (*Beta vulgaris* L.) products: Changes in antioxidant properties and bioaccessibility. *Int. J. Mol. Sci.* **2016**, *17*, 858. [CrossRef] [PubMed]
145. Stagnari, F.; Galieni, A.; Speca, S.; Pisante, M. Water stress effects on growth, yield and quality traits of red beet. *Sci. Hortic.* **2014**, *165*, 13–22. [CrossRef]
146. Stagnari, F.; Galieni, A.; Cafiero, G.; Pisante, M. Application of photo-selective films to manipulate wavelenght of transmitted radiation and photosynthate composition in red beet (*Beta vulgaris* var. *conditiva* Alef.). *J. Sci. Food Agric.* **2014**, *94*, 713–720. [CrossRef] [PubMed]
147. Popa, A.; Moldovan, B.; David, L. Betanin from red beet (*Beta vulgaris* L.). *Rev. Chim.* **2015**, *66*, 413–416.
148. Escribano, J.; Pedreño, M.A.; Garcia-Carmona, F.; Muñoz, R. Characterization of the antiradical activity of betalains from *Beta vulgaris* L. roots. *Phytochem. Anal.* **1998**, *9*, 124–127. [CrossRef]
149. Gandía-Herrero, F.; Cabanes, J.; Escribano, J.; García-Carmona, F.; Jiménez-Atiénzar, M. Encapsulation of the most potent antioxidant betalains in edible matrixes as powders of different colors. *J. Agric. Food Chem.* **2013**, *61*, 4294–4302. [CrossRef] [PubMed]
150. Slavov, A.; Karagyozov, V.; Denev, P.; Kratchanova, M.; Kratchanov, C. Antioxidant activity of red beet juices obtained after microwave and thermal pretreatments. *Czech J. Food Sci.* **2013**, *31*, 139–147. [CrossRef]
151. Čanadanović-Brunet, J.M.; Savatović, S.S.; Ćetković, G.S.; Vulić, J.J.; Djilas, S.M.; Markov, S.L.; Cvetković, G.S. Antioxidant and antimicrobial activities of beet root pomace extracts. *Czech J. Food Sci.* **2011**, *29*, 575–585. [CrossRef]
152. Vulić, J.J.; Čanadanović-Brunet, J.; Cvetković, G.; Tumbas, V.; Djilas, S.; Četojević-Simin, D.; Čanadanović, V. Antioxidant and cell growth activities of beet root pomace extracts. *J. Funct. Food.* **2012**, *4*, 570–578. [CrossRef]
153. Bucur, L.; Tarălungă, G.; Schroder, V. The betalains content and antioxidant capacity of red beet (*Beta vulgaris* L. subsp. *vulgaris*) root. *Farmacia* **2016**, *64*, 198–201.
154. Pitalua, E.; Jimenez, M.; Vernon-Carter, E.J.; Beristain, C.I. Antioxidantive activity of microcapsules with beetroot juice using gum Arabic as wall material. *Food Bioprod. Process.* **2010**, *88*, 253–258. [CrossRef]
155. Schliemann, W.; Cai, Y.; Degenkolb, T.; Schmidt, J.; Corke, H. Betalains of *Celosia argentea*. *Phytochemistry* **2001**, *58*, 159–165. [CrossRef]
156. Iamonico, D. About the circumscription of *Celosia argentea* (*Amaranthaceae*) and the related Linnaean taxa. *Phytotaxa* **2013**, *90*, 61–64. [CrossRef]
157. Chaturvedi, M.; Datta, K.; Nath, P.; Pal, M. Cytopalynology of *Celosia* L. *Grana* **1993**, *32*, 169–175. [CrossRef]
158. Feng, N.; Xue, Q.; Guo, Q.; Zhao, R.; Guo, M. Genetic diversity and population structure of *Celosia argentea* and related species revealed by SRAP. *Biochem. Genet.* **2009**, *47*, 521–532. [CrossRef] [PubMed]
159. Grant, W.F. A cytological study of *Celosia argentea*, *C. argentea* var. *cristata* and their hybrids. *Bot. Gaz.* **1954**, *115*, 323–336. [CrossRef]
160. Grant, W.F. Speciation and basic chromosome number in the genus *Celosia*. *Can. J. Bot.* **1961**, *39*, 45–50. [CrossRef]
161. Grant, W.F. Speciation and nomenclature in the genus *Celosia*. *Can. J. Bot.* **1962**, *40*, 1355–1363. [CrossRef]
162. Nath, P.; Phri, D.; Pal, M. Nuclear DNA content in *Celosia* (*Amaranthaceae*). *Plant Syst. Evol.* **1992**, *182*, 253–257. [CrossRef]
163. Nath, P.; Phri, D.; Jha, S.S.; Pal, M. Seed protein electrophoresis of wild and cultivated species of *Celosia* (*Amaranthaceae*). *Genet. Resour. Crop Evol.* **1997**, *44*, 241–245. [CrossRef]
164. Mastuti, R.; Arumingtyas, E.L.; Fatinah, A.A. Genetic diversity of *Celosia* variants in East Java based on polyphenol oxidase—PPO genes. *Procedia Chem.* **2015**, *14*, 361–366. [CrossRef]
165. Surse, S.N.; Shrivastava, B.; Sharma, P.; Gide, P.S.; Attar, S. *Celosia cristata*: Potent pharmacotherapeutic herb—A review. *Int. J. Pharm. Phytopharm. Res.* **2014**, *3*, 444–446.
166. Nidavani, R.B.; Mahalakshmi, A.M.; Shalawadi, M. Towards a better understanding of an updated of ethnopharmacology of *Celosia argentea* L. *Int. J. Pharm. Pharm. Sci.* **2013**, *5* (Suppl. 3), 54–59.
167. Cai, Y.; Sun, M.; Schliemann, W.; Corke, H. Chemical stability and colorant properties of betaxanthin pigments from *Celosia argentea*. *J. Agric. Food Chem.* **2001**, *49*, 4429–4435. [CrossRef] [PubMed]

168. Molehin, O.R.; Adefegha, S.A.; Oboh, G.; Saliu, J.A.; Athayde, M.L.; Boligon, A.A. Comparative study on the phenolic content, antioxidant properties and HPLC fingerprinting of three varieties of *Celosia* species. *J. Food Biochem.* **2014**, *38*, 575–583. [CrossRef]
169. Odukoya, O.A.; Inya-Agha, S.I.; Segun, F.I.; Sodifiya, M.O.; Ilori, O.O. Antioxidant activities of selected Nigerian green leafy vegetables. *Am. J. Food Technol.* **2007**, *2*, 169–175. [CrossRef]
170. Rehman, A.; Imran, M.; Mehboob, S.; Khan, N.A.; Alam, W.; Riaz, K. Etiology, pathogenicity and management of collar rot in cockscomb (*Celosia argentea*). *Int. J. Agric. Biol.* **2015**, *17*, 9–14.
171. Bakar, D.A.; Ahmed, B.A.; Taha, R.M. In vitro callus induction and plant regeneration of *Celosia argentea*—An important medicinal plant. *Braz. Arch. Biol. Technol.* **2014**, *57*, 860–866. [CrossRef]
172. Rub, R.A.; Pati, M.J.; Siddiqui, A.A.; Moghe, A.S.; Shaikh, N.N. Characterization of anticancer principles of *Celosia argentea* (*Amaranthaceae*). *Pharmacogn. Res.* **2016**, *8*, 97–104. [CrossRef] [PubMed]
173. Tang, Y.; Xin, H.-L.; Guo, M.L. Review on research of the phytochemistry and pharmacological activities of *Celosia argentea*. *Braz. J. Pharmacogn.* **2016**, *26*, 787–796. [CrossRef]
174. Wu, Q.B.; Wang, Y.; Liang, L.; Jiang, Q.; Guo, M.L.; Zhang, J.J. Novel triterpenoid saponins from the seeds of *Celosia argentea* L. *Nat. Prod. Res.* **2013**, *27*, 1353–1360. [CrossRef] [PubMed]
175. Saritha, P.; Sreeramulu, A. Allelopathic effects of *Celosia argentea* L. root extracts on crop plant seed germination. *Int. J. Life Sci. Biotechnol. Pharma Res.* **2013**, *2*, 142–154.
176. Perveen, S.; Yousaf, M.; Zahoor, A.F.; Rasool, N.; Jabber, A. Extraction, isolation and identification of various environment friendly components from cock's comb (*Celosia argentea*) leaves for allelopathic potential. *Toxicol. Environ. Chem.* **2014**, *96*, 1523–1534. [CrossRef]
177. Gnanamani, A.; Priya, K.S.; Radhakrishan, N.; Babu, M. Antibacterial activity of two plant extracts on eight burn pathogens. *J. Ethnopharmacol.* **2003**, *86*, 59–61. [CrossRef]
178. Wiart, C.; Mogana, S.; Khalifah, S.; Mahan, M.; Ismail, S.; Buckle, M.; Narayana, A.K.; Sulaiman, M. Antimicrobial screening of plants used for traditional medicine in the sate of Perak, Peninsular Malaysia. *Fitoterapia* **2004**, *75*, 68–73. [CrossRef] [PubMed]
179. Bhujbal, S.S.; Chitlange, S.S.; Suralkar, A.A.; Shinde, D.B.; Patil, M.J. Anti-inflammatory activity of an isolated flavonoid fraction from *Celosia argentea* Linn. *J. Med. Plant Res.* **2008**, *2*, 52–54.
180. Hase, K.; Kadota, S.; Basnet, P.; Takahashi, T.; Namba, T. Protective effect of celosian, an acidic polysaccharide, on chemically and immunologically induced liver injuries. *Biol. Pharm. Bull.* **1996**, *19*, 567–572. [CrossRef] [PubMed]
181. Hase, K.; Kadota, S.; Basnet, P.; Takahashi, T.; Namba, T. Hepatoprotective effects of traditional medicines. Isolation of the active constituent from seeds of *Celosia argentea*. *Phytother. Res.* **1996**, *10*, 387–392. [CrossRef]
182. Hayakawa, Y.; Fujii, H.; Hase, K.; Ohnishi, Y.; Sakukawa, R.; Kadota, S.; Namba, T.; Saiki, I. Anti-metastatic and immunomodulating properties of the water extract from *Celosia argentea* seeds. *Biol. Pharm. Bull.* **1998**, *21*, 1154–1159. [CrossRef] [PubMed]
183. Rub, R.A.; Patil, M.J.; Shaikh, N.N.; Haikh, T.; Ahmed, J.; Siddiqui, A.A. Immunomodulatory profile of *Celosia argentea*–Activity of isolated compounds I and II. *Int. J. Adv. Biotechnol. Res.* **2015**, *6*, 270–277.
184. Vetrichelvan, T.; Jegadeesan, M.; Devi, B.A.U. Anti-diabetic activity of alcoholic extract of *Celosia argentea* Linn. seeds in rats. *Biol. Pharm. Bull.* **2002**, *25*, 526–528. [CrossRef] [PubMed]
185. Shen, S.; Ding, X.; Ouyang, M.-A.; Wu, Z.-J.; Xie, L.-H. A new phenolic glycoside and cytotoxic constituents from *Celosia argentea*. *J. Asian Nat. Prod. Res.* **2010**, *12*, 821–827. [CrossRef] [PubMed]
186. Guo, W.-Z.; Di, H.; Bao, R.; Chu, G.-H.; Tang, X.-H.; Feng, M.; Diao, L.-J.; Lu, L. The healing effect of *Celosia argentea* leaf extract on burn wounds: An in vivo and in vitro evaluation. *Int. J. Clin. Exp. Med.* **2016**, *9*, 21018–21027.
187. Priya, K.S.; Arumugam, G.; Rathinam, B.; Wells, A.; Babu, M. *Celosia argentea* Linn. leaf extract improves wound healing in a rat burn wound model. *Wound Repair Regen.* **2004**, *12*, 618–625. [CrossRef] [PubMed]
188. Telagari, M.; Hullatti, K. In vitro α-amylase and α-glucosidase inhibitory activity of *Adiantum caudatum* Linn. and *Celosia argentea* Linn. Extracts and fractions. *Indian J. Pharmacol.* **2015**, *47*, 425–429. [PubMed]
189. Saqib, F.; Janbaz, K.H.J.; Sherwani, M.K. In vitro inhibitory potential of methanolic extract of *Celosia argentea* var. *cristata* on tyrosinase, acetylcholinesterase and butyrylcholinesterase enzymes. *Bangladesh J. Pharmacol.* **2015**, *10*, 449–454.
190. Xue, Q.; Sun, Z.L.; Guo, M.L.; Wang, Y.; Zhang, G. Two new compounds from Semen Celosiae and their protective effects against CCl_4-induced hepatotoxity. *Nat. Prod. Res.* **2011**, *25*, 772–780. [CrossRef] [PubMed]

191. Malomo, S.O.; Ore, A.; Yakubu, M.T. In vitro and in vivo antioxidant activities ofthe aqueous extract of *Celosia argentea* leaves. *Indian J. Pharmacol.* **2011**, *43*, 278–285. [PubMed]
192. Iwalewa, E.O.; Adewunni, C.O.; Omisone, N.O.A.; Adebanji, O.A.; Azike, C.K.; Adigun, A.O.; Adesina, O.A.; Olowoyo, O.G. Pro- and antioxidant effects and cytoprotective potentials of nine edible vegetables in Southwest Nigeria. *J. Med. Food* **2005**, *8*, 539–544. [CrossRef] [PubMed]
193. Prakash, D.; Nath, P.; Pal, M. Composition and variation in vitamin C, carotenoids, protein, nitrate and oxalate contents in *Celosia* leaves. *Plant Food Hum. Nutr.* **1995**, *47*, 221–226. [CrossRef]
194. Suzuki, H.; Morita, H.; Iwasaki, S.; Kobayashi, J. New antimitotic bicyclic peptides, celogentins D-H and J, from the seeds of *Celosia argentea*. *Tetrahedron* **2003**, *59*, 5307–5315. [CrossRef]
195. Morita, H.; Takeya, K. Bioactive cyclic peptides from higher plants. *Heterocycles* **2010**, *80*, 739–764. [CrossRef]
196. Zhang, S.-M.; Wang, X.-F.; Feng, J.; Sun, Z.-L. Chemical constituents of the seeds of *Celosia cristata*. *Chem. Nat. Prod.* **2016**, *52*, 827–829. [CrossRef]
197. Morita, H.; Suzuki, H.; Kobayashi, J. Celogenamide A, a new cyclic peptide from the seeds of *Celosia argentea*. *J. Nat. Prod.* **2004**, *67*, 1628–1630. [CrossRef] [PubMed]
198. Morita, H.; Shimbo, K.; Shigemori, H.; Kobayashi, J. Antimitotic activity of moroidin, a bicyclic peptide from the seeds of *Celosia argentea*. *Bioorg. Med. Chem. Lett.* **2000**, *10*, 469–471. [CrossRef]
199. Suzuki, H.; Morita, H.; Shiro, M.; Kobayashi, J. Celogentin K, a new cyclic peptide from the seeds of *Celosia argentea* and X-ary strucutre of moroidin. *Tetrahedron* **2004**, *60*, 2489–2495. [CrossRef]
200. Bobayashi, J.; Suzuki, H.; Shimbo, K.; Takeya, K.; Morita, H. Celogentins A–C, new antimitotic bicyclic peptides from the seeds of *Celosia argentea*. *J. Org. Chem.* **2001**, *66*, 6626–6633. [CrossRef]
201. Piattelli, M.; Minale, L. Pigments of *Centrospermae* II. Distribution of betacyanins. *Phytochemistry* **1964**, *3*, 547–557. [CrossRef]
202. Cai, Y.; Sun, M.; Corke, H. HPLC characterization of betalains from plants in the *Amaranthaceae*. *J. Chromatogr. Sci.* **2005**, *43*, 454–460. [CrossRef] [PubMed]
203. Guadarrama-Flores, B.; Rodríguez-Monroy, M.; Cruz-Sosa, F.; García-Carmona, F.; Gandía-Herrero, F. Production of dihydroxylated betalains and dopamine in cell suspension cultures of *Celosia argentea* var. *plumosa*. *J. Agric. Food Chem.* **2015**, *63*, 2741–2749. [CrossRef] [PubMed]
204. Nicola, M.G.; Amico, V.; Piatteli, M. Effect of white amd far-red light on betalain formation. *Phytochemistry* **1974**, *13*, 439–442. [CrossRef]
205. Rink, E.; Böhm, H. Effect of DOPA feeding on betaxanthins in various species of *Centrospermae*. *Phytochemistry* **1991**, *30*, 1109–1112. [CrossRef]
206. Singh, O.S.; Chhabra, N. Effect of plant growth regulators on betacyanin synthesis in *Celosia argentea* var. *cristata* in the dark. *Z. Pflanzenphysiol.* **1976**, *78*, 189–196. [CrossRef]
207. Bodhipadma, K.; Noichinda, S.; Yadbuntung, I.; Buaeiam, W.; Leung, D.W.M. Comparison of in vitro and in vivo inflorescence of common cockscomb (*Celosia argentea* var. *cristata*). *Sci. Asia* **2010**, *36*, 68–71. [CrossRef]
208. Taha, R.M.; Wafa, S.N. Plant regeneration and cellular behaviour studies in *Celosia cristata* grown in vivo and in vitro. *Sci. World J.* **2012**, *2012*. [CrossRef] [PubMed]
209. Yaacob, J.S.; Saleh, A.; Elias, H.; Abdullah, S.; Mahmad, N.; Mohamed, N. In vitro regeneration and acclimatization protocols of selected ornamental plants (*Agapanthus praecox*, *Justicia betonica* and *Celosia cristata*). *Sains Malays.* **2014**, *43*, 715–722.
210. Corio-Costet, M.F.; Chapuis, L.; Delbecque, J.P. *Chenopodium album* L. (Fat Hen): In vitro cell culture and production of secondary metabolites (phytosterols and ecdysteroids). In *Biotechnology in Agriculture and Forestry, vol 41. Medicinal and Aromatic Plants X*; Bajaj, Y.P.S., Ed.; Springer: Berlin, Germany, 1998; pp. 97–112.
211. Filho, A.M.M.; Pirozi, M.R.; Borges, J.T.S.; Sant'Ana, H.M.P.; Chaves, J.B.P.; Coimbra, J.S.R. Quinoa: Nutritional, functional and antinutritional aspects. *Crit. Rev. Food Sci. Nutr.* **2017**, *57*, 1618–1630. [CrossRef] [PubMed]
212. Nowak, V.; Du, J.; Charrondière, U.R. Assessment of the nutritional composition of quinoa (*Chenopodium quinoa* Willd.). *Food Chem.* **2016**, *193*, 47–54. [CrossRef] [PubMed]
213. Ruiz, K.B.; Biondi, S.; Oses, R.; Acuña-Rodríguez, I.S.; Antognoni, F.; Martinez-Mosqueira, E.A.; Coulibaly, A.; Canahua-Murillo, A.; Pinto, M.; Zurita-Silva, A.; et al. Quinoa biodiversity and sustainability for food security under climate change. A review. *Agron. Sustain. Dev.* **2014**, *34*, 349–359. [CrossRef]
214. Tang, Y.; Li, X.; Zhang, B.; Chen, P.X.; Liu, R.; Tsao, R. Characterisation of phenolics, betanins and antioxidant activities in seeds of three *Chenopodium quinoa* Willd. genotypes. *Food Chem.* **2015**, *166*, 380–388. [CrossRef] [PubMed]

215. Escribano, J.; Cabanes, J.; Jiménez-Atiénzar, M.; Ibañez-Tremolada, M.; Gómez-Pando, L.R.; García-Carmona, F.; Gandía-Herrero, F. Characterization of betalains, saponins and antioxidant power in differently colored quinoa (*Chenopodium quinoa*) varieties. *Food Chem.* **2017**, *234*, 285–294. [CrossRef] [PubMed]
216. Adolf, V.I.; Jacobsen, S.-E.; Shabala, S. Salt tolerance mechanisms in quinoa (*Chenopodium quinoa* Willd.). *Environ. Exper. Bot.* **2013**, *92*, 43–54. [CrossRef]
217. Jacobsen, S.J.; Sørensen, M.; Pedersen, S.M.; Weiner, J. Feeding the world: Genetically modified crops versus agricultural biodiversity. *Agron. Sustain. Dev.* **2013**, *33*, 651–662. [CrossRef]
218. Zurita-Silva, A.; Fuentes, F.; Zamora, P.; Jacobsen, S.-E.; Schwember, A.R. Breeding quinoa (*Chenopodium quinoa* Willd.): Potential and perspectives. *Mol. Breed.* **2014**, *34*, 13–30. [CrossRef]
219. Koyro, H.-W.; Eisa, S.S. Effects of salinity on composition, viability and germination of seeds of *Chenopodium quinoa* Willd. *Plant Soil* **2008**, *302*, 79–90. [CrossRef]
220. Bazile, D.; Martínez, E.A.; Fuentes, F. Diversity of quinoa in a biogeographical Island: A review of constraints and potential from arid to temperate regions of Chile. *Not. Bot. Horti Agrobot.* **2014**, *42*, 289–298. [CrossRef]
221. Jacobsen, S.-E. The worldwide potential for quinoa (*Chenopodium quinoa* Willd.). *Food Rev. Int.* **2003**, *19*, 167–177. [CrossRef]
222. Ruiz, K.B.; Biondi, S.; Martínez, E.A.; Orsini, F.; Antognoni, F.; Jacobsen, S.-E. Quinoa—A model crop for understanding salt-tolerance mechanisms in halophytes. *Plant Biosyst.* **2016**, *150*, 357–371. [CrossRef]
223. Ng, S.-C.; Anderson, A.; Coker, J.; Ondrus, M. Characteerization of lipid oxidation products in quinoa (*Chenopodium quinoa*). *Food Chem.* **2007**, *101*, 185–192. [CrossRef]
224. Wang, S.; Zhu, F. Formulation and quality attributes of quinoa food products. *Food Bioproc. Technol.* **2016**, *9*, 49–68. [CrossRef]
225. Comino, I.; Moreno, M.L.; Real, A.; Rodríguez-Herrera, A.; Barro, F.; Sousa, C. The gluten-free diet: Testing alternative cereals tolerated by celiac patients. *Nutrients* **2013**, *5*, 4250–4268. [CrossRef] [PubMed]
226. Jancurová, M.; Minarovičová, L.; Dandar, A. Quinoa—A review. *Czeck J. Food Sci.* **2009**, *27*, 71–79. [CrossRef]
227. Zevallos, V.F.; Ellis, H.J.; Suligoj, T.; Herencia, L.I.; Ciclitira, P.J. Variable activation of immune response by quinoa (*Chenopodium quinoa* Wild.) prolamins in celiac disease. *Am. J. Clin. Nutr.* **2012**, *96*, 337–344. [CrossRef] [PubMed]
228. Mujica, A. Andean grains and legumes. In *Neglected Crops: 1492 from a Different Perspective*; Hernando Bermujo, J.E., Leon, J., Eds.; FAO: Rome, Italy, 1994; Volume 26, pp. 131–148. Available online: http://www.hort.purdue.edu/newcrop/1492/grains.html (accessed on 25 August 2017).
229. Szakiel, A.; Paczkawski, C.; Henry, M. Influence of environmental abiotic factors on the content of saponins in plants. *Phytochem. Rev.* **2011**, *10*, 471–491. [CrossRef]
230. Vega-Gálvez, A.; Miranda, M.; Vergara, J.; Uribe, E.; Puente, L.; Martínez, E.A. Nutritions facts and functional potential of quinoa (*Chenopodium quinoa* Willd.), an ancient Andean grain: A review. *J. Sci. Food Agric.* **2010**, *90*, 2541–2547. [CrossRef] [PubMed]
231. Gómez-Caravaca, A.M.; Iafelice, G.; Lavini, A.; Pulvento, C.; Caboni, M.F.; Marconi, E. Phenolic compounds and saponins in quinoa samples (*Chenopodium quinoa* Willd.) grown under different saline and ninsaline irrigation regimens. *J. Agric. Food Chem.* **2012**, *60*, 4620–4627. [CrossRef] [PubMed]
232. Tang, Y.; Tsao, R. Phytochemicals in quinoa and amaranth grains and their antioxidant, anti-inflammatory and potential health beneficial effects: A review. *Mol. Nutr. Food Res.* **2017**, *61*, 1600767. [CrossRef] [PubMed]
233. Repo-Carrasco-Valencia, R.; Hellström, J.K.; Pihlava, J.-M.; Mattila, P.H. Flavonoids and other phenolic compounds in Andean indigenous grains: Quinoa (*Chenopodium quinoa*), kañiva (*Chenopodium pallidicaule*) and kiwicha (*Amaranthus caudatus*). *Food Chem.* **2010**, *120*, 128–133. [CrossRef]
234. Pasko, P.; Baiton, H.; Zagrodzki, P.; Gorinstein, S.; Fołta, M.; Zachwieja, Z. Anthocyanins, total polyphenols and antioxidant activity in amaranth and quinoa seeds and sprouts during their grow. *Food Chem.* **2009**, *115*, 994–998. [CrossRef]
235. Abderrahim, F.; Huanatico, E.; Segura, R.; Arribas, S.; Gonzalez, M.C.; Condezo-Hoyos, L. Physical features, phenolic compounds, betalains and total antioxidant capacity for coloured quinoa seeds (*Chenopodium quinoa* Willd.) from Peruvian Altiplano. *Food Chem.* **2015**, *183*, 83–90. [CrossRef] [PubMed]
236. Alvarez-Jubete, L.; Wijngaard, H.; Arendt, E.K.; Gallagher, E. Polyphenol composition and in vitro antioxidant activity of amaranth, quinoa buckwheat and wheat as affected by sprouting and baking. *Food Chem.* **2010**, *119*, 770–778. [CrossRef]

237. Miranda, M.; Vega-Gálvez, A.; Uribe, E.; López, J.; Martínez, E.; Rodriguez, M.J.; Quispe, I.; di Scala, K. Physico-chemical analysis, anrioxidant capacity and vitamins of six ecotypes of Chilean quinoa (*Chenopodium quinoa* Willd.). *Procedia Food Sci.* **2011**, *1*, 1439–1446. [CrossRef]
238. Yao, Y.; Yang, X.; Shi, Z.; Ren, G. Anti-inflammatory activity of saponins from quinoa (*Chenopodium quinoa* Willd.) seeds in lipopolysaccharide-stimulated RAW 264.7 macrophage cells. *J. Food Sci.* **2014**, *79*, H1018–H1023. [CrossRef] [PubMed]
239. Farinazzi-Machado, F.M.V.; Barbalho, S.M.; Oshiiwa, M.; Goulart, R.; Pessan Junior, O. Use of cereal bars with quinoa (*Chenopodium quinoa* W.) to reduce risk factors related to cardiovascular diseases. *Food Sci. Technol.* **2012**, *32*, 239–244. [CrossRef]
240. De Carvalho, F.G.; Ovidio, P.P.; Padovan, G.J.; Jordao Junior, A.A.; Marchini, J.S.; Navarro, A.M. Metabolic parameters of postmenopausal women after quinoa or corn flakes intake-a prospective and double-blind study. *Int. J. Food Sci. Nutr.* **2014**, *65*, 380–385. [CrossRef] [PubMed]
241. Navruz-Varli, N.; Sanlier, N. Nutritional and health benefits of quinoa (*Chenopodium quinoa* Willd.). *J. Cereal Sci.* **2016**, *69*, 371–376. [CrossRef]
242. Dinan, L.; Lanfort, L.R. Effects and applications of arthropod steroid hormones (ecdysteroids) in mammals. *J. Endocrinol.* **2006**, *191*, 1–8. [CrossRef] [PubMed]
243. Foucault, A.S.; Even, P.; Lafont, R.; Dioh, W.; Veillet, S.; Tome, D.; Huneau, J.F.; Herman, W.H. Quinoa extract enriched in 20-hydroxyecdysone affects energy homeostasis and intestinal fat absorption in mice fed a high-fat diet. *Physiol. Behav.* **2014**, *128*, 226–231. [CrossRef] [PubMed]
244. Wang, Z.Q.; Yu, Y.; Zhang, X.H.; Ribnicky, D.; Cefalu, W.T. Ecdysterone enhances muscle insulin signaling by modulating acylcarnitine profile and mitochondrial oxidative phosphorylation complexes in mice fed a high-fat diet. *Diabetes* **2011**, 1–10. [CrossRef]

4

Anti-Oxidant and Anti-Inflammatory Activity of Ketogenic Diet: New Perspectives for Neuroprotection in Alzheimer's Disease

Alessandro Pinto [1,*], Alessio Bonucci [2], Elisa Maggi [2], Mariangela Corsi [2] and Rita Businaro [2]

1 Department of Experimental Medicine, Sapienza University of Rome, 00161 Roma, Italy
2 Department of Medico-Surgical Sciences and Biotechnologies, Sapienza University of Rome, 04100 Latina, Italy; bonucci.alessio@libero.it (A.B.); elisa.maggi@biologo.onb.it (E.M.); mariangela.corsi@uniroma1.it (M.C.); rita.businaro@uniroma1.it (R.B.)
* Correspondence: alessandro.pinto@uniroma1.it

Abstract: The ketogenic diet, originally developed for the treatment of epilepsy in non-responder children, is spreading to be used in the treatment of many diseases, including Alzheimer's disease. The main activity of the ketogenic diet has been related to improved mitochondrial function and decreased oxidative stress. B-Hydroxybutyrate, the most studied ketone body, has been shown to reduce the production of reactive oxygen species (ROS), improving mitochondrial respiration: it stimulates the cellular endogenous antioxidant system with the activation of nuclear factor erythroid-derived 2-related factor 2 (Nrf2), it modulates the ratio between the oxidized and reduced forms of nicotinamide adenine dinucleotide (NAD^+/NADH) and it increases the efficiency of electron transport chain through the expression of uncoupling proteins. Furthermore, the ketogenic diet performs anti-inflammatory activity by inhibiting nuclear factor kappa-light-chain-enhancer of activated B cells (NF-kB) activation and nucleotide-binding domain, leucine-rich-containing family, pyrin domain-containing-3 (NLRP3) inflammasome as well as inhibiting histone deacetylases (HDACs), improving memory encoding. The underlying mechanisms and the perspectives for the treatment of Alzheimer's disease are discussed.

Keywords: Ketogenic diet; Alzheimer's disease; neuroprotection; inflammation; oxidative stress

---

1. Introduction

According to the World Alzheimer Report 2016, there are 47 million people worldwide suffering from dementia, and this number will rise to 131 million by 2050 due to population aging. This data also implies a great economic impact, which is expected to be one billion dollars worldwide by 2018. Despite of recent progress in understanding the neurobiology and pathophysiology of Alzheimer's disease (AD), no resolutive pharmacological treatments but only a few symptomatic drugs are currently available to patients. Based on this consideration, much effort is aimed at the development of effective prevention lines: so far many non-pharmacological treatments have been proposed, including lifestyle interventions such as targeted nutritional protocols, caloric restriction and exercise, as well as mental challenges and socialization [1].

Moreover, although the effects of diet in aging and neurodegeneration is becoming well-established, the evidence regarding the effect of diet on cognition in neurological disorders has not been proved yet. This is surprising because preservation of cognition is often a predominant concern for patients with neurological disorders, perhaps due to the substantial impact on occupation, social relationships, activities of daily living, and quality of life [2].

Alzheimer's disease etiopathogenesis has been linked to oxidative stress, neuroinflammation, mitochondrial impairment, hypometabolism and blood-brain barrier (BBB) disruption [3–6].

The proved effectiveness of the ketogenic diet in childhood refractory epilepsy and the early metabolic dysfunction observed in mild cognitive impairment (MCI), which usually precedes the onset of AD, paved the way to evaluate the possible therapeutic role of dietary metabolic approaches to AD and other neurodegenerative diseases. The brain hypometabolism was associated to a reduced glucose utilization, detected by fluorodeoxyglucose positron emission tomography (FDG-PET), but several alteration in amino acids and lipids metabolic pathways have been recently identified through modern metabolomics techniques [7–11].

Chronic inflammation and oxidative stress are considered two key factors in the development of Alzheimer's disease, underlying neurotoxic mechanisms leading to neuronal death occurring in the brain areas responsible for memory and cognitive processes [12]. A bulk of studies have shown that the blood-brain barrier is impaired in Alzheimer's disease resulting in an altered expression of some transporters, including the down-regulation of glucose transporter. The primary fuel for the brain is glucose that must be taken from the blood and transported across the BBB by the specific glucose transporters (GLUTs) due to the inability of neurons to synthesize or store it. When there is a decreased expression of these transporters, as it has been shown in AD, Ketone Bodies (KBs) become the alternative energy source to glucose for the brain due to their ability to cross the BBB carried by specific transporters that are not down-regulated during AD. For all these reasons many studies have been performed to verify if the induction of a mild ketosis may favor the trophism of neuronal cells in the course of AD.

In the last few years the number of publications about the ketogenic diet (KD) and neurological disease have been progressively increasing. The beneficial effects of these diets for enhancing cellular metabolism and mitochondrial function, inducing a shift in energy metabolism, have been described in more detail, although the specific effects on cognition have not been analyzed in such depth [13,14]. The aim of this review is to summarize the current evidence regarding KD and AD with specific reference to antioxidant and anti-inflammatory mechanisms, as well as their effects on cognitive processes.

2. Ketone Bodies as Alternative Fuel for the Brain

The adult brain represents about 2% of body weight, but it consumes about 20–23% of whole-body energy expenditure, mostly in the form of glucose. Indeed, during episodic period of starvation or low-carbohydrates intake, the KBs metabolism becomes the main source of alternative energy as a results of carbohydrate deficiency and increased availability of fatty acids from lipolysis [15]. β-hydroxybutyrate (βHB) and acetoacetate (AcAc) can replace glucose in the brain, whereas acetone, produced by spontaneous decarboxylation of AcAc, is rapidly eliminated through urine and lungs. Under human physiological condition plasma KBs concentration fluctuate between 100 and 250 mM, increased to ~1 mM after prolonged exercise or 24 h of fasting and to 6–8 mM during a prolonged fast without giving rise to clinically hazardous acidosis. In diabetic ketoacidosis, plasma concentration of KBs can exceed 20 mM [16,17]. The human liver produces up to 300 g of ketone bodies per day which contribute between 5% and 20% of total energy expenditure in fed, fasted, and starved states [15].

3. Ketogenic Diets

The classic KD was designed in 1923 for the treatment of epilepsy by Dr. Russell Wilder at the Mayo Clinic. Ketogenic diets are composed of high amount of fat and low carbohydrates, typically at a macronutrient ratio of fat to protein plus carbs equal to 3–4:1 (4 grams of fat to 1 gram of protein and carbohydrate combined) which approximately results in 90% of total calories intake from fat, 6% from protein, and 4% from carb (because fat has 9 calories per gram, while both protein and carb have just 4 calories per gram). The moderate protein intake avoids amino acids induced gluconeogenesis and promotes KBs formation. The resulting metabolic profile is characterized by a slight reduction of blood glucose concentration with increasing KBs and mimics the fasting state with the brain beginning to use KBs to generate cellular energy. The very low carbohydrate intake of classic KD is difficult to maintain and consequently at least five main variants of the KD were published in medical literature as treatments for diseases that have an underlying metabolic dysregulation, such as epilepsy, cancer, and Alzheimer's disease. All KDs are a variation of the classic KD, the main difference being the macronutrient ratio: the Modified Ketogenic Diet (2:1–1:1), the Modified Atkins Diet (MAD; 1:1), and more recently the Medium-Chain Triglyceride (MCT) oil diet (1.9:1), Low Glycemic Index Treatment (LGIT) and Intermittent Fasting [2,6]. Usually, fat type and chain length are not specified, but typically a ketogenic diet includes mostly saturated fats, which have 16–20 carbon atoms. In the last few years the alternative medium-chain triglyceride (MCT) ketogenic diet was developed, comprising about 60% octanoic acid (an eight-carbon fatty acid) and about 40% decanoic acid (a ten-carbon fatty acid). The quick metabolism of the shorter fatty acids results in more efficient generation of ketone bodies allowing to assume a greater proportion of carbohydrates with only about 45% of lipid energy intake [2,6].

A key issue is the potential occurrence of adverse effects in course of KD treatment. The incidence of adverse effects is primarily associated with the KD model applied, with the classic KD (4:1 ratio) burdened by a lower tolerance when compared with the 3:1 ratio KD or MAD, and it is significantly reduced by the current availability of specific dietary supplements or formulas. The most common adverse events are the gastrointestinal symptoms, including vomiting, constipation and diarrhea; moreover, weight loss and hyperlipidemia are potential side effects whereas the major adverse events (dehydration, electrolyte alteration, arrythmias) are uncommon. During the first few days and weeks after KD initiation, mild side effects such as headaches, fatigue, can occur. The pathological ketoacidosis due to a lack of insulin in type 1 diabetes is not possible as result of dietary changes alone. The frequency evaluation of KD side effects in patients with AD is difficult due to the small number of available clinical trials and the heterogeneity of KD model applied [18–21].

Although several clinical trials were carried out on childhood refractory epilepsy, adverse events have not been consistently reported [22]. As well as children, elderly people subjected to long-term KD treatment require a close monitoring for adverse events by a neurologist, nutritionist and dietitian, and they should be subjected to a periodic dual energy X-ray absorptiometry (DEXA) screening for body composition health (bone, fat free mass, muscle mass and fat mass).

4. Mechanisms Underlying the Beneficial Effects of Ketogenic Diet on Neurological

Despite the poor number of clinical trials experimenting on the effectiveness of different types of ketogenic diets on Alzheimer's cognitive impairment (summarized in Table 1), a growing body of biological mechanisms potentially able to explain the observed clinical effects have been proven in in vitro or in animal model studies.

The therapy of AD was primarily addressed to the prevention of the specific histological injures (amyloid plaques, neurofibrillary tangles) but the lack of success moved the focus of research to functional dysregulation of brain metabolism, mitochondrial homeostasis and excitatory and inhibitory neuronal signaling, laying the foundation for the development of a "metabolic therapy".

Before describing more extensively the activity of ketogenic diet associated to the decrease of the oxidative damage and to the modulation of inflammatory status, the main mechanisms reported in the scientific literature are briefly summarized.

The putative neuroprotective effects of ketone bodies have been associated with the following mechanisms:

- increasing intracellular adenosine triphosphate (ATP) availability;
- reducing ROS generation by mitochondrial complex I;
- inhibiting mitochondrial permeability transition;
- stimulating mitochondrial biogenesis, resulting in stabilized synaptic function;
- altering metabolism of neurotransmitters such as glutamate and gamma-amino butyric acid (GABA);
- activating energy-sensing signaling pathways such as the peroxisome proliferator activated receptor (PPAR), mammalian target of rapamycin (mTOR), and adenosine monophosphate-(AMP)-activated kinase (AMPK) pathways.

Table 1. Clinical trials experimenting on the effectiveness of different types of ketogenic diets on Alzheimer's cognitive impairment.

Authors	Objective	Subjects	Procedures	Results	Authors' Comments
Reger et al. [23]	to explore, in individuals with memory disorders, whether hyperketonemia improves cognitive functioning (change from baseline in the Alzheimer's disease (AD) Assessment Scale-Cognitive subscale, ADAS-Cog).	20 individuals, mean age 74.7 (S.D. = 6.7), with probable AD (n = 15; National Institute of Neurological and Communicative Disorders and Stroke and the Alzheimer's Disease and Related Disorders Association (NINCDS-ADRDA criteria; 9 = ε4+) or amnestic mild cognitive impairment (n = 5; 1 = ε4+); mildly to moderately cognitively impaired with a mean Mini-Mental State Examination (MMSE) of 22.0 (S.D. = 5.5).	double-blind placebo controlled design with two study visits; during each visit, subjects received one of two isocaloric conditions (690 calories) in a randomized order: emulsified medium chain triglycerides (MCTs), or emulsified long chain triglycerides as a placebo.	significant increases in levels of the ketone body β-hydroxybutyrate (β-OHB) were observed 90 min after treatment (p = 0.007) when cognitive tests were administered; MCT treatment facilitated performance on the ADAS-Cog for ε4− subjects, but not for ε4+ subjects (p = 0.04).	β-OHB elevations were moderated by apolipoprotein E (APOE) genotype (p = 0.036).
Henderson et al. [24].	to assess whether 90-day daily dosing of the oral ketogenic product AC-1202 (medium chain triglyceride composed of glycerin and caprylic acid, C8:0) improve cognitive performance; additional outcomes included how cognitive scores were influenced by APOE4 genotype status.	152 subjects diagnosed with mild to moderate AD according to NINCDS-ADRDA criteria and Diagnostic and Statistical Manual of mental disorders-IV (DSM-IV) criteria, with a MMSE score of between 14 and 24 (inclusive) at screen (86, age 76.9 ± 8.9 years, were allocated to AC-102, and 66, age 76.8 ± 7.4 years, to placebo).	AC-1202 was compared to Placebo in a randomized, double-blind, placebo-controlled, parallel-group study; subjects were on a normal diet and continued taking approved AD medications; pre- and post-dosing serum β-hydroxybutyrate (β-OHB) levels were evaluated. Cognitive performance change from baseline was assessed after 90 days by ADAS-Cog and AD Cooperative Study—Clinical Global Impression of Change (ADCS-CGIC).	AC-1202 rapidly elevated serum ketone bodies in AD patients and resulted in significant differences in ADAS-Cog scores compared to the Placebo after 45 and 90 days of treatment. Effects were most notable in APOE4(-) subjects who were dosage compliant.	adverse events were more frequently observed in participants receiving AC-1202 and concerned mainly transient, mild to moderate gastrointestinal effects; this medium-chain triglyceride preparation of fractionated coconut oil (caprylic trigyceride) has been approved for the treatment of AD in the USA.
Krikorian et al. [25]	the primary outcomes included measures of executive ability, long term memory, and mood obtained at pretreatment baseline and after the 6-week of the intervention: high carbohydrate or very low carbohydrate diet.	23 (10 men, 13 women) older adults with mild cognitive impairment (Clinical Dementia Rating, CDR), age 70.1 ± 6.2 years.	the subjects were randomly assigned to the 6-week dietary interventions consisted of high carbohydrate (50% of calories) and very low carbohydrate (5% to 10% of calories) diets, the latter intended to induce ketosis; all subjects also provided urine samples at the baseline and final visits for urinary ketone assessment; working memory and set switching aspects of executive ability was evaluated by The Trail Making Test part B, secondary or long term memory with the Verbal Paired Associate Learning and mood with the Geriatric Depression Scale; waist circumference, fasting serum glucose and insulin level were analyzed.	ketone levels were positively correlated with memory performance (p = 0.04); the primary finding indicated improved secondary memory performances for the low carbohydrate subjects; there was no effect of the intervention on the Trail Making Test part B and Geriatric Depression Scale; there were significant changes in anthropometric and metabolic values and in dietary parameters; after the intervention, weight, waist circumference, fasting glucose and insulin value were lower for the low carbohydrate but not high carbohydrate group.	these preliminary data provide evidence that dietary ketosis by means of carbohydrate restriction can provide neurocognitive benefit for older adults with early memory decline and increased risk for neurodegeneration. Correction of hyperinsulinemia and other mechanisms associated with ketosis such as reduced inflammation and enhanced energy metabolism also may have contributed to improved neurocognitive function; a prominent issue will be duration of the effects and whether there is persistence of benefit beyond the period of active intervention.

Table 1. *Cont.*

Authors	Objective	Subjects	Procedures	Results	Authors' Comments
Rebello et al. [26]	to evaluated the effect of the daily consumption of an oil, composed of medium chain triglycerides (MCTs) for 24 weeks on serum ketone body concentrations (β-hydroxybutyrate [βHB]) and cognitive performance.	6 individuals ≥50 (58–78) years, with mild cognitive impairment (MCI).	pilot and feasibility, randomized double blind placebo-controlled parallel trial; participants received 56 g/day of either medium chain triglycerides (MCTs) or placebo for 24 weeks; serum β-hydroxybutyrate concentrations, apolipoprotein-E4 status, and cognitive assessments (Alzheimer's Disease Assessment Scale-Cognitive subscale (ADAS-Cog), Trail Making Test, and Digit Symbol Test) were carried out.	intake of MCT oil increased serum ketone bodies and improved memory, only in subjects with mild Alzheimer's disease who did not have an APOE ε4 allele while intake of placebo did not show improvement in any of the cognitive measures tested.	Due to the small number of participants only the raw scores were examined. Consumption of 56 g/day of MCTs for 24weeks increases serum ketone concentrations and appears to be a candidate for larger randomized control trials in the future
Ota et al. [27]	to examine the effects of a single MCT supplemented ketogenic meal serving on cognition in elderly non-demented subjects	subjects were 19 non-demented elderly adults over 60 years old (13 females; mean age: 66.1 ± 2.9 years)	subjects underwent neurocognitive tests 90 and 180 min after oral intake of a ketogenic meal (Ketonformula®) containing 20 g of MCTs and an socaloric placebo meal without MCTs on separate days.	elevation of plasma ketone concentration after intake of a single ketogenic meal containing 20 g of MCTs was confirmed (all $p < 0.001$); as for cognition, improvements were observed in the digit span test, Trail-Making Test B, and the global score ($Z = -2.4$, $p = 0.017$) following the ketogenic meal and the change in the executive functioning score was positively correlated with that of the plasma β-hydroxybutyrate level; the cognition-enhancing effect was observed predominantly for individuals who had a relatively low global score at baseline ($Z = -2.8$, $p = 0.005$), compared to individuals with a high global score ($Z = -0.7$, $p = 0.51$).	plasma levels of ketone bodies were successfully increased after intake of the ketogenic meal; the ketogenic meal was suggested to have positive effects on working memory, visual attention, and task switching in non-demented elderly; the study is limited by the small sample size which may have resulted in false-positive and -negative results of the effect of the ketogenic meal in some cognitive tests.
Ohnuma et al. [28]	This clinical trial, carried out in Japan, analyzed the effect of 90-day administration of a ketogenic meal "Axona" (40 g of powder containing 20 g of caprylic triglycerides) on cognitive function in mild-to-moderate Alzheimer's disease (AD) patients.	22 Japanese patients with sporadic AD at a mild-to-moderate stage (ten females, 12 males), mean age (± standard deviation) 63.9 (± 8.5) years, Mini-Mental State Examination (MMSE) score, 10–25, seven patients were ApoE4-positive.	prospective, open-label, observational study; Axona was administered for 3 months using an indurating, four-step dose-titration method (from 10 to 40 g per day) for 7 days before the trial, and examined the tolerance and adverse effects of this intervention; blood tests included: haemogram, alanine aminotransferase and aspartate aminotransferase, creatinine and urea nitrogen, glucose, glycohaemoglobin A1C, low-density lipoprotein and high-density lipoprotein, triacylglycerol, albumin, and total protein, and sodium, chloride, and potassium; serum total ketone bodies (acetoacetic acid and β-hydroxybutyric acid); the effect on cognitive function was assessed using the MMSE and Alzheimer's Disease Assessment Scale (ADAS) cognitive subscale, Japanese version (ADAS-Jcog); *ApoE* genotypes were determined.	the tolerance of Axona was good, without severe gastrointestinal adverse effects; Axona did not improve cognitive function in our sample of AD patients, even in those patients without the ApoE4 allele; however, some ApoE4-negative patients with baseline MMSE score ≥14 showed improvement in their cognitive functions.	the modified dose-titration method, starting with a low dose of Axona, decreased gastrointestinal adverse effects in Japanese patients. Axona might be effective for some relatively mildly affected patients with AD (with cognitive function MMSE score of ≥14 and lacking the ApoE4 allele).

Table 1. *Cont.*

Authors	Objective	Subjects	Procedures	Results	Authors' Comments
Taylor et al. [29]	The primary objective of Ketogenic Diet Retention and Feasibility Trial (KDRAFT) was to address the feasibility of implementing a very high-fat ketogenic diet (VHF-KD) intervention in AD participants; secondary objectives included evaluating the effects of a VHF-KD on cognition.	15 participants with AD. Individuals were eligible to the study if they had a clinical dementia rating (CDR) of very mild AD (CDR 0.5), mild AD (CDR 1), or moderate AD (CDR 2).	single-arm, pilot clinical study enrolled 15 participants with AD and required participants to maintain an MCT-supplemented KD for 3 months and then to resume a normal diet for 1 month (washout period). KD included 70% of energy as fat (including the MCT), 20% as protein, and carbohydrate less than 10% of energy; ketogenic ratio (lipid grams to non lipid grams) of 1:1 or better. MCT oil supplement (Now Foods, USA) contained a combination of C8:0 and C10:0 fatty acids; participants self-monitored urine ketones daily; serum electrolytes, renal function tests, liver function tests, and glucose levels were measured at the baseline and month 3 visits. Serum β-hydroxybutyrate (βHB) and insulin levels were measured at baseline, month 1, month 2, month 3, and washout, Homeostatic Model Assessment Index 2-Insulin Resistance (HOMA2-IR) values were calculated; Dual energy X-ray absorptiometry was used to assess body composition; MMSE, to identify cognitive impairment, and ADAS-cog, to measure changes in memory, language, praxis, and attention, were administered at baseline, at the end of the intervention (month 3), and after the 1-month washout.	7 CDR0.5, 4 CDR1, and 4 CDR2 participants were enrolled; 10 completers achieved ketosis; among the completers, the mean of the Alzheimer's Disease Assessment Scale-cognitive subscale score improved by 4.1 points during the diet (P 5.02) and reverted to baseline after the washout. Only one participant's ADAS-cog score declined while following the diet protocol. Serum βHB levels were significantly elevated at months 1, 2, and 3 compared with that of baseline and returned to the normal range at the end of thewashout period (0.12 mmol/L).	Because of small sample size and single-arm design, any interpretationp of this study's cognitive performance data requires caution; the pilot trial justifies KD studies in mild Alzheimer's disease.

The advances in understanding of the mechanisms of action of medium-chain fatty acids (e.g., decanoic acid and octanoic acid) have more recently shifted attention away from ketone bodies to the direct role of fatty acids as a therapeutic effectors, paving the way for novel dietary and drug therapies for epilepsy and other disorders, as comprehensively described in Augustin's recent review. According to this review medium-chain fatty acids are able to cross the blood–brain barrier reaching in the brain a concentrations more than 50% greater than the plasma one, providing an alternative energy source for brain neurons and astrocytes. Octanoic acid seems to undergo β-oxidation in astrocytes more easily than decanoic acid and readily produces ketone bodies; decanoic acid instead stimulates glycolysis producing lactate available as fuel for the brain cells [6].

5. The Antioxidant Activity of the Ketogenic Diet: An Insight into Molecular Mechanism

Mitochondria are the main source of energy in the cell, implicated in ATP production through oxidative phosphorylation. They play a key role in apoptosis and production of reactive oxygen species (ROS) as a result of escape of electrons during the transfer along the electron transport chain (ETC). Accumulation of ROS, primarily derived from mitochondrial complexes I and III [30,31], damages proteins, lipids and nucleic acids. Oxidative stress causes mitochondrial dysfunction which enhances ROS production in a pathological positive feedback loop.

KBs metabolism reduces oxidative stress compared to glycolysis, hypothesizing a further neuroprotective mechanism carried out by these compounds [32].

β-Hydroxybutyrate (β-HOB), the most studied KB, has been shown to reduce the production of ROS improving mitochondrial respiration and bypassing the complex I dysfunction [33,34].

(a) The ketogenic diet (KD) stimulates the cellular endogenous antioxidant system with the activation of nuclear factor erythroid-derived 2 (NF-E2)-related factor 2 (Nrf2), the major inducer of detoxification genes.

Nrf2 is a member of the cap "n" collar (Cnc) family of transcription factors, a 605 amino acid protein, with six functional domains termed Nrf2-erythroid-derived cap'n'collar homolog (ECH) homologues (Neh). Under homeostatic conditions, Nrf2 is sequestered and inhibited in the cytoplasm by kelch-like ECH associated protein 1 (Keap1) interacting with Neh2 domains of Nrf2 [35,36]. Keap 1 is a substrate adaptor for different ubiquitin ligase systems, Cullin 3 (Cul3) RING-box 1 (RBX1) E3 ubiquitin ligase complex being the most studied [37]. They constantly ubiquitinate Nrf2 which is then degraded by the proteasome [38,39].

Nrf2-Keap 1 can be considered a sensor of cellular redox status since Keap 1 is a cysteine-rich protein. When distinct cysteine residues (Cys273 and Cys288) are oxidized, a conformational change takes place in Keap1 and so Nrf2 is able to translocate to the nucleus [40,41]. The translocation of Nrf2 is also possible if protein kinase C δ (PKCδ) phosphorylates Ser40 on Nrf2 and if Cys151 on Keap1 gets oxidized [42].

Once into the nucleus Nrf2 constitutes a heterodimer with small Mafs [43] and binds to the antioxidant responsive element (ARE) [44,45]. ARE is an enhancer element in the promoter region of cytoprotective genes such as proteins with thiol (-SH) group like glutathione (GSH), thioredoxin (TXN) and piroxiredoxin (PRDN) or detoxification enzymes like superoxide dismutase (SOD), catalase, hem oxygenase-1 (HO-1) and glutamate cysteine ligase (CGL) ([46–48]. Nrf2 is able to induce glutathione reductase, thioredoxin and peroxiredoxin, fundamental enzymes implicated in the regeneration of active form of endogenous antioxidants [49].

Moreover, β-HB is an endogenous inhibitor of class I and class IIa histone deacetylases (HDACs). The inhibition of HDACs (1–5,7,8,9) upregulates the transcription of detoxifying genes including catalase, mitochondrial superoxide dismutase (mn-SOD) and metallothionein 2 in order to counteract oxidative stress [50,51].

Hippocampus of rats fed a KD for up 3 week showed Nrf2 activation and nuclear translocation [52,53]. CGL subunits (GCLC and CGLM) have antioxidant-response elements (ARE)-like sequences: in this work CGL biosynthesis increases as well as glutathione but there is a decrease in the mitochondrial level of ROS. How KD activates the Nrf2-ARE pathway is not completely understood, Milder et al. [53] have showed that in hippocampal mitochondria of KD-fed rats there is an acute increase of H_2O_2 level after only 1 day. The first boost of H_2O_2 production is in contrast with the reduction of its level after 3 week of diet. Probably H_2O_2 acts as a redox signal which initiates signaling cascade. Interestingly H_2O_2 enhances DNA binding of Nrf2 to the ARE [54]. Nrf2 activation is assisted by lipid peroxidation: for example arachidonic and linolenic acid during mitochondrial dysfunction may react with reactive nitrogen species (RNS) and ROS to produce 4-hydroxy-2-nonenal (4-HNE), an α, β-unsaturated aldehyde. Acute increase of H_2O_2 and 4-HNE during the first days of diet activates the release of Nrf2 from Keap 1 to produce an adaptive antioxidant response [52,55].

(b) A further mechanism explaining the protective activity of the ketogenic diets against oxidative stress is the intracellular modulation of the $NAD^+/NADH$ ratio. An increased $NAD^+/NADH$ ratio protects against ROS and plays an important role in cellular respiration, mitochondrial biogenesis and redox reactions [56]. Nicotinamide adenine dinucleotide (NAD) presents two forms: the oxidized form (NAD^+) and the reduced form (NADH). During the glycolytic pathway glucose reduces 4 molecules of NAD^+, while, on the contrary, the complete mitochondrial oxidation of β-HOB and acetoacetate (AcAc) reduces respectively 1 and none molecule of NAD^+ [57]. In hippocampus and cerebral cortex of KD-fed rats a significant increase in the $NAD^+/NADH$ ratio was detected not only after 3 weeks but also after 2 days [58]. The fully oxidation of KBs and its product ATP inhibits glycolytic pathway which leads to a further accumulation of NAD^+. A high $NAD^+/NADH$ ratio may influence gene expression through Sirtuin 1 (SIRT1), a type 3 histone deacetylase [59]. SIRT1 is a 747 amino acid NAD^+ dependent enzyme with a globular highly conserved catalytic domain [60], it also possess a nuclear export signals and may translocate between the nucleus and the cytoplasm [61]. Tumor suppressor hypermethylated in cancer 1 (HIC1) together with C term binding protein (CtBP) can suppress SIRT1 gene expression. This suppressor complex dissociates when the glycolytic pathway is inhibited and $NAD^+/NADH$ ratio heightens (interestingly similar condition occurs during KD). When it happens, SIRT1 protein levels increase [62]. Even DNA damage, forkhead transcription factor (FOXO3A) [63], starvation with the cAMP response-element-binding protein (CREB) activation [64] might enhance the transcription of SIRT1. SIRT1 is implicated in many biological processes deacetylating histone and non-histone targets [65] and many of them seem to be associated with antioxidant properties of KD. Additionally, SIRT1 might exercise other functions to limit oxidative stress, such as improving synthesis of heat shock proteins, increasing antioxidant defenses, promoting DNA repairing activity of p53 and FOXO factors [66,67] and deacetylating Nrf2 [68].

(c) Ketone metabolism increases the efficiency of electron transport chain (ETC) through the expression of uncoupling proteins (UCP) [69]. UCP reduces the mitochondrial membrane potential and diminishes the production of ROS and reactive oxygen nitrogen species (RONS) [70,71]. UCP4 and UCP5 are increased in brains of ketone ester-supplemented rats [72]. The KD inductive effect on UCP2, 4 and 5 expression could be a consequence of SIRT1 activation [73].

(d) SIRT1 activation, mediated by KD, could offset mitochondrial dysfunction enhancing mitochondrial biogenesis [74]. In the cell there is a constant balance between the mitophagy of damaged mitochondria and the biogenesis to renew mitochondria population [75]. The major regulator of the biogenesis process is the Peroxisome proliferator-activated receptor Gamma Coactivator-1α (PCG-1α) whose transcription is triggered by Nrf2 [76,77]. SIRT1 plays a key role in deacetylase PCG-1α [78] which co-activates the transcription of Nuclear Respiratory Factor (NRF). NRF 1 and NRF 2 lead to the transcription of mitochondrial transcription factor A (TFAM), subsequently TFAM drives the replication of mitochondrial DNA and the mitochondrial biogenesis [79].

(e) At last, ROS and reactive nitrogen species (RNS) can also open the mitochondrial permeability transition pore (mPTP). mPTP releases cytochrome c (Cytc) and apoptosis inducing factor (AIF) which activate caspases 3 and 9 that finally initiate the apoptotic pathway [80–82]. Mitochondrial ATP-sensitive potassium channels (mitoKATP channels) in the inner mitochondrial membrane are implicated in modulation of ETC and calcium buffering through enhancing K+ efflux [83]. During oxidative stress KBs can activate mitoKATP channels, improving the efficiency of ETC [84] and inhibiting mPT [85–87].

6. The Anti-Inflammatory Activity of Ketogenic Diet: An Insight into Molecular Mechanism

Several neurodegenerative diseases are interconnected by shared neurotoxic mechanisms related to inflammatory mechanisms such as cytokine release, neurotrophin synthesis inhibition, release of NO and CO, which are potentially harmful to surrounding tissues, and so on. Against this the cells provide endogenous mechanisms tending to neutralize the molecules responsible for inflammatory damage [12].

A winning strategy to attempt to block neuroinflammation may consist in the enhancement of endogenous anti-inflammatory programs. One of the most promising approaches seems to be the ketogenic diet that was set up in the first decade of the last century to treat refractory epilepsy and then applied with success to treat other neurological diseases [88].

A great interest has been focusing on the use of KD in the treatment of AD for two main reasons: (i) KD was shown to decrease the production of Amyloid Precursor Protein (APP) and therefore the βamyloid peptide; and (ii) KD was related to the activation of peroxisome proliferator-activated receptor gamma (PPARγ) and then to the decrease of systemic inflammation [89,90].

βHB, one of the main KB detected in the blood after the supply of a ketogenic diet, is able to cross the BBB thanks to the specific expression of its transporter MCT1 on endothelial cells. But after its entrance into the brain, β-hydroxybutyrate (βHB) not only provides energy but activates the receptor hydroxy-carboxylic acid receptor 2 (HCA2), lowering neuroinflammation [91].

HCA2, a G-protein coupled receptor, is expressed on macrophages, dendritic cells and microglia [92]. βHB which is the main endogenous ligand of HCA2, activates human HCA2 with an half maximal effective concentration (EC50) of about 700 mM, a concentration attained only after feeding a ketogenic diet [91]. HCA2 may elicit anti-inflammatory effects through the inhibition of NF-kB activation [93]. HCA2 activation induces a neuroprotective macrophage phenotype related to Prostaglandin D2 (PGD2) production by Cyclooxygenase 1 (COX1), that helps to resolve inflammation [94] and has neuroprotective effects [95]. A metabolite of PGD2 inhibits the main activator of NF-kB which is IKB kinase (IKK). As a consequence HCA2 activation inhibits NF-kB in macrophages [93]. The activation of HCA2 by ketogenic diet was shown to induce a neuroprotective phenotype in bone-marrow derived macrophages that infiltrate the brain [92].

HDACs are a group of proteins that are able to regulate gene expression by deacetylating lysine residues on histone proteins. It is known that hyperacetylation of histones is associated with the activation of gene expression and therefore HDACs with their action on histone proteins may suppress gene expression. Some studies in animal models have highlighted the role of HDACs inhibitors in enhancing mnesic processes suggesting their potential use in the treatment of cognitive diseases.

HDAC plays an important role in the pathogenesis of AD by altering chromatin structure and accessibility [96]. βHB inhibits HDACs 1, 3 and 4 (class I and IIa) in vitro [97]. Reducing HDAC2 in a mouse model for amyloid deposition via RNA interference was able to improve memory function and synaptic plasticity [98]. HDAC3 negatively regulates spatial memory in APP/Presenilin 1 (PS1) mice and HDAC3 inhibition might represent a potential therapy for the treatment of AD [99]. Reducing HDAC6 levels is mechanistically linked to tubulin-acetylation and improved mitochondria transport [100].

βHB mediated the inhibition of NLRP3 inflammasome in lipopolysaccharides (LPS)-stimulated human monocytes leading to a reduced production of interleukin-1beta (IL-1beta) and interleukin-18

(IL-18) without significantly affecting tumor necrosis factor-alpha (TNF-alpha) levels [101]. βHB dose-dependently inhibited IL-1beta and IL-18 secretion blocking NLRP3 inflammasome activation by limiting K^+ efflux from cells [101]. Several experiments have ruled out a hypothetic role for mitochondrial ROS in the effects of ketone bodies on the inflammasome.

Since 2008 it has become clear that a low carbohydrate diet causes an increase of KB serum levels, paralleled by a reduction in several inflammatory parameters [102], and that KD allows neuroprotection for brain injuries and neurodegenerative diseases [103].

A randomized controlled dietary intervention trial was done on 40 overweight subjects aged 18–55 years, fed with a diet very low in carbohydrate or an isocaloric diet low in fat for 12 weeks. Subjects fed with KD developed a mild ketosis and showed weight loss, decreased adiposity, and an improved glycemic control as well as an improved insulin sensitivity. Both diets significantly decreased the concentration of several serum inflammatory markers, but there was an overall greater anti-inflammatory effect associated with KD: a larger reduction was observed in TNF-alpha, interleukin-8 (IL-8), monocyte chemoattractant protein (MCP-1), plasminogen activator inhibitor-1 (PAI-1), E-selectin, intercellular adhesion molecule-1 (ICAM-1), while these markers showed a little change in the subjects fed with a low fat diet, suggesting that it is the macronutrient composition, not the weight loss or the caloric reduction the real responsible for the anti-inflammatory activity [102].

Basic research provides evidence that KD play a neuroprotective role in some acute or chronic neurodegenerative diseases. Rats fed a KD for 3–4 weeks showed a reduced peripheral inflammatory response after the injection of Freund's complete adjuvant in their paw, compared to animal fed a standard diet. Ketone metabolism results in decreased production of reactive oxygen species, known to contribute to inflammation. Moreover polyunsaturated polyunsaturated fatty acids activate PPAR which inhibit NF-kB and AP-1 [104].

KD neuroprotective activity has been analyzed previously, based on its anti-inflammatory effects.

In a model of experimental autoimmune encephalomyelitis KD reverted the increased expression of inflammatory cytokines, as well as the production of reactive oxygene species [105].

In a mouse model of Parkinson's disease, where substantia nigra dopaminergic neurons dysfunction is induced by mPTP treatment, KD was shown to inhibit the proinflammatory activation induced by mPTP [106]. Activated microglia produce relevant proinflammatory citokines, including IL-1beta, IL-6, TNF-alpha which were associated to dying or damaged dopaminergic neurons [107]. In the study by Yang et al. [106] KD was able to decrease the activation of microglia and its products IL-1beta, IL-6, TNF-alpha, sparing at the same time tyrosine hydroxylase (TH)-positive neurons in substantia nigra, compared to control animals fed a standard diet. Moreover, the deficit of motor function induced by mPTP was partially but significantly recovered by KD pre-treatment. A study focused on Parkinson's disease patients showed that a KD supplied for 28 days induced a significant improvement in symptoms [108].

7. Conclusions

The results obtained so far by applying the ketogenic diet to the treatment of several neurological diseases seem to be particularly interesting for the recovery of cognitive functions, although they are numerically limited. Different studies conducted on animal models have proposed a causal role for KD, although they do not always reflect with precision the pathogenesis underlying the development of neurological diseases. The few studies conducted on humans available so far are based on a pre/post design but without a reference control group and without randomization. Of particular interest were the RCTs that correlated the introduction of KD to an improvement of verbal receptive vocabulary and of reaction time in children affected by epilepsy, as well as an improvement in attention and memory in patients affected by multiple sclerosis. The results demonstrated causal evidence and stressed the need to increase the number of studies to demonstrate that 4:1 KD induces a cognitive improvement in neurological diseases.

The metabolomics techniques and the network-based integration methodologies will allow us to investigate the interaction among multiple genes, epigenetics and environmental factors, in order to better understand the pathogenesis of AD, to study and to monitor the activity and the efficacy of new therapeutic approaches such as KD and, finally, to develop a personalized management of the disease.

Funding: This study was supported by Sapienza University of Rome "Ricerche Universitarie" (No. C26A15FHES) to Rita Businaro.

Conflicts of Interest: The authors declare no conflict of interest.

References

1. Mendiola-Precoma, J.; Berumen, L.C.; Padilla, K.; Garcia-Alcocer, G. Therapies for Prevention and Treatment of Alzheimer's Disease. *Biomed. Res. Int.* **2016**, *2016*, 2589276. [CrossRef] [PubMed]
2. Francis, H.M.; Stevenson, R.J. Potential for diet to prevent and remediate cognitive deficits in neurological disorders. *Nutr. Rev.* **2018**, *76*, 204–217. [CrossRef] [PubMed]
3. Stafstrom, C.E.; Rho, J.M. The Ketogenic Diet as a Treatment Paradigm for Diverse Neurological Disorders. *Front. Pharmacol.* **2012**, *9*, 3–59. [CrossRef] [PubMed]
4. Johri, A.; Beal, M.F. Mitochondrial dysfunction in neurodegenerative diseases. *J. Pharmacol. Exp. Ther.* **2012**, *342*, 619–630. [CrossRef] [PubMed]
5. Müller, W.E.; Eckert, A.; Kurz, C.; Eckert, G.P.; Leuner, K. Mitochondrial dysfunction: Common final pathway in brain aging and Alzheimer's disease-therapeutic aspects. *Mol. Neurobiol.* **2010**, *41*, 159–171. [CrossRef] [PubMed]
6. Augustin, K.; Khabbush, A.; Williams, S.; Eaton, S.; Orford, M.; Cross, J.H.; Heales, S.J.R.; Walker, M.C.; Williams, R.S.B. Mechanisms of action for the medium-chain triglyceride ketogenic diet in neurological and metabolic disorders. *Lancet Neurol.* **2018**, *17*, 84–93. [CrossRef]
7. Wilkins, J.M.; Trushina, E. Application of Metabolomics in Alzheimer's Disease. *Front. Neurol.* **2018**, *8*, 719. [CrossRef] [PubMed]
8. Zachariou, M.; Minadakis, G.; Oulas, A.; Afxenti, S.; Spyrou, G.M. Integrating multi-source information on a single network to detect disease-related clusters of molecular mechanisms. *J. Proteom.* **2018**. [CrossRef] [PubMed]
9. Yi, L.; Liu, W.; Wang, Z.; Ren, D.; Peng, W. Characterizing Alzheimer's disease through metabolomics and investigating anti-Alzheimer's disease effects of natural products. *Ann. N. Y. Acad. Sci.* **2017**, *1398*, 130–141. [CrossRef] [PubMed]
10. Kaddurah-Daouk, R.; Zhu, H.; Sharma, S.; Bogdanov, M.; Rozen, S.G.; Matson, W.; Oki, N.O.; Motsinger-Reif, A.A.; Churchill, E.; Lei, Z.; et al. Pharmacometabolomics Research Network. Alterations in metabolic pathways and networks in Alzheimer's disease. *Transl. Psychiatry* **2013**, *3*, e244. [CrossRef] [PubMed]
11. Xu, X.H.; Huang, Y.; Wang, G.; Chen, S.D. Metabolomics: A novel approach to identify potential diagnostic biomarkers and pathogenesis in Alzheimer's disease. *Neurosci. Bull.* **2012**, *28*, 641–648. [CrossRef] [PubMed]
12. Verdile, G.; Keane, K.N.; Cruzat, V.F.; Medic, S.; Sabale, M.; Rowles, J.; Wijesekara, N.; Martins, R.N.; Fraser, P.E.; Newsholme, P. Inflammation and Oxidative Stress: Molecular Connectivity between Insulin Resistance, Obesity, and Alzheimer's Disease. *Mediat. Inflamm.* **2015**, *2015*, 105828. [CrossRef] [PubMed]
13. Gano, L.B.; Patel, M.; Rho, J.M. Ketogenic diets, mitochondria, and neurological diseases. *J. Lipid Res.* **2014**, *55*, 2211–2228. [CrossRef] [PubMed]
14. Gasior, M.; Rogawski, M.A.; Hartman, A.L. Neuroprotective and disease-modifying effects of the ketogenic diet. *Behav. Pharmacol.* **2006**, *17*, 431–439. [CrossRef] [PubMed]
15. Puchalska, P.; Crawford, P.A. Multi-dimensional Roles of Ketone Bodies in Fuel Metabolism, Signaling, and Therapeutics. *Cell. MeTable* **2017**, *25*, 262–284. [CrossRef] [PubMed]
16. Hashim, S.A.; VanItallie, T.B. Ketone body therapy: From the ketogenic diet to the oral administration of ketone ester. *J. Lipid Res.* **2014**, *55*, 1818–1826. [CrossRef] [PubMed]
17. Laffel, L. Ketone bodies: A review of physiology, pathophysiology and application of monitoring to diabetes. *Diabetes Metab. Res. Rev.* **1999**, *15*, 412–426.

18. Martin, K.; Jackson, C.F.; Levy, R.G.; Cooper, P.N. Ketogenic diet and other dietary treatments for epilepsy. *Cochrane Database Syst. Rev.* **2016**, *2*, CD001903. [CrossRef] [PubMed]
19. Cervenka, M.C.; Henry, B.J.; Felton, E.A.; Patton, K.; Kossoff, E.H. Establishing an adult epilepsy diet center: Experience, efficacy and challenges. *Epilepsy Behav.* **2016**, *58*, 61–68. [CrossRef] [PubMed]
20. Langea, K.W.; Langeb, K.M.; Makulska-Gertrudaa, E.; Nakamuraa, Y.; Reissmanna, A.; Kanayac, S.; Hauser, J. Ketogenic diets and Alzheimer's disease. *Food Sci. Hum. Wellness* **2017**, *6*, 1–9. [CrossRef]
21. Roehl, K.; Sewak, S.L. Practice Paper of the Academy of Nutrition and Dietetics: Classic and Modified Ketogenic Diets for Treatment of Epilepsy. *J. Acad. Nutr. Diet.* **2017**, *117*, 1279–1292. [CrossRef] [PubMed]
22. Kossoff, E.H.; Zupec-Kania, B.A.; Amark, P.E.; Ballaban-Gil, K.R.; Christina Bergqvist, A.G.; Blackford, R.; Buchhalter, J.R.; Caraballo, R.H.; Helen Cross, J.; Dahlin, M.G.; et al. Optimal clinical management of children receiving the ketogenic diet: Recommendations of the International Ketogenic Diet Study Group. *Epilepsia* **2009**, *50*, 304–317. [CrossRef] [PubMed]
23. Reger, M.A.; Henderson, S.T.; Hale, C.; Cholerton, B.; Baker, L.D.; Watson, G.S.; Hyde, K.; Chapman, D.; Craft, S. Effects of beta-hydroxybutyrate on cognition in memory-impaired adults. *Neurobiol. Aging* **2004**, *25*, 311–314. [CrossRef]
24. Henderson, S.T.; Vogel, J.L.; Barr, L.J.; Garvin, F.; Jones, J.J.; Costantini, L.C. Study of the ketogenic agent AC-1202 in mild to moderate Alzheimer's disease: A randomized, double-blind, placebo-controlled, multicenter trial. *Nutr. Metab. (Lond.)* **2009**, *6*, 31. [CrossRef] [PubMed]
25. Krikorian, R.; Shidler, M.D.; Dangelo, K.; Couch, S.C.; Benoit, S.C.; Clegg, D.J. Dietary ketosis enhances memory in mild cognitive impairment. *Neurobiol. Aging* **2012**, *33*, e19–e27. [CrossRef] [PubMed]
26. Rebello, C.J.; Keller, J.N.; Liu, A.G.; Johnson, W.D.; Greenway, F.L. Pilot feasibility and safety study examining the effect of medium chain triglyceride supplementation in subjects with mild cognitive impairment: A randomized controlled trial. *BBA Clin.* **2015**, *3*, 123–125. [CrossRef] [PubMed]
27. Ota, M.; Matsuo, J.; Ishida, I.; Hattori, K.; Teraishi, T.; Tonouchi, H.; Ashida, K.; Takahashi, T.; Kunugi, H. Effect of a ketogenic meal on cognitive function in elderly adults: Potential for cognitive enhancement. *Psychopharmacology (Berl.)* **2016**, *233*, 3797–3802. [CrossRef]
28. Ohnuma, T.; Toda, A.; Kimoto, A.; Takebayashi, Y.; Higashiyama, R.; Tagata, Y.; Ito, M.; Ota, T.; Shibata, N.; Arai, H. Benefits of use, and tolerance of, medium-chain triglyceride medical food in the management of Japanese patients with Alzheimer's disease: A prospective, open-label pilot study. *Clin. Interv. Aging* **2016**, *1*, 29–36. [CrossRef] [PubMed]
29. Taylor, M.K.; Sullivan, D.K.; Mahnken, J.D.; Burns, J.M.; Swerdlow, R.H. Feasibility and efficacy data from a ketogenic diet intervention in Alzheimer's disease. *Alzheimer's Dement. Transl. Res. Clin. Interv.* **2018**, *4*, 28–36. [CrossRef]
30. Kushnareva, Y.; Murphy, A.N.; Andreyev, A. Complex I-mediated reactive oxygen species generation: Modulation by cytochrome c and NAD(P)+ oxidation-reduction state. *Biochem. J.* **2002**, *368 Pt 2*, 545–553. [CrossRef] [PubMed]
31. Andreyev, A.Y.; Kushnareva, Y.E.; Starkov, A.A. Mitochondrial metabolism of reactive oxygen species. *Biochemistry (Mosc.)* **2005**, *70*, 200–214. [CrossRef] [PubMed]
32. Prins, M.L. Cerebral metabolic adaptation and ketone metabolism after brain injury. *J. Cereb. Blood Flow MeTable* **2008**, *28*, 1–16. [CrossRef] [PubMed]
33. Tieu, K.; Perier, C.; Caspersen, C.; Teismann, P.; Wu, D.C.; Yan, S.D.; Naini, A.; Vila, M.; Jackson-Lewis, V.; Ramasamy, R.; et al. D-beta-hydroxybutyrate rescues mitochondrial respiration and mitigates features of Parkinson disease. *J. Clin. Investig.* **2003**, *112*, 892–901. [CrossRef] [PubMed]
34. Achanta, L.B.; Rae, C.D. β-Hydroxybutyrate in the Brain: One Molecule, Multiple Mechanisms. *Neurochem. Res.* **2017**, *42*, 35–49. [CrossRef] [PubMed]
35. Itoh, K.; Wakabayashi, N.; Katoh, Y.; Ishii, T.; Igarashi, K.; Engel, J.D.; Yamamoto, M. Keap1 represses nuclear activation of antioxidant responsive elements by Nrf2 through binding to the amino-terminal Neh2 domain. *Genes Dev.* **1999**, *13*, 76–86. [CrossRef] [PubMed]
36. Holland, R.; Fishbein, J.C. Chemistry of the cysteine sensors in Kelch-like ECH-associated protein 1. *Antioxid. Redox Signal.* **2010**, *13*, 1749–1761. [CrossRef] [PubMed]
37. Zhang, D.D.; Lo, S.C.; Cross, J.V.; Templeton, D.J.; Hannink, M. Keap1 is a redox-regulated substrate adaptor protein for a Cul3-dependent ubiquitin ligase complex. *Mol. Cell. Biol.* **2004**, *24*, 10941–10953. [CrossRef] [PubMed]

38. Baird, L.; Llères, D.; Swift, S.; Dinkova-Kostova, A.T. Regulatory flexibility in the Nrf2-mediated stress response is conferred by conformational cycling of the Keap1-Nrf2 protein complex. *Proc. Natl. Acad. Sci. USA* **2013**, *110*, 15259–15264. [CrossRef] [PubMed]
39. Baird, L.; Swift, S.; Llères, D.; Dinkova-Kostova, A.T. Monitoring Keap1-Nrf2 interactions in single live cells. *Biotechnol. Adv.* **2014**, *32*, 1133–1144. [CrossRef] [PubMed]
40. Zhang, D.D.; Hannink, M. Distinct cysteine residues in Keap1 are required for Keap1-dependent ubiquitination of Nrf2 and for stabilization of Nrf2 by chemopreventive agents and oxidative stress. *Mol. Cell. Biol.* **2003**, *23*, 8137–8151. [CrossRef] [PubMed]
41. Eggler, A.L.; Liu, G.; Pezzuto, J.M.; van Breemen, R.B.; Mesecar, A.D. Modifying specific cysteines of the electrophile-sensing human Keap1 protein is insufficient to disrupt binding to the Nrf2 domain Neh2. *Proc. Natl. Acad. Sci. USA* **2005**, *102*, 10070–10075. [CrossRef] [PubMed]
42. Niture, S.K.; Jain, A.K.; Jaiswal, A.K. Antioxidant-induced modification of INrf2 cysteine 151 and PKC-delta-mediated phosphorylation of Nrf2 serine 40 are both required for stabilization and nuclear translocation of Nrf2 and increased drug resistance. *J. Cell Sci.* **2009**, *122*, 4452–4464. [CrossRef] [PubMed]
43. Motohashi, H.; Katsuoka, F.; Engel, J.D.; Yamamoto, M. Small Maf proteins serve as transcriptional cofactors for keratinocyte differentiation in the Keap1-Nrf2 regulatory pathway. *Proc. Natl. Acad. Sci. USA* **2004**, *101*, 6379–6384. [CrossRef] [PubMed]
44. Nguyen, T.; Sherratt, P.J.; Pickett, C.B. Regulatory mechanisms controlling gene expression mediated by the antioxidant response element. *Annu. Rev. Pharmacol. Toxicol.* **2003**, *43*, 233–260. [CrossRef] [PubMed]
45. Rushmore, T.H.; Morton, M.R.; Pickett, C.B. The antioxidant responsive element. Activation by oxidative stress and identification of the DNA consensus sequence required for functional activity. *J. Biol. Chem.* **1991**, *266*, 11632–11639. [PubMed]
46. Tebay, L.E.; Robertson, H.; Durant, S.T.; Vitale, S.R.; Penning, T.M.; Dinkova-Kostova, A.T.; Hayes, J.D. Mechanisms of activation of the transcription factor Nrf2 by redox stressors, nutrient cues, and energy status and the pathways through which it attenuates degenerative disease. *Free Radic. Biol. Med.* **2015**, *88 Pt B*, 108–146. [CrossRef] [PubMed]
47. Kumar, H.; Lim, H.W.; More, S.V.; Kim, B.W.; Koppula, S.; Kim, I.S.; Choi, D.K. The role of free radicals in the aging brain and Parkinson's Disease: Convergence and parallelism. *Int. J. Mol. Sci.* **2012**, *13*, 10478–10504. [CrossRef] [PubMed]
48. Hayes, J.D.; Dinkova-Kostova, A.T. The Nrf2 regulatory network provides an interface between redox and intermediary metabolism. *Trends Biochem. Sci.* **2014**, *39*, 199–218. [CrossRef] [PubMed]
49. Chorley, B.N.; Campbell, M.R.; Wang, X.; Karaca, M.; Sambandan, D.; Bangura, F.; Xue, P.; Pi, J.; Kleeberger, S.R.; Bell, D.A. Identification of novel NRF2-regulated genes by ChIP-Seq: Influence on retinoid X receptor alpha. *Nucleic Acids Res.* **2012**, *40*, 7416–7429. [CrossRef] [PubMed]
50. Shimazu, T.; Hirschey, M.D.; Newman, J.; He, W.; Shirakawa, K.; Le Moan, N.; Grueter, C.A.; Lim, H.; Saunders, L.R.; Stevens, R.D.; et al. Suppression of oxidative stress by β-hydroxybutyrate, an endogenous histone deacetylase inhibitor. *Science* **2013**, *339*, 211–214. [CrossRef] [PubMed]
51. Newman, J.C.; Verdin, E. Ketone bodies as signaling metabolites. *Trends Endocrinol. MeTable* **2014**, *25*, 42–52. [CrossRef] [PubMed]
52. Jarrett, S.G.; Milder, J.B.; Liang, L.P.; Patel, M. The ketogenic diet increases mitochondrial glutathione levels. *J. Neurochem.* **2008**, *106*, 1044–1051. [CrossRef] [PubMed]
53. Milder, J.B.; Liang, L.P.; Patel, M. Acute oxidative stress and systemic Nrf2 activation by the ketogenic diet. *Neurobiol. Dis.* **2010**, *40*, 238–244. [CrossRef] [PubMed]
54. Wilson, L.A.; Gemin, A.; Espiritu, R.; Singh, G. ets-1 is transcriptionally up-regulated by H_2O_2 via an antioxidant response element. *FASEB J.* **2005**, *19*, 2085–2087. [CrossRef] [PubMed]
55. Chen, Z.H.; Saito, Y.; Yoshida, Y.; Sekine, A.; Noguchi, N.; Niki, E. 4-Hydroxynonenal induces adaptive response and enhances PC12 cell tolerance primarily through induction of thioredoxin reductase 1 via activation of Nrf2. *J. Biol. Chem.* **2005**, *280*, 41921–41927. [CrossRef] [PubMed]
56. Yang, Y.; Sauve, A.A. NAD+ metabolism: Bioenergetics, signaling and manipulation for therapy. *Biochim. Biophys. Acta* **2016**, *1864*, 1787–1800. [CrossRef] [PubMed]
57. Cotter, D.G.; Schugar, R.C.; Crawford, P.A. Ketone body metabolism and cardiovascular disease. *Am. J. Physiol. Heart Circ. Physiol.* **2013**, *304*, H1060–H1076. [CrossRef] [PubMed]

58. Elamin, M.; Ruskin, D.N.; Masino, S.A.; Sacchetti, P. Ketone-Based Metabolic Therapy: Is Increased NAD+ a Primary Mechanism? *Front. Mol. Neurosci.* **2017**, *10*, 377. [CrossRef] [PubMed]
59. Chen, D.; Bruno, J.; Easlon, E.; Lin, S.J.; Cheng, H.L.; Alt, F.W.; Guarente, L. Tissue-specific regulation of SIRT1 by calorie restriction. *Genes Dev.* **2008**, *22*, 1753–1757. [CrossRef] [PubMed]
60. Davenport, A.M.; Huber, F.M.; Hoel, A. Structural and functional analysis of human SIRT1. *J. Mol. Biol.* **2014**, *426*, 526–541. [CrossRef] [PubMed]
61. Tanno, M.; Sakamoto, J.; Miura, T.; Shimamoto, K.; Horio, Y. Nucleocytoplasmic shuttling of the NAD+-dependent histone deacetylase SIRT1. *J. Biol. Chem.* **2007**, *282*, 6823–6832. [CrossRef] [PubMed]
62. Zhang, Q.; Wang, S.Y.; Fleuriel, C.; Leprince, D.; Rocheleau, J.V.; Piston, D.W.; Goodman, R.H. Metabolic regulation of SIRT1 transcription via a HIC1:CtBP corepressor complex. *Proc. Natl. Acad. Sci. USA* **2007**, *104*, 829–833. [CrossRef] [PubMed]
63. Nemoto, S.; Fergusson, M.M.; Finkel, T. Nutrient availability regulates SIRT1 through a forkhead-dependent pathway. *Science* **2004**, *306*, 2105–2108. [CrossRef] [PubMed]
64. Noriega, L.G.; Feige, J.N.; Canto, C.; Yamamoto, H.; Yu, J.; Herman, M.A.; Mataki, C.; Kahn, B.B.; Auwerx, J. CREB and ChREBP oppositely regulate SIRT1 expression in response to energy availability. *EMBO Rep.* **2011**, *12*, 1069–1076. [CrossRef] [PubMed]
65. North, B.J.; Marshall, B.L.; Borra, M.T.; Denu, J.M.; Verdin, E. The human Sir2 ortholog, SIRT2, is an NAD+ -dependent tubulin deacetylase. *Mol. Cell* **2003**, *11*, 437–444. [CrossRef]
66. Zelin, E.; Freeman, B.C. Lysine deacetylases regulate the heat shock response including the age-associated impairment of HSF1. *J. Mol. Biol.* **2015**, *427*, 1644–1654. [CrossRef] [PubMed]
67. Hori, Y.S.; Kuno, A.; Hosoda, R.; Horio, Y. Regulation of FOXOs and p53 by SIRT1 modulators under oxidative stress. *PLoS ONE.* **2013**, *8*, e73875. [CrossRef] [PubMed]
68. Kawai, Y.; Garduño, L.; Theodore, M.; Yang, J.; Arinze, I.J. Acetylation-deacetylation of the transcription factor Nrf2 (nuclear factor erythroid 2-related factor 2) regulates its transcriptional activity and nucleocytoplasmic localization. *J. Biol. Chem.* **2011**, *286*, 7629–7640. [CrossRef] [PubMed]
69. Sullivan, P.G.; Rippy, N.A.; Dorenbos, K.; Concepcion, R.C.; Agarwal, A.K.; Rho, J.M. The ketogenic diet increases mitochondrial uncoupling protein levels and activity. *Ann. Neurol.* **2004**, *55*, 576–580. [CrossRef] [PubMed]
70. Harper, M.E.; Bevilacqua, L.; Hagopian, K.; Weindruch, R.; Ramsey, J.J. Ageing, oxidative stress, and mitochondrial uncoupling. *Acta Physiol. Scand.* **2004**, *182*, 321–331. [CrossRef] [PubMed]
71. Andrews, Z.B.; Diano, S.; Horvath, T.L. Mitochondrial uncoupling proteins in the CNS: In support of function and survival. *Nat. Rev. Neurosci.* **2005**, *6*, 829–840. [CrossRef] [PubMed]
72. Kashiwaya, Y.; Pawlosky, R.; Markis, W.; King, M.T.; Bergman, C.; Srivastava, S.; Murray, A.; Clarke, K.; Veech, R.L. A ketone ester diet increases brain malonyl-CoA and Uncoupling proteins 4 and 5 while decreasing food intake in the normal Wistar Rat. *J. Biol. Chem.* **2010**, *285*, 25950–25956. [CrossRef] [PubMed]
73. Wang, S.J.; Zhao, X.H.; Chen, W.; Bo, N.; Wang, X.J.; Chi, Z.F.; Wu, W. Sirtuin 1 activation enhances the PGC-1α/mitochondrial antioxidant system pathway in status epilepticus. *Mol. Med. Rep.* **2015**, *11*, 521–526. [CrossRef] [PubMed]
74. Bough, K.J.; Wetherington, J.; Hassel, B.; Pare, J.F.; Gawryluk, J.W.; Greene, J.G.; Shaw, R.; Smith, Y.; Geiger, J.D.; Dingledine, R.J. Mitochondrial biogenesis in the anticonvulsant mechanism of the ketogenic diet. *Ann. Neurol.* **2006**, *60*, 223–235. [CrossRef] [PubMed]
75. Peterson, C.M.; Johannsen, D.L.; Ravussin, E. Skeletal muscle mitochondria and aging: A review. *J. Aging Res.* **2012**, *2012*, 194821. [CrossRef] [PubMed]
76. Cheng, A.; Wan, R.; Yang, J.L.; Kamimura, N.; Son, T.G.; Ouyang, X.; Luo, Y.; Okun, E.; Mattson, M.P. Involvement of PGC-1α in the formation and maintenance of neuronal dendritic spines. *Nat. Commun.* **2012**, *3*, 1250. [CrossRef] [PubMed]
77. Puigserver, P.; Spiegelman, B.M. Peroxisome proliferator-activated receptor-gamma coactivator 1 alpha (PGC-1 alpha): Transcriptional coactivator and metabolic regulator. *Endocr. Rev.* **2003**, *24*, 78–90. [CrossRef] [PubMed]
78. Olmos, Y.; Sánchez-Gómez, F.J.; Wild, B.; García-Quintans, N.; Cabezudo, S.; Lamas, S.; Monsalve, M. SirT1 regulation of antioxidant genes is dependent on the formation of a FoxO3a/PGC-1α complex. *Antioxid. Redox Signal.* **2013**, *19*, 1507–1521. [CrossRef] [PubMed]

79. Aquilano, K.; Baldelli, S.; Pagliei, B.; Ciriolo, M.R. Extranuclear localization of SIRT1 and PGC-1α: An insight into possible roles in diseases associated with mitochondrial dysfunction. *Curr. Mol. Med.* **2013**, *13*, 140–154. [CrossRef] [PubMed]
80. Abeti, R.; Abramov, A.Y. Mitochondrial Ca^{2+} in neurodegenerative disorders. *Pharmacol. Res.* **2015**, *99*, 377–381. [CrossRef] [PubMed]
81. Halestrap, A.P. Mitochondrial calcium in health and disease. *Biochim. Biophys. Acta* **2009**, *1787*, 1289–1290. [CrossRef] [PubMed]
82. Azarashvili, T.; Stricker, R.; Reiser, G. The mitochondria permeability transition pore complex in the brain with interacting proteins-promising targets for protection in neurodegenerative diseases. *Biol. Chem.* **2010**, *391*, 619–629. [CrossRef] [PubMed]
83. Busija, D.W.; Lacza, Z.; Rajapakse, N.; Shimizu, K.; Kis, B.; Bari, F.; Domoki, F.; Horiguchi, T. Targeting mitochondrial ATP-sensitive potassium channels—A novel approach to neuroprotection. *Brain Res. Brain Res. Rev.* **2004**, *46*, 282–294. [CrossRef] [PubMed]
84. Kim, D.Y.; Abdelwahab, M.G.; Lee, S.H.; O'Neill, D.; Thompson, R.J.; Duff, H.J.; Sullivan, P.G.; Rho, J.M. Ketones prevent oxidative impairment of hippocampal synaptic integrity through KATP channels. *PLoS ONE* **2015**, *10*, e0119316. [CrossRef] [PubMed]
85. Teshima, Y.; Akao, M.; Li, R.A.; Chong, T.H.; Baumgartner, W.A.; Johnston, M.V.; Marbán, E. Mitochondrial ATP-sensitive potassium channel activation protects cerebellar granule neurons from apoptosis induced by oxidative stress. *Stroke* **2003**, *34*, 1796–1802. [CrossRef] [PubMed]
86. Nagy, K.; Kis, B.; Rajapakse, N.C.; Bari, F.; Busija, D.W. Diazoxide preconditioning protects against neuronal cell death by attenuation of oxidative stress upon glutamate stimulation. *J. Neurosci. Res.* **2004**, *76*, 697–704. [CrossRef] [PubMed]
87. Robin, E.; Simerabet, M.; Hassoun, S.M.; Adamczyk, S.; Tavernier, B.; Vallet, B.; Bordet, R.; Lebuffe, G. Postconditioning in focal cerebral ischemia: Role of the mitochondrial ATP-dependent potassium channel. *Brain Res.* **2011**, *1375*, 137–146. [CrossRef] [PubMed]
88. Paoli, A.; Bianco, A.; Damiani, E.; Bosco, G. Ketogenic diet in neuromuscular and neurodegenerative diseases. *Biomed. Res. Int.* **2014**, *2014*, 474296. [CrossRef] [PubMed]
89. Cullingford, T.E. The ketogenic diet; fatty acids, fatty acid-activated receptors and neurological disorders. *Prostag. Leukotr.* **2004**, *70*, 253–264. [CrossRef] [PubMed]
90. Jeong, E.A.; Jeon, B.T.; Shin, H.J.; Kim, N.; Lee, D.H.; Kim, H.J.; Kang, S.S.; Cho, G.J.; Choi, W.S.; Roh, G.S. Ketogenic diet-induced peroxisome proliferator-activated receptor-γ activation decreases neuroinflammation in the mouse hippocampus after kainic acid-induced seizures. *Exp. Neurol.* **2011**, *232*, 195–202. [CrossRef] [PubMed]
91. Taggart, A.K.; Kero, J.; Gan, X.; Cai, T.Q.; Cheng, K.; Ippolito, M.; Ren, N.; Kaplan, R.; Wu, K.; Wu, T.J.; et al. (D)-beta-Hydroxybutyrate inhibits adipocyte lipolysis via the nicotinic acid receptor PUMA-G. *J. Biol. Chem.* **2005**, *280*, 26649–26652. [CrossRef] [PubMed]
92. Rahman, M.; Muhammad, S.; Khan, M.A.; Chen, H.; Ridder, D.A.; Müller-Fielitz, H.; Pokorná, B.; Vollbrandt, T.; Stölting, I.; Nadrowitz, R.; et al. The β-hydroxybutyrate receptor HCA2 activates a neuroprotective subset of macrophages. *Nat. Commun.* **2014**, *5*, 3944. [CrossRef] [PubMed]
93. Zandi-Nejad, K.; Takakura, A.; Jurewicz, M.; Chandraker, A.K.; Offermanns, S.; Mount, D.; Abdi, R. The role of HCA2 (GPR109A) in regulating macrophage function. *FASEB J.* **2013**, *27*, 4366–4374. [CrossRef] [PubMed]
94. Rajakariar, R.; Hilliard, M.; Lawrence, T.; Trivedi, S.; Colville-Nash, P.; Bellingan, G.; Fitzgerald, D.; Yaqoob, M.M.; Gilroy, D.W. Hematopoietic prostaglandin D2 synthase controls the onset and resolution of acute inflammation through PGD2 and 15-deoxyDelta12 14 PGJ2. *Proc. Natl. Acad. Sci. USA* **2007**, *104*, 20979–20984. [CrossRef] [PubMed]
95. Taniguchi, H.; Mohri, I.; Okabe-Arahori, H.; Aritake, K.; Wada, K.; Kanekiyo, T.; Narumiya, S.; Nakayama, M.; Ozono, K.; Urade, Y.; et al. Prostaglandin D_2 protects neonatal mouse brain from hypoxic ischemic injury. *J. Neurosci.* **2007**, *27*, 4303–4312. [CrossRef] [PubMed]
96. Peixoto, L.; Abel, T. The role of histone acetylation in memory formation and cognitive impairments. *Neuropsychopharmacology* **2013**, *38*, 62–76. [CrossRef] [PubMed]
97. Newman, J.C.; Verdin, E. β-hydroxybutyrate: Much more than a metabolite. *Diabetes Res. Clin. Pract.* **2014**, *106*, 173–181. [CrossRef] [PubMed]

98. Gräff, J.; Rei, D.; Guan, J.S.; Wang, W.Y.; Seo, J.; Hennig, K.M.; Nieland, T.J.; Fass, D.M.; Kao, P.F.; Kahn, M.; et al. An epigenetic blockade of cognitive functions in the neurodegenerating brain. *Nature* **2012**, *483*, 222–226. [CrossRef] [PubMed]
99. Zhu, X.; Wang, S.; Yu, L.; Jin, J.; Ye, X.; Liu, Y.; Xu, Y. HDAC3 negatively regulates spatial memory in a mouse model of Alzheimer's disease. *Aging Cell* **2017**, *16*, 1073–1082. [CrossRef] [PubMed]
100. Govindarajan, N.; Rao, P.; Burkhardt, S.; Sananbenesi, F.; Schlüter, O.M.; Bradke, F.; Lu, J.; Fischer, A. Reducing HDAC6 ameliorates cognitive deficits in a mouse model for Alzheimer's disease. *EMBO Mol. Med.* **2013**, *5*, 52–63. [CrossRef] [PubMed]
101. Youm, Y.H.; Nguyen, K.Y.; Grant, R.W.; Goldberg, E.L.M.; Kim, D.; D'Agostino, D.; Planavsky, N.; Lupfer, C.; Kanneganti, T.D.; Kang, S.; et al. The ketone metabolite β-hydroxybutyrate blocks NLRP3 inflammasome-mediated inflammatory disease. *Nat. Med.* **2015**, *21*, 263–269. [CrossRef] [PubMed]
102. Forsythe, C.E.; Phinney, S.D.; Fernandez, M.L.; Quann, E.E.; Wood, R.J.; Bibus, D.M.; Kraemer, W.J.; Feinman, R.D.; Volek, J.S. Comparison of low fat and low carbohydrate diets on circulating fatty acid composition and markers of inflammation. *Lipids* **2008**, *43*, 65–77. [CrossRef] [PubMed]
103. Prins, M.L.; Fujima, L.S.; Hovda, D.A. Age-dependent reduction of cortical contusion volume by ketones after traumatic brain injury. *J. Neurosci. Res.* **2005**, *82*, 413–420. [CrossRef] [PubMed]
104. Ruskin, D.N.; Kawamura, M.; Masino, S.A. Reduced pain and inflammation in juvenile and adult rats fed a ketogenic diet. *PLoS ONE* **2009**, *4*, e8349. [CrossRef] [PubMed]
105. Kim, D.Y.; Hao, J.; Liu, R.; Turner, G.; Shi, F.D.; Rho, J.M. Inflammation-mediated memory dysfunction and effects of a ketogenic diet in a murine model of multiple sclerosis. *PLoS ONE.* **2012**, *7*, e35476. [CrossRef] [PubMed]
106. Yang, X.; Cheng, B. Neuroprotective and anti-inflammatory activities of ketogenic diet on MPTP-induced neurotoxicity. *J. Mol. Neurosci.* **2010**, *42*, 145–153. [CrossRef] [PubMed]
107. Liu, B.; Hong, J.S. Role of microglia in inflammation-mediated neurodegenerative diseases: Mechanisms and strategies for therapeutic intervention. *J. Pharmacol. Exp. Ther.* **2003**, *304*, 1–7. [CrossRef] [PubMed]
108. Vanitallie, T.B.; Nonas, C.; Di Rocco, A.; Boyar, K.; Hyams, K.; Heymsfield, S.B. Treatment of Parkinson disease with diet-induced hyperketonemia: A feasibility study. *Neurology* **2005**, *64*, 728–730. [CrossRef] [PubMed]

5

The Effects of Beta-Hydroxy-Beta-Methylbutyrate-Free Acid Supplementation and Resistance Training on Oxidative Stress Markers

Hamid Arazi [1,*], Abbas Asadi [1] and Katsuhiko Suzuki [2]

[1] Department of Exercise Physiology, Faculty of Sports Sciences, University of Guilan, Rasht 1438, Iran; Abbas_asadi1175@yahoo.com
[2] Faculty of Sport Sciences, Waseda University, Tokorozawa 359-1192, Japan; katsu.suzu@waseda.jp
* Correspondence: Hamidarazi@yahoo.com

Abstract: The aim of this study was to investigate the effects of 6-week beta-hydroxy-beta methylbutyrate-free acid (HMB-FA) supplementation on oxidative stress and biochemical variables in responses to resistance training. Sixteen healthy young males participated in this study and were randomly assigned to a HMB-FA supplementation group ($n = 8$) or a placebo supplementation group ($n = 8$). The resistance training program was applied for 6 weeks with two sessions per week. Blood samples were collected before and after training, and 8-hydroxy-2-deoxyguanosine (8-OHdG), malondialdehyde (MDA), protein carbonyl (PC), and biochemical variables, such as alanine transaminase (ALT), aspartate aminotransferase (AST), alkaline phosphatase (ALP), and the numbers of total white blood cells (WBC), neutrophils, lymphocytes, and monocytes were analyzed. Following intervention, both the HMB-FA and placebo supplementation groups showed significant decreases in MDA (effect size [ES]; −0.39, −0.33) and PC (ES; −1.37, −1.41), respectively. However, 8-OHdG did not change after 6 weeks of training in any of the groups. In addition, both groups showed similar training effects on biochemical variables after 6 weeks of intervention. It was concluded that HMB-FA supplementation during resistance training did not add further adaptive changes related to oxidative stress markers.

Keywords: leucine; strength training; free radicals; oxidative stress

---

1. Introduction

It has been well documented that both aerobic and anaerobic exercise result in neutrophil translocation to the active skeletal muscle, subsequently resulting in oxidative stress [1]. Although an acute bout of exercise could result in activation of several systems of free radical generation (i.e., burst of neutrophils) [2], regular exercise training promotes antioxidant defenses and exerts anti-inflammatory effects (i.e., resting redox status) on the blood and skeletal muscle [3].

Most of the experimental studies that have investigated the effects of exercise training on oxidative stress have used endurance training, and only a few studies have investigated the effects of resistance training on oxidative stress adaptations, showing that long term resistance training has protective effects, including the enhancement of defense systems (i.e., superoxide dismutase) [4–7].

It is well known that antioxidant supplementation can inhibit the induction of endogenous antioxidant capacity in response to exercise training [6,7]. On the other hand, antioxidant supplementation among athletes is common; however, there is little information regarding whether amino acid supplementation protects against the negative health consequences of reactive oxygen species (ROS), such as oxidative DNA damage, lipid peroxidation, and protein modification caused by resistance training in men [8].

Leucine, a branched-chain amino acid, is a potent stimulus for translation initiation and protein synthesis [9]. Leucine is also believed to have immunomodulatory effects [10] which may be mediated by its metabolites [11]. Beta-hydroxy-beta-methylbutyrate (HMB) is an intermediate of leucine metabolism and has been shown to increase protein synthesis while simultaneously decreasing muscle proteolysis [11]. It has been well documented that HMB supplementation decreases muscle damage, cytokine and inflammatory responses to exercise and chronic HMB supplementation has positive effects on muscle mass, body composition, and strength [11,12]. However, other studies have reported conflicting results and the results are controversial [13–15]. For example, different authors have demonstrated no change [16] or an increase in immune function in humans and an attenuation of catabolism and muscle damage via HMB supplementation [11,12,17,18]. Regarding the effects of HMB supplementation on immune cells, no studies have directly examined the effects of HMB supplementation on oxidative stress responses to resistance training.

To the best of our knowledge, the majority of the studies have used a commercially available calcium salt form of HMB (HMB-Ca) for supplementation; however, a new free acid form of HMB (HMB-FA) has been found to yield higher plasma concentrations over a shorter period of time compared to the calcium salt form (36 vs. 131 min) [17]. The greater bioavailability of HMB-FA may provide greater benefits regarding its efficacy as a nutrient supplement used to enhance training adaptations and can promote the actions of defense system against oxidative stress and may play an important role in attenuating oxidative damage following exercise training. However, this is the first study to evaluate the effects of resistance training and HMB-FA supplementation on oxidative stress and biochemical variables in response to exercise training. Given the limited available information and few studies about the effects of HMB-FA supplementation in humans, especially the role of HMB-FA on oxidative stress following resistance training, the objective of this study was to evaluate the effects of chronic HMB-FA supplementation on oxidative stress markers and biochemical variables in response to 6 weeks of resistance training.

2. Materials and Methods

2.1. Experimental Design

This study had a placebo-controlled, double-blind, randomized design. All subjects were familiarized with the training program two weeks prior to the initiation of the study. Then, the subjects were recruited to the human performance laboratory to standardize training procedures. One week later the subjects were again recruited to laboratory for assessment of age, height and weight. For the prescription of the resistance training program, one repetition maximum test in each exercise was assessed on two non-consecutive days (i.e., leg press, bench press, knee extension and cable biceps curl on one day and knee flexion, lat pull-down, shoulder press, and triceps push down on another day, 48 h apart) at the same time of day, by the same investigators, using the Kraemer and Fry procedure [19]. Finally, forty-eight hours prior to the initiation of the training period, blood samples were taken in order to determine resting oxidative stress and biochemical variables. Forty-eight hours after the completion of the six-week training period, blood draws were again completed to determine the resting oxidative stress and biochemical variables.

2.2. Participants

Initially, twenty healthy men volunteered to participate in this study. To be included in the final analyses, subjects were required to complete all of the training sessions and attend all assessment sessions. As a result of these requirements, four subjects were excluded from the study.

Therefore, 16 men were included in the final analyses (Figure 1). For the final study subjects, the two study groups were as follows: beta-hydroxy-beta-methylbutyrate-free acid (HMB-FA) supplementation ($n = 8$, age = 21.5 ± 0.5 years, height = 181.7 ± 4.1 cm, body weight = 79.2 ± 13.0 kg, and BMI = 23.9 ± 3.2 kg/m^2) and placebo supplementation ($n = 8$, age = 21.3 ± 0.9 years, height = 179.5 ± 4.5 cm, body weight = 78.9 ± 13.3 kg, and BMI = 24.4 ± 4 kg/m^2). The subjects fulfilled the following inclusion criteria: (1) at least 1 year of resistance training experience determined by questionnaire and/or self-reported history by subjects; (2) had not used any drugs or supplements that could affect the results for 6 months before the initiation of study and throughout the study period; (3) 6 months with the absence of musculoskeletal injury or any orthopedic problems which could affect the efficiency of resistance training; and (4) no participation in other competitive sport activity aside from resistance training during the intervention period. Moreover, the subjects were familiar with the selected exercises in the resistance training program in their training routine and were asked to maintain their physical and diet habits throughout the experiment. The subjects were informed about the experimental procedures and possible risks and benefits associated with participation in the study, and they signed an informed consent before the start of the study. The study was conducted in accordance with the Declaration of Helsinki and was approved by the ethics committee of the University (DT-167908).

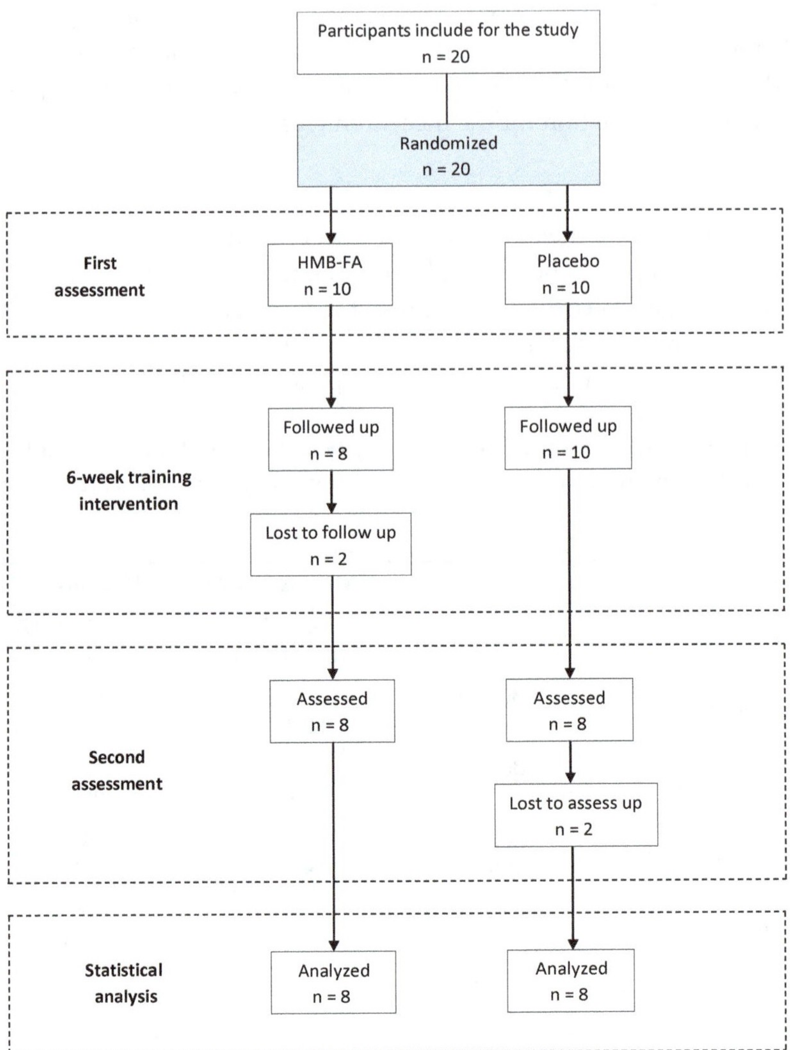

Figure 1. Study flow.

2.3. Measurements

Height was measured using a wall mounted stadiometer (Seca 222, Terre Haute, IN, USA) recorded to the nearest 0.5 cm; body weight was measured to the nearest 0.1 kg using a digital scale (Tanita, BC-418MA, Tokyo, Japan); and body mass index was calculated (kg/m^2).

2.4. Blood Sampling

Blood samples were collected after 10 h of fasting, between 8 and 9 a.m., 48 h before, and 48 h after, the 6-week training intervention. A total of 10 mL of whole blood was drawn from the antecubital vein. The blood was collected into EDTA-containing tubes and centrifuged immediately at 1500× g for 10 min at 4 °C. The blood was allowed to clot at room temperature for 30 min, and the resulting serum was frozen at −80 °C for further analyses.

2.5. Biochemical Analyses

Serum 8-hydroxy-2-deoxyguanosine (8-OHdG), malondialdehyde (MDA), and protein carbonyl (PC) were analyzed using commercially available, enzyme-linked immunosorbent assays (ELISA) kits (ZellBio GmbH Veltlinerweg 29, 89075, Ulm, Germany). Serum alanine transaminase (ALT), aspartate aminotransferase (AST), and alkaline phosphatase (ALP) activities were measured using an automated analyzer (Model 747-400, Hitachi, Tokyo, Japan). Complete blood count analyses were conducted using an automated hematology analyzer (pocH-100i, Sysmex, Kobe, Japan), including the numbers of white blood cells (WBC), neutrophils, lymphocytes, and monocytes. All the assays were conducted in duplicate. The coefficient of variation for the measurements was less than 7%.

2.6. Diet Control

In order to examine whether dietary changes influenced oxidative stress variables, 3 consecutive days of diet recall were completed before beginning the training protocol [4,12]. At the end of the training period, subjects again recorded food intake for 3 consecutive days (before blood sampling). The mean daily calories, protein, carbohydrate, fat, vitamin C and vitamin E intakes during the 3 days assessed before and after the training intervention are presented in Table 1.

Table 1. Dietary intake assessed for the beta-hydroxy-beta methylbutyrate-free acid (HMB-FA) and placebo supplementation groups before and after the training period. Data are presented as means ± SDs.

Diet Variables	Time	HMB-FA (n = 8)	Placebo (n = 8)
Energy intake (kcal)	Before	2532 ± 210	2421 ± 176
	After	2891 ± 198	2782 ± 215
Carbohydrate (g)	Before	260 ± 23	259 ± 29
	After	282 ± 31	278 ± 41
Fat (g)	Before	75 ± 11	79 ± 13
	After	84 ± 14	81 ± 17
Protein (g)	Before	98 ± 19	93 ± 21
	After	119 ± 22	115 ± 34
Vitamin E (mg)	Before	8.9 ± 1.0	9.0 ± 2.0
	After	10.0 ± 2.0	9.5 ± 1.6
Vitamin C (mg)	Before	65 ± 22	67 ± 17
	After	77 ± 18	78 ± 15

2.7. Supplementation

The HMB-FA supplement consisted of one gram of beta-hydroxy-beta-methylbutyrate in the free acid gel form (BetaTor, Body Attack, GmbH & Co., KG, Waldhofstrabe 19, 25474, Ellerbek, Germany). Each serving of placebo contained one gram of polydextrose. On training days, one serving of HMB-FA or placebo was consumed 30 min prior to the exercise session. Two servings were given with the breakfast and supper meals. On the non-training days, participants were instructed to consume one serving with each of three separate meals throughout the day. Subjects were required to return all used and unused packets at the end of each week.

2.8. Training Programe

The resistance training protocol consisted of a 6-week hypertrophic program involving 2 sessions per week. Each training session lasted 80 min, including 10 min of standard warm-up, 65 min of main training and 5 min of cool down. Subjects performed 3 sets of 8 to 12 repetitions with 75 to 85% of 1 RM (leg press, knee extension, knee flexion, lat pull-down, bench press, shoulder press, cable biceps curl and triceps push down) per session. The 2 and 3 min resting intervals were assigned between sets and exercises, respectively. All training sessions was monitored by Certified Conditioning Specialists in order to ensure that all exercises were performed correctly, with the appropriate amount of effort.

2.9. Statistical Analysis

Data are presented as means $\pm$ SDs. The distribution of each variable was examined using the Shapiro–Wilk test. The dependent variables were analyzed using 2 (group) $\times$ 2 (time) analysis of variance (ANOVA). Effect sizes (ES) were calculated to determine training effects. The magnitude of the ES statistics was considered trivial <0.20; small, 0.20–0.50; medium, 0.5–0.80; large, 0.8–1.30; or very large >1.30 [20]. The effect size is reported in conjunction with the 95% confidence interval (CI) for all analyzed measures. The significance level was set at $p \leq 0.05$.

3. Results

The energy, carbohydrate, lipid, and protein intakes did not differ between the before and after intervention measurements for the HMB-FA and placebo groups (Table 1). There were also no significant differences between groups in age, height, body mass and BMI.

Changes in the serum 8-OHdG, MDA and PC are presented in Figure 2. No significant time or group by time changes in 8-OHdG were observed after 6 weeks of training.

The serum MDA decreased significantly (p = 0.01) in the HMB-FA supplementation (from 14.4 $\pm$ 7 to 12.2 $\pm$ 4.5 nmol/mL; ES = 0.39, 95% CI = −0.62 to 1.35) and placebo supplementation (from 14.2 $\pm$ 4.5 to 12.5 $\pm$ 5.1 nmol/mL; ES = 0.33, 95% CI = −0.66 to 1.31) groups after 6 weeks of training. Both groups showed very large, significant (p = 0.05) decrements in the serum PC levels (HMB-FA: from 89.9 $\pm$ 9.1 to 77.9 $\pm$ 8.4 ng/mL; ES = −1.37, 95% CI = 0.22 to −2.37; placebo: from 92.8 $\pm$ 10.2 to 78.8 $\pm$ 9.6 ng/mL; ES = −1.41, 95% CI = 0.25 to −2.42) after training. No statistically significant group $\times$ time interactions in MDA (p = 0.61) or PC (p = 0.37) were observed after the training intervention.

The HMB-FA and placebo groups demonstrated large, significant (p = 0.05) decreases in ALT after 6 weeks of training. In addition, both groups showed medium decrements (p = 0.04) in AST (HMB-FA group, ES = −0.59; placebo group, ES = −0.58) and trivial to small changes (HMB-FA group, ES = −0.02, p = 0.1; placebo group, ES = 0.29, p = 0.04) in ALP after 6 weeks of training. For WBC, the HMB-FA and placebo groups achieved small to trivial significant decreases. Trivial to medium changes in neutrophils, lymphocytes, and monocytes were observed after resistance training for the HMB-FA and placebo groups (Table 2). No statistically significant group $\times$ time interactions in biochemical variables (p > 0.05) were observed after the training intervention.

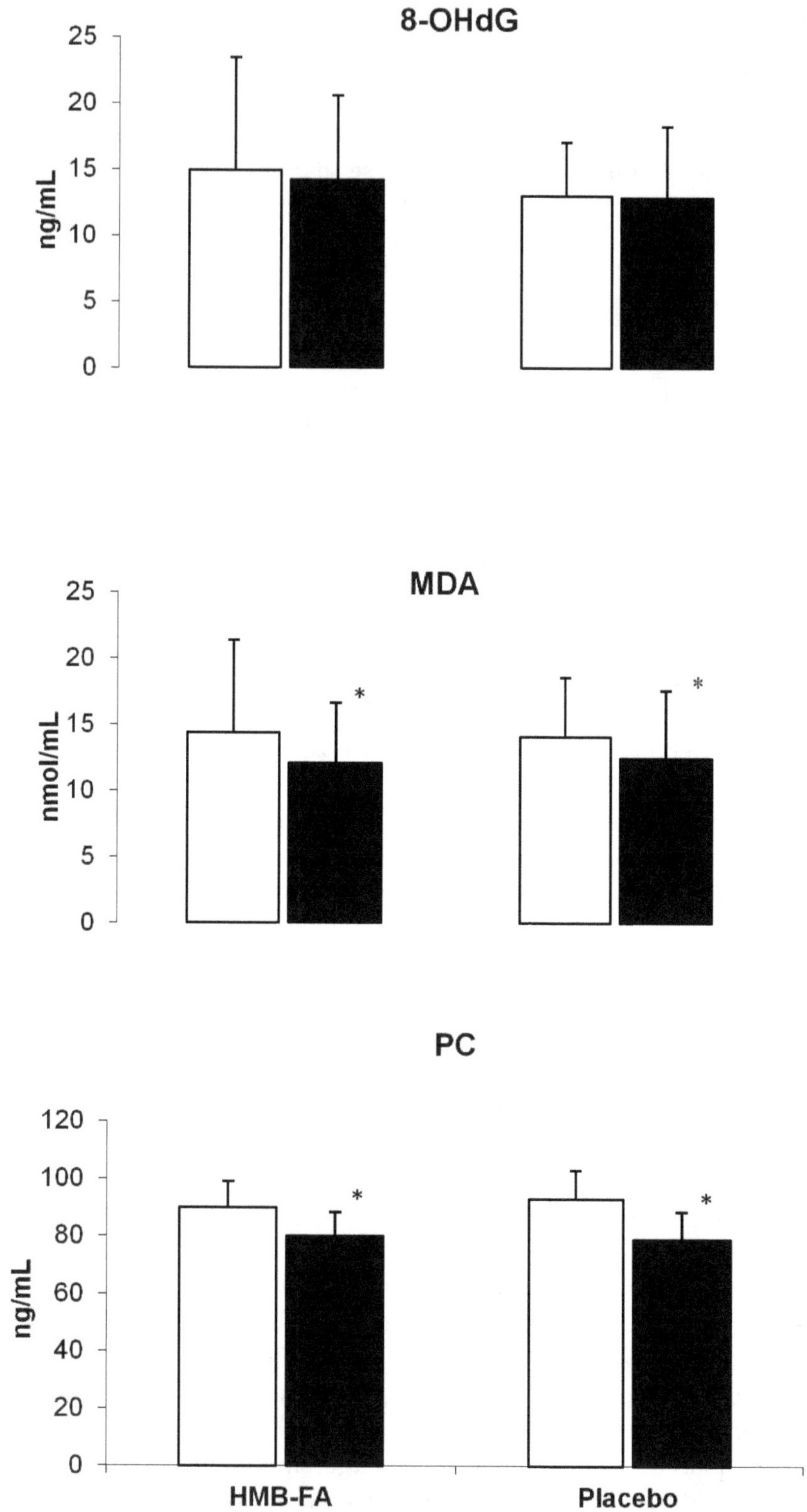

Figure 2. Changes in oxidative stress markers following 6 weeks of a training intervention (means ± SDs).*: denotes significant differences between baseline and post training values ($p \leq 0.05$); (□ pre-test, ■ post-test); 8-OHdG: 8-hydroxy-2-deoxyguanosine; MDA: malondialdehyde; PC: protein carbonyl.

Table 2. Changes in biochemical variables following 6 weeks of a training intervention.

Blood Variables		HMB-FA Group Mean ± SD		Placebo Group Mean ± SD	
ALT (U/L)	Pre	31.1 ± 14.2		34.5 ± 19.8	
	Post	20.1 ± 8.2	*	20.4 ± 7.3	*
	Effect size	−0.94 (−1.92, 0.14)	Large	−0.95 (−1.92, 0.13)	Large
AST (U/L)	Pre	30.2 ± 13.2		30.8 ± 12.2	
	Post	23.7 ± 8.5	*	24.7 ± 8.4	*
	Effect size	−0.59 (−1.56, 0.44)	Medium	−0.58 (−1.55, 0.45)	Medium
ALP (U/L)	Pre	166.0 ± 29.3		164.2 ± 36	
	Post	165.3 ± 49.0		174.6 ± 36.1	*
	Effect size	−0.02 (−1.00, 0.96)	Trivial	0.29 (−0.71, 1.26)	Small
WBC (μ/L)	Pre	8312.5 ± 1817.7		8400.0 ± 900.8	
	Post	7600.0 ± 1033.7	*	8062.5 ± 1924.2	*
	Effect size	−0.48 (−1.45, 0.54)	Small	−0.19 (−1.20, 0.77)	Trivial
Neutrophils (%)	Pre	51.4 ± 10.3		49.5 ± 8.6	
	Post	52.3 ± 9.5		54.5 ± 9.0	*
	Effect size	0.09 (−0.89, 1.07)	Trivial	0.57 (−0.46, 1.53)	Medium
Lymphocytes (%)	Pre	35.8 ± 9.4		35.7 ± 6.5	
	Post	35.0 ± 8.4		34.5 ± 5.7	
	Effect size	0.09 (−0.89, 1.07)	Trivial	−0.02 (−1.17, 0.8)	Trivial
Monocytes (%)	Pre	9.0 ± 1.5		8.9 ± 1.2	
	Post	8.2 ± 1.1	*	7.9 ± 1.6	*
	Effect size	−0.61 (−1.57, 0.43)	Medium	−0.71 (−1.68, 0.34)	Medium

Notes: ALT = alanine transaminase; AST = aspartate aminotransferase; ALP = alkaline phosphatase; WBC = white blood cells; * = significant difference compared to pre-training ($p \leq 0.05$); effect sizes are presented with 95% confidence intervals.

4. Discussion

The aim of this study was to investigate the effects of 6 weeks of resistance training, together with HMB-FA supplementation, on oxidative stress and biochemical variables in humans. The results of this study demonstrate that 6 weeks of resistance training can attenuate oxidative stress and biochemical variables after resistance training and HMB-FA supplementation does not induce further adaptive changes in oxidative stress markers.

In the present study, serum 8-OHdG did not change after training for both the HMB-FA and placebo groups. In contrast, MDA and PC levels significantly decreased after 6 weeks of training in both groups. This finding demonstrates that HMB-FA supplementation with resistance training can result in possible decreases in MDA. Very few studies have examined the effects of resistance training on MDA levels [4–6] and to the authors knowledge, no studies have investigated the influence of HMB-FA supplementation on MDA changes following long duration training. In accordance with our findings, Cakir-Atabek et al. [21] reported that 6 weeks of resistance training reduced resting MDA levels. In addition, Azizbeigi et al. [4] demonstrated that 8 weeks of progressive resistance training induced significant decreases in resting MDA levels in men. A potential mechanism for the resistance training-induced reduction of MDA could include contraction-induced antioxidant enzyme upregulation [22]. Moreover, the antioxidant effects of exercise may not only be mediated by increased expression of antioxidant enzymes, but may also include reduced expression of pro-oxidant enzymes [23]. Regarding the minimal differences between the HMB-FA and placebo groups in terms of MDA decrement (ES; 0.39, 15.3% vs. 0.33, 12%) after resistance training, it seems that, the Cholesterol Synthesis Hypothesis (CSH) could be proposed as a possible mechanism [23]. However, in this study we did not measure any variables related to the CSH, although Nissen et al. [23] reported that muscle cell damage after resistance exercise may cause cells to lack the capacity to produce adequate amounts of cholesterol to maintain sarcolemma integrity. This is important for muscle tissue. Cholesterol is formed from acetyl-CoA, catalyzed by the enzyme, HMG-CoA reductase. The majority of HMB is converted into HMG-CoA reductase [23]. Therefore, supplementation with HMB-FA may increase the intramuscular HMB concentration and may provide greater available substrate for cholesterol synthesis, which is needed to stabilize the sarcolemma and inhibit cell membrane breakdown and consequently, prohibit MDA production in the blood serum.

The amount of protein carbonyl (PC) was decreased for both the HMB-FA and placebo groups after 6 weeks of resistance training (ES; −1.37 vs. −1.41). This finding is in line with previous studies which have reported decrements in protein carbonylation after long term resistance training [4,7]. The physiological consequences of the carbonylation of proteins are dependent on the kind of protein affected by oxidation [5]. Training-induced protein oxidation might also be triggered by iron-containing protein disruption [24]. A calcium homeostasis imbalance may also cause ROS generation through activation of phospholipase and proteolytic enzymes [24]. However, it is difficult to say which proteins and pathways are associated, since proteins may differ greatly in their susceptibility to oxidative damage and carbonylation of proteins. In this study, we used hypertrophic-type resistance training, and this type of training could improve antioxidant levels in the body [4,7] resulting in a decrement of PC. Regarding the lower changes in PC levels for the HMB-FA compared with the placebo group, it seems that HMB supplementation may inhibit intracellular protein degradation and decrease the ubiquitin–proteasome proteolysis pathway [23,25], resulting in a restriction of the carbonylation of proteins.

For the biochemical variables, the HMB-FA and placebo groups exhibited similar decrements in ALT and AST (large to medium ES), while the placebo group showed a greater increase in ALP after 6 weeks of resistance training (ES; 0.29 vs. −0.02). Although both groups showed significant decreases in WBC, the HMB-FA group indicated greater training effects than the placebo group (ES; −0.49 vs. −0.19). The 6 weeks of resistance training did not induce any significant effects in neutrophils or lymphocytes for the HMB-FA group, while the placebo group showed significant increases in neutrophils after 6 weeks. In monocytes, both groups showed slight decrements after 6 weeks of training. A possible potential mechanism(s) for the resistance training-induced reduction of biochemical variables could be due to upregulation of antioxidant enzymes following chronic resistance training and decrements in the expression of pro-oxidant enzymes [4,7].

These findings reveal that supplementation with HMB does not induce enough protective effects for biochemical variables and further studies are needed to determine the long-term effects of HMB-FA supplementation on inflammation after resistance training.

5. Conclusions

In conclusion, the results of this study demonstrated that 6 weeks of resistance training could decrease oxidative stress markers in men. Separately, HMB-FA supplementation has a similar effect on the inhibition of oxidative stress markers and biochemical variables; however, regarding ES, the HMB-FA group exhibited greater training effects than the placebo group. Resistance training can be considered an effective therapeutic intervention to reduce oxidative stress, and HMB-FA supplementation during resistance training does not add further adaptive changes related to oxidative stress markers.

Author Contributions: The authors' contributions were as follows: All authors designed the research. A.A. conducted the research including sample analysis. A.A. and H.A. analyzed the data and wrote the paper. All authors read and approved the final manuscript.

Acknowledgments: We gratefully thank Asghar Abbasi from the University of California, Irvine, for English editing.

Conflicts of Interest: The authors declare no conflict of interest.

References

1. Bloomer, R.J.; Goldfarb, A.H.; Wideman, L.; Mckenzie, M.J.; Consitt, L.A. Effects of acute aerobic and anaerobic exercise on blood markers of oxidative stress. *J. Strength Cond. Res.* **2005**, *19*, 276–285. [PubMed]
2. Bloomer, R.J.; Goldfarb, A.H. Anaerobic exercise and oxidative stress: A review. *Can. J. Appl. Physiol.* **2004**, *29*, 245–263. [CrossRef] [PubMed]
3. Shephard, R.J.; Shek, P.N. Association between physical activity and susceptibility to cancer: Possible mechanisms. *Sports Med.* **1998**, *26*, 293–315. [CrossRef] [PubMed]
4. Azizbeigi, K.; Azarbayjani, M.A.; Peeri, M. The effect of progressive resistance training on oxidative stress and antioxidant enzyme activity in erythrocytes in untrained men. *Int. J. Sport Nutr. Exerc. Metabol.* **2013**, *23*, 230–238. [CrossRef]
5. Margoins, K.; Fatouros, I.G.; Jamurtas, A.Z.; Nikolaidis, M.G.; Douroudos, I.; Chatzinikolaou, A. Oxidative stress biomarkers responses to physical overtraining: Implications for diagnosis. *Free Radic. Biol. Med.* **2007**, *43*, 901–910. [CrossRef] [PubMed]
6. Bobeuf, F.; Labonte, M.; Dionne, I.J. Combined effect of antioxidant supplementation and resistance training on oxidative stress markers, muscle and body composition in an elderly population. *J. Nutr. Health Aging* **2011**, *15*, 883–889. [CrossRef] [PubMed]
7. Atashak, S.; Peeri, M.; Azarbayjani, M.A.; Azizbeigi, K. Effects of ginger supplementation and resistance training on some blood oxidative stress markers in obese men. *J. Exerc. Sci. Fit.* **2014**, *12*, 26–30. [CrossRef]
8. Rahimi, R. Creatine supplementation decreases oxidative DNA damage and lipid peroxidation induced by a single bout of resistance exercise. *J. Strength Cond. Res.* **2011**, *25*, 3448–3455. [CrossRef] [PubMed]
9. Blomstrand, E.; Eliasson, J.; Karlsson, H.K. Branched-chain amino acids activate key enzymes in protein synthesis after physical exercise. *J. Nutr.* **2006**, *136* (Suppl. 1), 269S–273S. [CrossRef] [PubMed]
10. Calder, P.C. Branched-chain amino acids and immunity. *J. Nutr.* **2006**, *136* (Suppl. 1), 288S–293S. [CrossRef] [PubMed]
11. Panton, L.B.; Rathmacher, J.A.; Baier, S. Nutritional supplementation of the leucine metabolite beta-hydroxy-beta-methylbutyrate (HMB) during resistance training. *Nutrition* **2000**, *16*, 734–739. [CrossRef]
12. Wilson, J.M.; Lowery, R.P.; Joy, J.M.; Andersen, J.C.; Wilson, S.M.; Stout, J.R.; Duncan, N.; Fuller, J.C.; Baier, S.M.; Naimo, M.A.; et al. The effects of 12 weeks of beta-hydroxy-beta-methylbutyrate free acid supplementation on muscle mass, strength and power in resistance-trained individuals: A randomized, double-blind, placebo-controlled study. *Eur. J. Appl. Physiol.* **2014**, *114*, 1217–1227. [CrossRef] [PubMed]
13. Thomson, J.; Watson, P.E.; Rowlands, D.S. Effects of nine weeks of β-Hydroxy-β-Methylbutyrate supplementation on strength and body composition in resistance trained men. *J. Strength Cond. Res.* **2009**, *23*, 827–835. [CrossRef] [PubMed]
14. Manjarrez-Montes-de-Oca, R.; Torres-Vaca, M.; González-Gallego, J.; Alvear-Ordenes, I. El β-Hidroxi-β-Metilbutirato (HMB) como suplemento nutricional (I): Metabolismo y toxicidad. *Nutr. Hosp.* **2015**, *31*, 590–596.
15. Drummond, M.J.; Fry, C.S.; Glynn, E.L.; Dreyer, H.C.; Dhanani, S.; Timmerman, K.L.; Volpi, E.; Rasmussen, B.B. Rapamycin administration in humans blocks the contraction-induced increase in skeletal muscle protein synthesis. *J. Physiol.* **2009**, *587*, 1535–1546. [CrossRef] [PubMed]
16. Gonzalez, A.M.; Stout, J.R.; Jajtner, A.R.; Townsend, J.R.; Wells, A.J.; Beyer, K.S.; Boone, C.H.; Pruna, G.J.; Mangine, G.T.; Scanlon, T.M.; et al. Effects of β-hydroxy-β-methylbutyrate free acid and cold water immersion on post-exercise markers of muscle damage. *Amino Acids* **2014**, *46*, 1501–1511. [CrossRef] [PubMed]
17. Fuller, J.C.; Sharp, R.L., Jr.; Angus, H.F.; Baier, S.M.; Rathmacher, J.A. Free acid gel form of beta-hydroxy-beta-methylbutyrate (HMB) improves HMB clearance from plasma in human subjects compared with the calcium HMB salt. *Br. J. Nutr.* **2011**, *105*, 367–372. [CrossRef] [PubMed]
18. Townsend, J.R.; Fragala, M.S.; Jajtner, A.R.; Gonzalez, A.M.; Wells, A.J.; Mangine, G.T.; Robinson IV, E.H.; McCormack, W.P.; Beyer, K.S.; Pruna, G.J.; Boone, C.H. β-hydroxy-β-methylbutyrate (HMB)-free acid attenuates circulating TNF-a and TNFr1 expression postresistance exercise. *J. Appl. Physiol.* **2013**, *115*, 1173–1182. [CrossRef] [PubMed]
19. Kraemer, W.J.; Fry, A.C. *Strength Testing: Development and Evaluation of Methodology*; Human Kinetics: Champaign, IL, USA, 1995.

20. Seitz, L.B.; Reyes, A.; Tran, T.T.; Saez de Villarreal, E.S.; Haff, G.G. Increases in lower-body strength transfer positively to sprint performance: A systematic review with meta-analysis. *Sport Med.* **2014**, *44*, 1693–1702. [CrossRef] [PubMed]
21. Cakir-Atabek, H.; Demir, S.; Pinarbasili, R.D. Effect of different resistance training intensity on indices of oxidative stress. *J. Strength Cond. Res.* **2010**, *24*, 2491–2497. [CrossRef] [PubMed]
22. Ramel, A.; Wagner, K.H.; Elmadfa, I. Plasma antioxidants and lipid oxidation after submaximal resistance exercise in men. *Eur. J. Nutr.* **2004**, *43*, 2–6. [CrossRef] [PubMed]
23. Nissen, S.; Sharp, R.L.; Panton, L.; Vukovich, M.; Trappe, S.; Fuller, J.C. β-Hydroxy-β-methylbutyrate (HMB) supplementation in human is safe and may decrease cardiovascular risk factors. *J. Nutr.* **2000**, *130*, 1937–1945. [CrossRef] [PubMed]
24. Jackson, M.J. Exercise and oxygen radical production by muscle. In *Handbook of Oxidants and Antioxidants in Exercise*; Sen, C.K., Packer, L., Hanninen, O., Eds.; Elsevier Science: Amsterdam, The Netherlands, 2000; pp. 57–68.
25. Fitschen, P.J.; Wilson, G.J.; Wilson, J.M.; Wilund, K.R. Efficacy of beta-hydroxy-beta-methylbutyrate supplementation in elderly and clinical populations. *Nutrition* **2013**, *29*, 29–36. [CrossRef] [PubMed]

6

Post-Irradiation Treatment with a Superoxide Dismutase Mimic, MnTnHex-2-PyP^{5+}, Mitigates Radiation Injury in the Lungs of Non-Human Primates after Whole-Thorax Exposure to Ionizing Radiation

John Mark Cline [1,*], Greg Dugan [1], John Daniel Bourland [2], Donna L. Perry [1,3], Joel D. Stitzel [4], Ashley A. Weaver [4], Chen Jiang [5], Artak Tovmasyan [6], Kouros Owzar [5], Ivan Spasojevic [7,8], Ines Batinic-Haberle [6] and Zeljko Vujaskovic [6,9]

1 Department of Pathology, Section on Comparative Medicine, Wake Forest University School of Medicine, Medical Center Boulevard, Winston-Salem, NC 27157-1040, USA; gdugan@wakehealth.edu (G.D.); perrydl@niaid.nih.gov (D.L.P.)
2 Department of Radiation Oncology, Wake Forest University School of Medicine, Medical Center Boulevard, Winston-Salem, NC 27157-1040, USA; bourland@wakehealth.edu
3 Integrated Research Facility, Division of Clinical Research, National Institute of Allergy and Infectious Disease, National Institutes of Health, Frederick, MD 21702, USA
4 Department of Biomedical Engineering, Wake Forest University School of Medicine, Biotech Place, 575 N. Patterson Ave., Winston-Salem, NC 21701, USA; jstitzel@wakehealth.edu (J.D.S.); asweaver@wakehealth.edu (A.A.W.)
5 Department of Biostatistics and Bioinformatics, Duke University Medical Center, Durham, NC 27708, USA; chen.jiang@duke.edu (C.J.); kouros.owzar@duke.edu (K.O.)
6 Department of Radiation Oncology, Duke University Medical Center, Durham, NC 27708, USA; artak.tovmasyan@duke.edu (A.T.); ibatinic@duke.edu (I.B.-H.); zvujaskovic@som.umaryland.edu (Z.V.)
7 Department of Medicine Duke University Medical Center, Durham, NC 27708, USA; ivan.spasojevic@duke.edu
8 Duke Cancer Institute, Pharmaceutical Research Shared Resource, PK/PD Core Laboratory, Duke University Medical Center, Durham, NC 27708, USA
9 Department of Radiation Oncology, University of Maryland School of Medicine, 655 W. Baltimore Street, Baltimore, MD 21201, USA
* Correspondence: jmcline@wakehealth.edu

Abstract: Radiation injury to the lung is the result of acute and chronic free radical formation, and there are currently few effective means of mitigating such injury. Studies in rodents indicate that superoxide dismutase mimetics may be effective in this regard; however, studies in humans or large animals are lacking. We hypothesized that post-exposure treatment with the lipophilic mitochondrial superoxide dismutase mimetic, MnTnHex-2-PyP^{5+} (hexyl), would reduce radiation-induced pneumonitis and fibrosis in the lungs of nonhuman primates. Rhesus monkeys (*Macaca mulatta*) received 10 Gy whole thorax irradiation, 10 Gy + hexyl treatment, sham irradiation, or sham irradiation + hexyl. Hexyl was given twice daily, subcutaneously, at 0.05 mg/kg, for 2 months. Animals were monitored daily, and respiratory rates, pulse oximetry, hematology and serum chemistry panels were performed weekly. Computed tomography scans were performed at 0, 2, and 4 months after irradiation. Supportive fluid therapy, corticosteroids, analgesics, and antibiotics were given as needed. All animals were humanely euthanized 4.5 months after irradiation, and pathologic assessments were made. Multifocal, progressive lung lesions were seen at 2 and 4 months in both irradiated groups. Hexyl treatment delayed the onset of radiation-induced lung lesions, reduced elevations of respiratory rate, and reduced pathologic increases in lung weight. No adverse effects of hexyl treatment were found. These results demonstrate (1) development of a nonhuman primate model of radiation-induced lung injury, (2) a significant mitigating effect of hexyl treatment on lung pathology in this model, and (3) no evidence for toxicity of hexyl at the dose studied.

Keywords: superoxide dismutase mimetic; MnTnHex-2-PyP^{5+}; irradiation; Macaca mulatta; lung injury

---

1. Introduction

Radiation-induced pulmonary injury causes substantial morbidity and mortality in both accidentally and therapeutically exposed individuals. Single-dose exposures of greater than 9 Gy in human patients induce a subacute inflammatory response (radiation pneumonitis) approximately 2–3 months after exposure, and a more chronic, irreversible syndrome of pulmonary interstitial fibrosis occurring months to years after exposure [1,2]. Among patients receiving fractionated radiotherapy for malignancies of the thorax, the likelihood of lung injury is increased by irradiation of the inferior thorax and by a higher mean dose for normal lungs [3]. The standard of treatment for radiation pneumonitis is high-dose corticosteroids [4]. There is currently no treatment for radiation-induced fibrosis. As mortality due to the hematopoietic syndrome has diminished due to bone marrow transplant and cytokine therapy, pulmonary injury has emerged as an increasingly relevant syndrome. Some survivors of the Chernobyl accident were successfully treated for acute hematopoietic syndrome, only to succumb to pulmonary disease [5].

Based on impressive therapeutic efficacy in different cellular and animal models of oxidative stress injury [6–34], high lipophilicity [6,29,35], high mitochondrial accumulation [6,36] and good safety/toxicity profile [6,7,9,35], the potent superoxide dismutase (SOD) mimetic and redox-active drug, manganese (III) *meso*-tetrakis (*N*-hexylpyridinium-2-yl) porphyrin, MnTnHex-2-PyP^{5+} (hexyl), was chosen as a mitigator in this nonhuman primate (NHP) model of pulmonary radiation injury (Figure 1). In a rat model of lung radiation injury, we have shown previously that MnTnHex-2-PyP^{5+} was superior to its ethyl analogs, Mn(III) *meso*-tetrakis(*N*-ethylpyridinium-2-yl)porphyrin, MnTE-2-PyP^{5+} (compound name: AEOL10113, BMX-010), as it mitigated radiation-induced lung injury when given at a 120-fold lower dose of 0.05 mg/kg/day for 2 weeks starting at 2 h after irradiation [27,28]. The reason for such dramatic difference in efficacy lies in the more than four orders of magnitude higher lipophilicity of hexyl relative to MnTE-2-PyP^{5+} [6,35,37,38], which, in turn, controls its higher biodistribution and mitochondrial accumulation; both analogs have very similar SOD-like activity [6,37]. The lipophilicity of hexyl is the highest within the class of water-soluble cationic *N*-alkylpyridylporphyrins presently explored [6,29,38]. Therefore, MnTnHex-2-PyP^{5+} distributes in all tissues thus far studied to higher levels than MnTE-2-PyP^{5+} [7,35,39], and is thus up to 120-fold more efficacious in different animal and cellular models, such as SOD-deficient *Escherichia coli* and *Saccharomyces cerevisiae*, yeast, pain, cerebral palsy, stroke, subarachnoid hemorrhage, ischemia/reperfusion models and ataxia telangiectasia (Figure 1) [6–34,37,40]. Such high efficacy allows for ~16-fold larger therapeutic window of MnTnHex-2-PyP^{5+} than of MnTE-2-PyP^{5+} (see details further below in Introduction) [6,9,35]. In addition to normal tissue radioprotection, the radiosensitization of brain, melanoma and breast tumors with hexyl was also demonstrated in mouse models [6,8]. Hexyl and its analogs accumulate in mitochondria [6,15,37] and there mimic the superoxide dismutase isoform, MnSOD [6,15,18,23,40,41]. High lipophilicity allows hexyl to accumulate in both heart and brain mitochondria; while MnTE-2-PyP^{5+} was found in brain [7,35,36,39] it was not found in brain mitochondria [6,29,36]. Hexyl readily crosses the blood–brain barrier [7,29,36] and is the only cationic Mn porphyrin that suppresses infarct volume in a rodent middle cerebral artery occlusion stroke model when given subcutaneously [13,16,29]. Such studies point to the critical role of bioavailability in the therapeutic effects of Mn porphyrins.

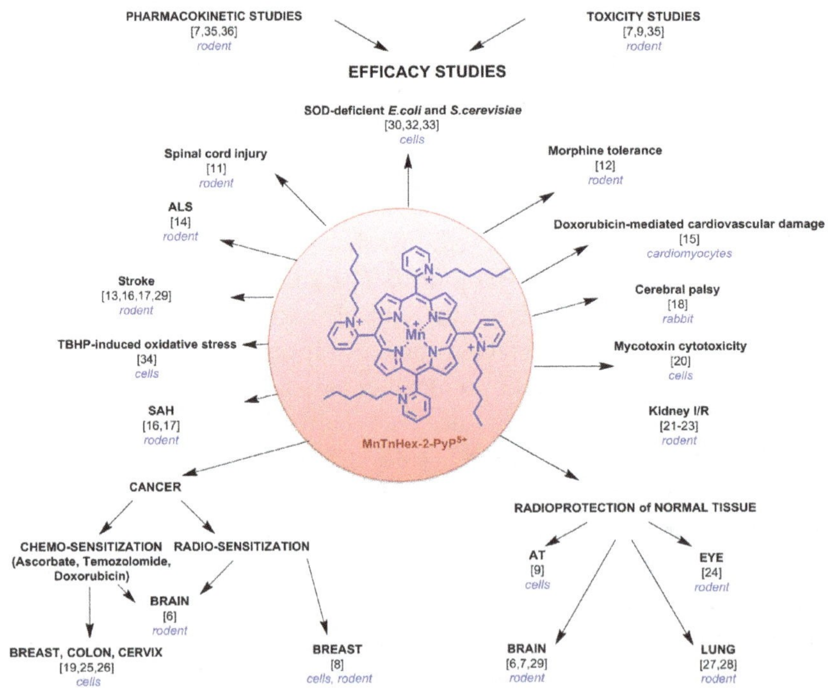

Figure 1. Structure and therapeutic effects of manganese (III) *meso*-tetrakis (*N*-hexylpyridinium-2-yl) porphyrin, MnTnHex-2-PyP^{5+} (hexyl). The therapeutic efficacy of hexyl was observed at the level of normal tissue injury and cancer. Hexyl protected normal tissue from oxidative stress injury, including radiation, at extremely low levels of 0.05 mg/kg. Yet, it did not protect cancer; moreover, it sensitized cancer towards radiation and chemotherapy. The therapeutic effects are detailed in text and summarized in references [6–34,37,40,42]. SAH—Subarachnoid Hemorrhage; I/R—Ischemia/Reperfusion; AT—Ataxia Telangiectasia; ALS—Amyotrophic Lateral Sclerosis; TSHP—*t*-butylhydroperoxide.

While MnTnHex-2-PyP^{5+} is a potent SOD mimetic, most recent studies point to its role and role of its porphyrin analogs (MnTE-2-PyP^{5+} and MnTnBuOE-2-PyP^{5+}) in the modification of the activity of transcription factors including nuclear factor kappa B (NF-κB) and nuclear factor E2-related factor 2 (Nrf2) [22,43–46] and different mitogen-activated protein kinases, such as extracellular signal-regulated kinase (ERK), c-Jun N-terminal kinase (JNK), protein kinase B (AKT) and p38 mitogen-activated protein kinase (p38-MAPK) [8,45,47]. Several studies provided evidence that this and other potent cationic porphyrin-based SOD mimics (such as MnTE-2-PyP^{5+} and MnTnBuOE-2-PyP^{5+}) modify protein cysteines of transcription factors [44–46], MAPK, and protein phosphatase 2A through their S-glutathionylation, thereby modifying their activities [45,47]. We have provided the evidence and the mechanistic basis that the SOD-like potency of Mn porphyrins is proportional to their ability to *S*-glutathionylate cysteines of proteins [6,29,47].

MnTnHex-2-PyP^{5+} exhibited therapeutic potential as a broadly applicable mitigator of oxidative stress injury and radioprotector of normal tissue, while demonstrating anticancer effects (Figure 1 and references therein). Its high lipophilicity allows it to cross the blood–brain barrier and accumulate in mitochondria [6,7,36]. Its impact on the radioprotection of lungs in a rat model was thoroughly explored [27,28]. MnTnHex-2-PyP^{5+} inhibited the hypoxia inducible factor 1-alpha (HIF-1α) pathway and its gene, vascular endothelial growth factor (VEGF), reduced oxidative stress and suppressed levels of transforming growth factor beta-1 (TGF-β1) [27,28]. Such data suggests that hexyl has the potential to suppress fibrotic processes. A prolonged dosing regimen is required as fibrosis is a late lung injury event. The inhibition of HIF-1α might have occurred via inhibition of NF-κB, which controls HIF-1α and is a major protein affected by Mn porphyrins (see above). In addition to lessening the normal tissue injuries, MnTnHex-2-PyP^{5+} is also an anticancer agent. It suppressed tumor growth, acting as a tumor radio- and chemo-sensitizer in a patient-derived glioblastoma multiforme subcutaneous xenograft mouse model [6]. $MnTnHex\text{-}2\text{-}PyP^{5+}$ also acted as a tumor radiosensitizer in 4T1 mouse breast and B16 mouse melanoma sc flank models [8].

In rodent safety/toxicity studies, the toxicity dose (TD_{50}), of $MnTnHex\text{-}2\text{-}PyP^{5+}$ was determined to be 12.5 mg/kg [9]. That dose causes shivers and hypotonia which is, in part, due to the blood pressure drop. Given its efficacy at a very low 0.05 mg/kg dose, $MnTnHex\text{-}2\text{-}PyP^{5+}$ (12.5/0.05 = 250) has a 16.3-fold (250/15.3) wider therapeutic window than clinically tested $MnTE\text{-}2\text{-}PyP^{5+}$. The TD_{50} of 91.5 mg/kg and efficacy dose of 6 mg/kg (91.5/6 = 15.3) were determined for $MnTE\text{-}2\text{-}PyP^{5+}$ in a parallel study [9]. In a mouse study, at the end of twice sc daily injections of 0.5–2.5 mg/kg for 4 weeks, we have seen the acute degeneration of hippocampal neurons, mild subcutaneous inflammation, degeneration and regeneration of subcutaneous muscles, and pigment accumulation in Kupffer cells of mice [7,35]. However, all mice recovered with no overt pathological changes four weeks after the injections of $MnTnHex\text{-}2\text{-}PyP^{5+}$ ceased [7,35].

The purpose of this study was to evaluate the efficacy and safety of $MnTnHex\text{-}2\text{-}PyP^{5+}$ in a novel nonhuman primate model of radiation induced lung injury. $MnTnHex\text{-}2\text{-}PyP^{5+}$ accumulates in lungs to a high level [35], and the mitigation of rat pulmonary radiation injury at 0.05 mg/kg/day justified the dosing schedule used in this study.

The high clinical prospects of the whole class of cationic Mn porphyrins is best evidenced in several ongoing clinical trials on two analogs of $MnTnHex\text{-}2\text{-}PyP^{5+}$. Mn(III) *meso*-tetrakis(*N*-n-butoxyethylpyridinium-2-yl)porphyrin, $MnTnBuOE\text{-}2\text{-}PyP^{5+}$ (BMX-001), is presently being tested as a radioprotector of normal tissue with glioma, head and neck, and anal cancer patients (National Institutes of Health Clinical Trial numbers NCT02655601, NCT02990468 and NCT03386500). $MnTE\text{-}2\text{-}PyP^{5+}$ (AEOL10113) is also in clinical development. Aeolus Pharmaceuticals is initiating Phase I trials on the di-imidazolyl analog, $MnTDE\text{-}2\text{-}ImP^{5+}$ (AEOL10150) as a pulmonary radioprotector [48,49]. Such clinical development further justifies the exploration of the therapeutic effects of Mn porphyrins and the studies of their mechanism of action.

The primate model developed for this study was chosen because the respiratory system of nonhuman primates (NHP) is anatomically and physiologically more similar to human beings than that of rodents; respiratory branching patterns are more complex in primates [50]. The resident inflammatory cell population also differs, with rodent lungs containing larger numbers of mast cells with the potential to release histamine and other inflammatory mediators. Primates also provide a large animal model, which allows more precise modeling and measurement of organ dosimetry. The relative sensitivity of mice, in particular, to pulmonary irradiation varies widely [51]. While rodent models allow a degree of genetic manipulation not possible in other species, NHP are a critical element of the late-stage translational application of promising interventions, particularly those that have a mechanism of action that may be primate specific. NHP provides the closest approximation in this regard with respect to the Food and Drug Administration's Animal Rule, for approval of novel agents which cannot be tested in human subjects [52]. They are also sufficiently long-lived and robust, to allow longitudinal assessment of an array of clinical outcomes, resulting in better pathophysiologic characterization of disease progression than is possible in rodent models.

2. Materials and Methods

2.1. Animals

Sixteen juvenile, Chinese-origin, male, rhesus macaques, weighing 3.3–5.7 (mean 3.9) kg, were obtained from a commercial vendor (AlphaGenesis, Yemassee, SC, USA). Animals were pre-screened to exclude simian retrovirus infection and tuberculosis, including quarantine under Centers for Disease Control guidelines. Animals were socially housed in pairs. All animal procedures were performed in accordance with the Guide for the Care and Use of Laboratory Animals [53] and followed protocols for avoidance of pain and discomfort and the assurance of environmental enrichment and psychological well-being, approved by the Wake Forest School of Medicine (WFSM) (Office for Protection from Research Risks #A-3391-01) Institutional Animal Care and Use Committee. WFSM is accredited by the Association for the Assessment and Accreditation of Laboratory Animal Care International and operates in compliance with the Animal Welfare Act.

2.2. Irradiation and Drug Treatment

Animals were randomized to treatment group based on body weight. Treatment groups included 10 Gy whole thorax irradiation (WTI)/sham drug treatment (10 Gy, $n = 5$), 10 Gy WTI with hexyl treatment (10 Gy + hexyl 0.05 mg/kg twice daily subcutaneously, $n = 5$), sham irradiation/sham drug treatment (Control, $n = 3$), and sham WTI with hexyl (Hexyl, $n = 3$). Hexyl was synthesized as previously described [54]. Each NHP to be irradiated was anesthetized with ketamine (5–15 mg/kg, subcutaneously) and dexmedetomidine (0.0075–0.015 mg/kg, subcutaneously) and placed supine with arms extended overhead and lightly restrained to prevent motion. A single fraction dose of 10 Gy was delivered, calculated for each beam at the midline (xiphoid process, nominal depth 4.5 cm), using high energy, 6 megavolt (MV) X rays from a clinical linear accelerator (Varian Medical Systems, Palo Alto, CA, USA). This dose was delivered using a pair of isocentric, equally weighted, parallel-opposed anterior and posterior beams with an asymmetric field size of 10×12.5 cm^2 and nominal dose rate of 200 cGy/min. The anterior beam included a 1-cm flexible slab of tissue-equivalent material on the anterior chest to ensure dose build-up to the anterior lung surface, and a 15-degree physical wedge with the thick end oriented to the superior, as a missing tissue compensator to provide better dose homogeneity at the midline of the mediastinum due to the slope of the anterior surface along the sagittal mid-plane. The central axis was placed through the xyphoid, and the irradiation geometry was confirmed for the anterior beam, which was then irradiated (5 Gy). Using isocentric gantry rotation, the opposed posterior field was set, confirmed and then irradiated (5 Gy). Dose calculations were performed for each beam, with the dose specified at the midline, assuming water-equivalency and without inhomogeneity corrections. Dose inhomogeneity in the lungs for 6 MV X rays is estimated to be a maximum of +10%, found along the greatest anterior–posterior lung diameter, compared to the midplane dose of 10 Gy in the mediastinum. The radiation field superior–inferior borders ranged from the thoracic inlet to 4 cm below the xyphoid process. The radiation field left–right borders flashed beyond the external skin surface of the thorax. Thus, the irradiated region included both lungs (superior to 4 cm below the xyphoid) and the contents of the thorax, including the heart and mediastinum and adjacent portions of the trachea, esophagus, and superior aspects of the liver and stomach.

Animals were given hexyl subcutaneously, twice daily, at a dose of 0.05 mg/kg/dose (0.1 mg/kg/day), for two months after irradiation. Treatment was initated two hours after irradiation by subcutaneous injection. After the initial loading dose, steady state concentrations were administered by subcutaneous implantation of an osmotic pump (Alzet, Durect Corporation, Cupertino, CA, USA). For this procedure, animals were sedated with ketamine, anesthetized with isoflurane, and pumps were placed in the subcutaneous tissues of the upper back using the aseptic surgical technique. Animals not treated with hexyl were given a sham implant or injection containing normal saline. Due to concerns regarding implant surgeries as a complicating factor for interpreting white blood cell counts, at week 6, all pumps were removed and hexyl was again given by twice-daily subcutaneous injection, on alternating sides in the subcutaneous tissue of the torso (to approximate the same physiological site as the injection pump), until the end of the 8-week dosing period.

2.3. Clinical Assessments

Animals were observed daily throughout the study. Respiratory rate and effort were evaluated daily. Treatment-induced morbidity was monitored and documented using a modification of the Children's Clinical Oncology Group toxicity criteria, customized for nonhuman primates [55]. Animals were lightly sedated with ketamine, weekly, for physical examination and blood collection for complete blood counts and serum chemistries (albumin, bicarbonate, globulin, total protein, electrolytes, triglycerides, bilirubin, hepatic and pancreatic enzymes, blood urea nitrogen, creatinine, creatine kinase, glucose, triglycerides, and cholesterol). Respiratory rates and oxygenation by pulse oximetry (Cardell Veterinary Monitor 9403, Midmark Corp, Versailles, OH, USA) were documented weekly. Normal respiratory rate was considered to be 50 breaths per minute (bpm). The most relevant thresholds for treatment or humane euthanasia were as follows: animals with respiratory rate (RR) >80 bpm were treated with corticosteroids (prednisone, 1 mg/kg/day, tapered). Animals with elevated neutrophil counts were treated with broad spectrum antibiotics (enrofloxacin 5 mg/kg and penicillin, 20,000–60,000 U/kg/day, for 5–8 days). Treatment decisions were made by a veterinary clinician (GD) blinded to treatment group. Animals with RR >100 bpm were euthanized. Veterinary consultation was provided for all animals showing signs of illness, and supportive fluid therapy, corticosteroids, analgesics, antibiotics, and other symptomatic care were given, as needed, based on clinical signs and clinical pathology findings.

2.4. Computed Tomography Imaging

All animals were evaluated by computed tomography (CT) imaging prior to irradiation, two months after irradiation, and 4 months after irradiation. Images were acquired on a 16-slice Siemens Biography computed tomography unit, without contrast, at a slice thickness of 0.5 cm, using a pediatric protocol. For this procedure, animals were sedated with ketamine and medetomidine, an endotracheal tube was placed, and anesthesia was induced and maintained with isoflurane. The lungs were fully inflated by manual pressure to the rebreathing bag for a brief breath-hold (approximately 10–20 s) during the scan to avoid motion artifacts. Regions of increased density in the lung were measured from image segmentations performed using Mimics v12.11 software (Materialise, Ann Arbor, MI, USA). A semiautomated method was used to isolate the volumes of air, normal lung tissue, and abnormally dense tissue within the lungs. Automatic thresholding, region growing, morphology, and Boolean operations were utilized, along with manual editing, to create masks representing each volume. Segmentations were performed by a single observer, blinded to treatment group. Three-dimensional reconstruction and volumetric calculations were used to determine the proportion of the lung occupied by air, normal lung tissue, and abnormally dense tissue [56–59].

2.5. Pathology

After 19 weeks of observation, all animals were humanely euthanized by intravenous pentobarbital overdose after sedation by intramuscular injection of ketamine. A complete necropsy examination was done for each animal, including gross and histologic examination of all major organ systems, organ weight measurements, and documentation of all abnormalities. Fixed and frozen tissue samples from right and left cranial, middle, and caudal lung lobes were collected. For tissues spanning the border of the radiation field (e.g., trachea, esophagus, skin, and spinal cord), tissues from within and outside the field were examined. Tissues for histology were fixed in 10% neutral buffered formalin, trimmed and embedded in paraffin, sectioned at a 5 micron thickness, and stained with hematoxylin and eosin. Lung sections were also stained with Masson's Trichrome stain for the identification of fibrosis, and by immunohistochemistry using the human alveolar macrophage marker, HAM56 (Dako, Carpinteria, CA, USA). Histologic examination of the lungs was done by an experienced veterinary pathologist (DLP), blinded to treatment group, and the distribution and amount of qualitative changes were estimated. Additionally, the histologic percentage of the lung parenchyma consisting of macrophages (% positive for the HAM56 macrophage marker by immunohistochemistry), and fibrosis (% section area positive using Masson's Trichrome stain) were measured on six sections from each animal (one per major lung lobe). Entire sections were measured using computer assisted color image analysis (Image Pro Plus, v. 5.1, Media Cybernetics, Silver Spring, MD, USA).

2.6. Statistical Considerations.

The study was analyzed as a 2 × 2 factorial design with irradiation and hexyl treatment as the independent variables. Dependent variables included respiratory rate, neutrophil count, body weight, lung weight, presence or absence of CT abnormalities, percentage of abnormally dense lung in CT images, and percentage area of macrophages and fibrosis in histologic sections. Parametric methods were used for analysis. For longitudinal data, change from baseline was analyzed, and a multivariate model with repeated measures was used. Fisher's exact test was used to test differences between groups in days to treatment. The R statistical environment [R] was used for conducting these analyses.

3. Results

3.1. Clinical Observations

During the course of the study, mean respiratory rates increased gradually in irradiated animals, reaching statistical significance by 4 months post-irradiation ($p < 0.009$, Welch two-sample t-test) (Figure 2A). Mean oxygenated hemoglobin measurements by pulse oximetry did not change over the course of the study (Figure 2B), suggesting successful compensation by an increased respiratory rate. Irradiated animals were more often treated with antibiotics or corticosteroids, and were treated sooner, more often, and for more total days than non-irradiated animals. The mean number of days to corticosteroid treatment was significantly prolonged for 10 Gy + hexyl-treated animals compared to 10 Gy alone (Table 1). One animal at 4 months crossed the predetermined respiratory rate threshold of 100 bpm, and euthanasia was elected slightly in advance of the remaining animals. No overt respiratory distress or cyanosis was seen in any animal. There were no significant treatment-related changes in body weight during the study (data not shown).

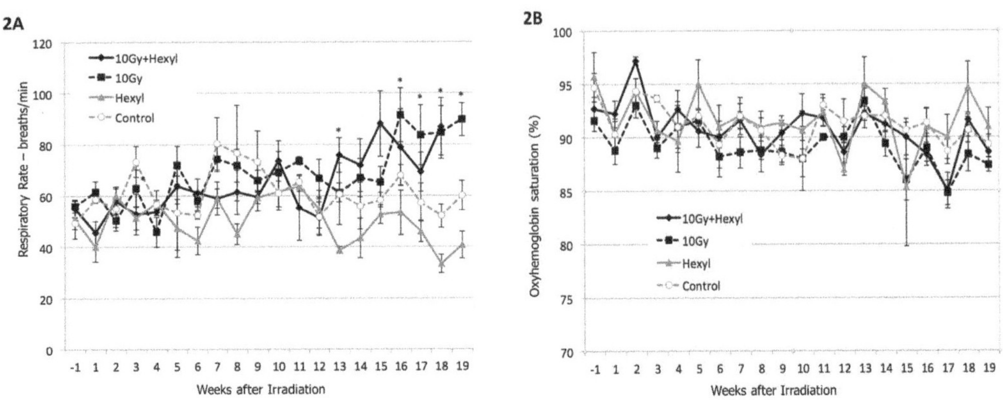

(A) (B)

Figure 2. Clinical assessments of pulmonary injury. (**A**) Respiratory rates; irradiated groups differ from non-irradiated animals ($p = 0.008$); * indicates individual time point differences at $p < 0.05$ (t-test). (**B**) Oxyhemoglobin saturation. Groups do not differ. Error bars are SEM (standard error of the mean).

Table 1. Patterns of antibiotic and corticosteroid treatment; median and range.

Group	Control	Hexyl	10 Gy	10 Gy + Hexyl	Significance *
Number of animals given antibiotics	2/3	2/3	4/5	5/5	nsd
Days to first antibiotic treatment	26 (26–26)	45 (41–48)	31 (26–47)	36 (26–77)	nsd
Number of antibiotic treatments	2 (0–3)	1 (0–1)	3 (0–5)	2 (1–4)	nsd
Total days of antibiotic treatment	11 (0–17)	5 (0–5)	18 (0–31)	12 (5–27)	nsd
Number of animals given prednisone	1/3	0/3	5/5	5/5	nsd

Table 1. *Cont.*

Group	Control	Hexyl	10 Gy	10 Gy + Hexyl	Significance *
Days to first prednisone treatment	47 (47–47)	NA	51 (26–77)	90 (51–103)	$p < 0.05$
Number of prednisone treatments	1 (NA)	0	2 (1–3)	1 (1–4)	nsd
Total days of prednisone treatment	9 (NA)	0	10 (5–14)	7 (4–21)	nsd

* Fisher's exact test; nsd = no significant difference; NA: not applicable.

3.2. Clinical Pathology

Elevations in total white blood cell (WBC) count were seen in both groups of irradiated animals, regardless of the presence of hexyl; this change was greater in irradiated animals that did not receive hexyl and reached a peak at about 6 weeks post-irradiation, followed by a decline (Figure 3A). This finding was interpreted as reflecting radiation-induced pneumonitis and consisted primarily of a neutrophilic response (Figure 3B). Lymphocyte counts were higher in the control group at baseline, and this difference persisted throughout the study. Declines in lymphocyte counts were seen in all animals, corresponding to the dates of monthly anesthesia for imaging or osmotic pump implantation (Figure 3C); this was interpreted as a transient stress response. In the final month of the study, eosinophil counts rose markedly in both irradiated groups (Figure 3D). No treatment-related changes were seen in any clinical chemistry parameters (Supplemental Table S1).

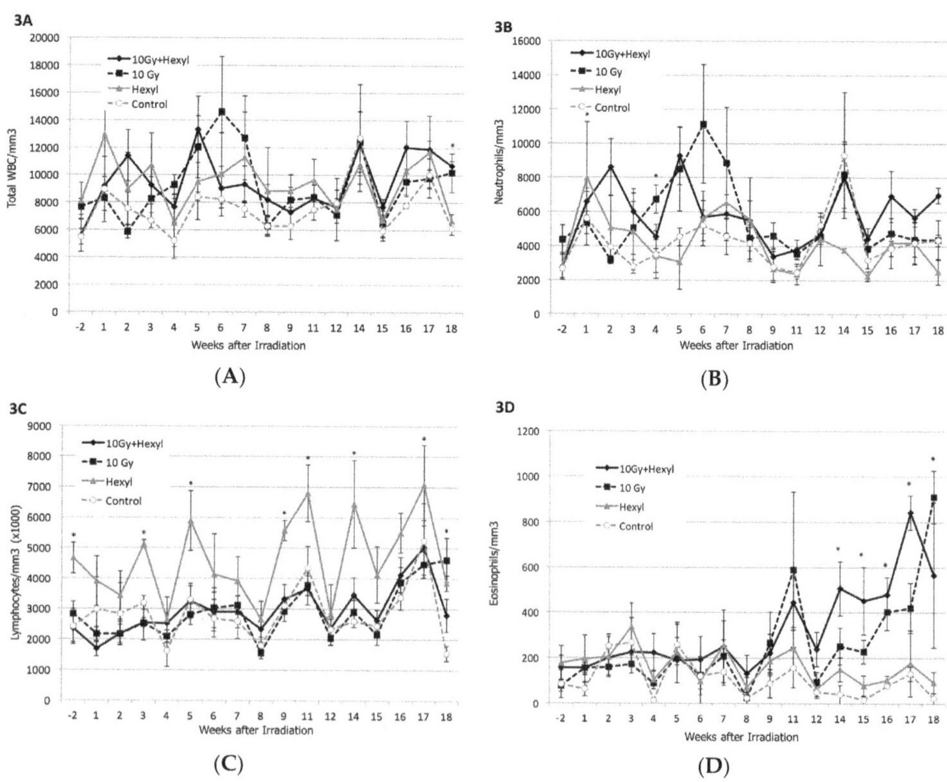

Figure 3. White blood cell changes. (**A**) Overall white blood cell count; (**B**) neutrophil count; (**C**) lymphocyte count; and (**D**) eosinophil count. White blood cell counts (primarily neutrophils) were elevated in irradiated animals 6 weeks after irradiation, coincident with the onset of clinical signs and computed tomography (CT) abnormalities. Lymphocyte counts were highest in non-irradiated hexyl-only animals, and decreased each month after sedation for physical examination. Eosinophil counts were elevated in months 3–5. Error bars are SEM; * = mean differs from control group ($p < 0.05$) (t-test).

3.3. CT Imaging

Imaging abnormalities, defined as abnormal radio-opacities exceeding 1% of the lung volume, were seen two months after irradiation in 2/5 animals given irradiation alone. Abnormalities were seen in all irradiated animals at 4 months. These consisted of multifocal, irregular, randomly distributed areas of increased radio-opacity in all lung lobes, which progressed in severity during the course of the study (Figures 4 and 5). The mean volumetric percentage of the lungs occupied by abnormally high density increased; it was minimal at two months and higher at 4 months in irradiated animals treated with hexyl (Figure 4D); this difference was not statistically significant. However, at the 4 month assessment, CT density correlated with elevated respiratory rate ($r = 0.629$, $p < 0.009$) (Figure 5B).

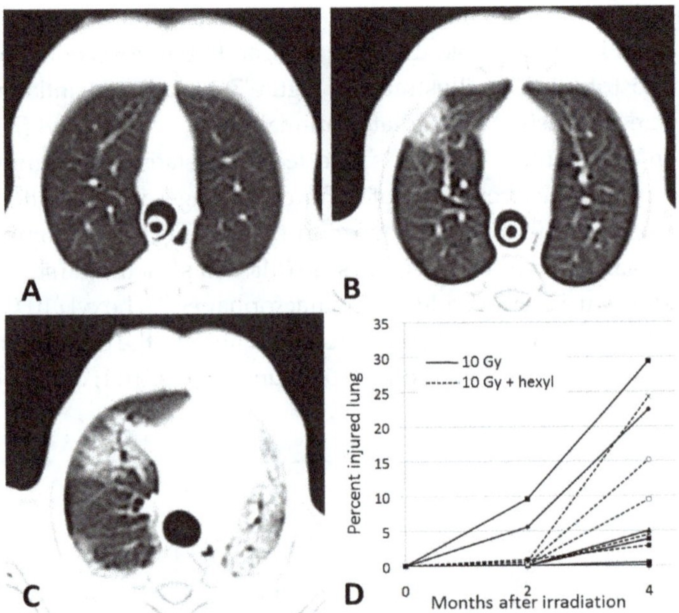

Figure 4. Computed tomography assessments of pulmonary injury. (**A–C**) Sequential images from a single animal from the irradiation-only group before irradiation (**A**), 2 months after irradiation (**B**), and 4 months after irradiation (**C**). (**D**) Percentage of injured lung by treatment group over the course of the study. Control and hexyl-alone groups are not shown (all values were <1%). CT abnormalities were seen at 2 and 4 months post-irradiation. The CT density area appears to be lower in hexyl-treated animals, particularly at 2 months, but there is no statistically significant difference.

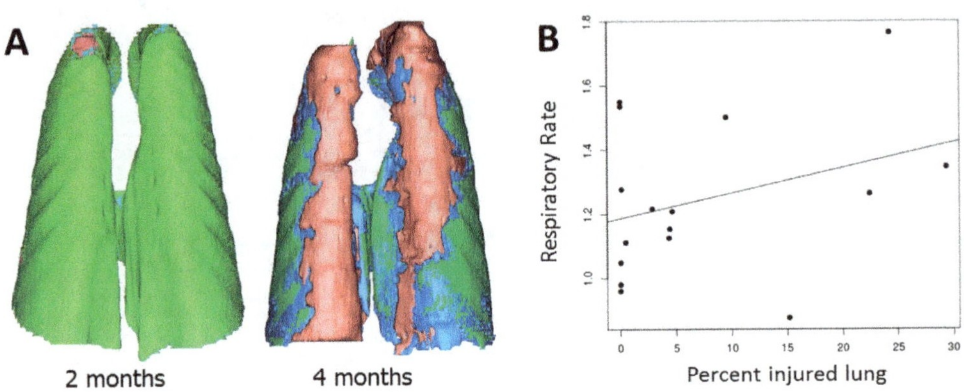

Figure 5. Three-dimensional reconstruction of pulmonary injury in the same animal illustrated in Figure 4 at two and four months after irradiation. The normal lung is green, the partially inflated lung is blue, and the fibrotic/consolidated lung is red (**A**), the dot plot of CT density and respiratory rate at 4 months post-irradiation with linear regression line ($r = 0.6289$) (**B**).

3.4. Pathology Findings

Gross abnormalities were limited to animals exposed to radiation, and consisted of increased lung weights, abnormally firm lung consistency on palpation, and multifocal to diffuse, gray to tan discoloration of the pulmonary parenchyma, involving up to approximately 90% of the lung parenchyma. Lung weights in irradiated animals were 77% higher than non-irradiated controls ($p < 0.0001$). These effects were somewhat mitigated by hexyl treatment; irradiated animals treated with hexyl had a 32% lower mean lung weight than those treated with radiation alone ($p = 0.02$; Figure 6).

Histologically, affected regions of the lung in irradiated animals contained four major changes: (1) interstitial and intra-alveolar infiltration of the lung parenchyma by macrophages and other inflammatory cells, (2) accumulation of proteinaceous fluid in alveolar spaces, (3) hyperplasia and hypertrophy of alveolar lining cells, leading to the replacement of the normal thin oxygen exchange layer of type I pneumocytes with a thicker layer of cuboidal Type II cells, and (4) fibrosis of the pulmonary interstitium. These changes and their distribution are illustrated in Figure 7. Notably, the inflammatory, exudative, and hyperplastic changes were diminished in irradiated animals treated with hexyl (Figure 7D), compared to animals given irradiation alone (Figure 7B); this is reflected in the statistically significant difference in lung weights (Figure 6). In contrast, the overall extent of fibrotic changes was not altered by hexyl treatment. Histomorphometric measurements of the proportion of the lung tissue composed of macrophages (HAM56 immunostaining) and fibrous connective tissue (Masson's Trichrome stain) are shown in Figure 8. While there was a trend towards reduced levels of macrophages by hexyl/10 Gy vs. 10 Gy, statistical significance was not reached. Within lung regions considered fibrotic, the proportion of the tissue occupied by collagen was 14%, compared to 3–5% in non-fibrotic lungs ($p = 0.0011$; data not shown).

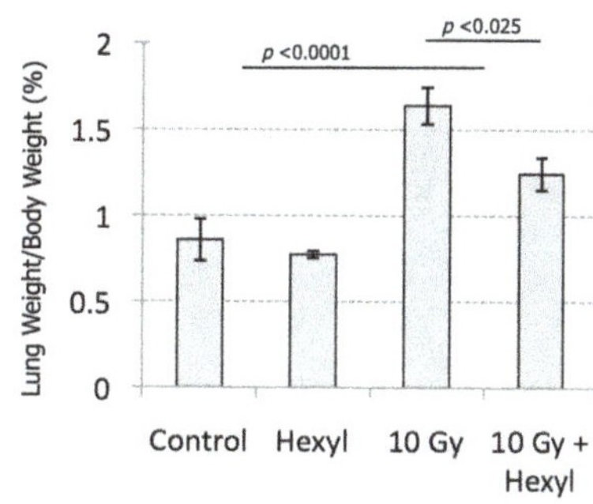

Figure 6. Mean lung weight at necropsy, by treatment group. The adverse main effect of irradiation is significant ($p < 0.0001$), as is the beneficial effect of hexyl treatment ($p = 0.02418$).

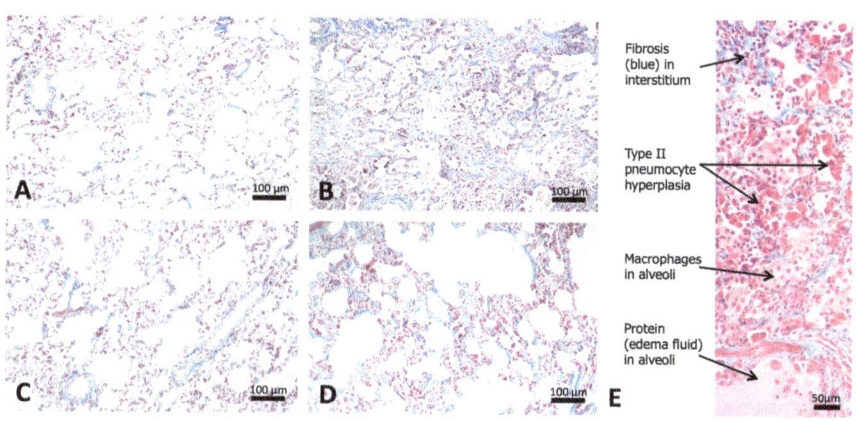

Figure 7. Histologic appearance of lung tissue in (**A**) sham-irradiated, saline-treated controls, (**B**) irradiated animals with no hexyl treatment, (**C**) sham-irradiated animals given hexyl treatment, and (**D**) irradiated animals given hexyl. Trichrome stain. (**E**) Higher-magnification photograph demonstrating specific histopathologic findings. Scale bars: A–D, 100 µm; E, 50 µm.

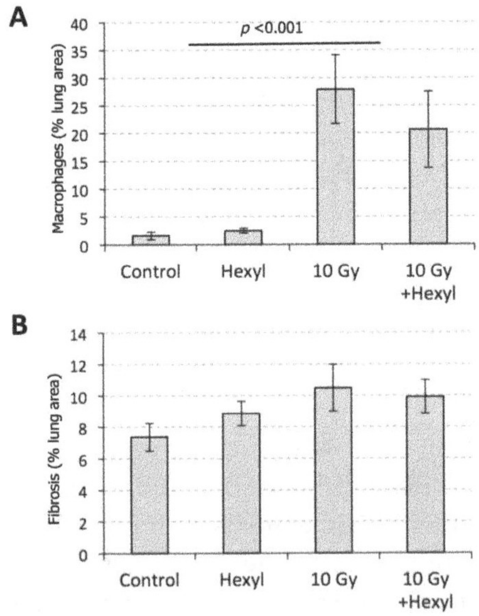

Figure 8. Pulmonary histomorphometry. (**A**) The main effect of radiation was significant ($p < 0.001$) for macrophages expressed as % area of the lung staining for human alveolar macrophage 56 (HAM56) antigen. (**B**) Pulmonary fibrosis was not statistically increased during the course of this experiment.

4. Discussion

Herein we described the effect of hexyl in a NHP model of radiation-induced lung injury, including an irradiation strategy that that reliably produces pneumonitis and fibrosis within a period of 2–4 months. This model allows longitudinal evaluation of the indicators of disease progression, including clinical evaluations, respiratory rate, oxyhemoglobin saturation, lung density, clinical pathology markers. A clinical and pathologic pattern of disease progression similar to the human disease was documented.

The major finding in this study was a statistically significant mitigating effect by hexyl treatment on the progression of radiation pneumonitis, as indicated by lung weight, which we attribute to diminished intrapulmonary inflammation and edema. The time course of this effect is interesting in that little or no increase in CT density was seen in hexyl-treated animals at the 2-month time point, whereas most hexyl-treated animals showed some pneumonitis and fibrosis at the final 4-month CT scan, and at 5 months at necropsy. Since treatment was discontinued at 2 months, it is possible that progressive pulmonary disease was, for that time, arrested by hexyl treatment, followed by progressive pneumonitis and fibrosis, beginning after treatment ended. Hexyl cleared from the mouse lungs within 10 days; the $t_{1/2}$ of the elimination of hexyl from the lungs after intraperitoneal injection was 58 h [35]. The mouse and monkey pharmacokinetics are similar (unpublished). We may thus safely assume that hexyl was absent in the lungs post 2 months of injections which would have, therefore, precluded the continuation of its radioprotective effects (observed during 2 months of dosing) and impact on fibrosis. Recently Oberley-Deegan's team reported the effect of an analogous compound, MnTE-2-PyP^{5+}, on the inhibition of a radiation-induced activation of mouse primary prostate fibroblasts via the TGF-β pathway [60]. TGF-β pathway was affected by hexyl and its analog, ethyl, in a mouse/rodent study (see Section 1. Introduction) [27,28]. Insight into the changes in the redox environments of lungs over 4 months of study is essential, as it would allow us to understand events at the molecular level, i.e., discuss the effects of hexyl on the redox-sensitive proteins, low molecular weight antioxidants (such as glutathione and ascorbate) and enzymes. Alternatively, hexyl treatment may have simply shifted the curve for progressive pneumonitis to the right, producing a delay but not an absolute prevention of the disease.

Due to slow clearance from all tissues [35], less frequent weekly dosing (post tissue loading) maintained throughout the study may prolong the beneficial effects obtained at 2 months post-radiation. Such dosing has been now adopted for the clinical trials on cancer patients for radioprotection of normal tissue with a similarly lipophilic and SOD-active, MnTnBuOE-2-PyP^{5+} [29,33,61,62]. Further work, with longer treatment, less frequent dosing and follow-up will be required to understand how to improve the mitigation of pulmonary injury.

Our findings in untreated NHP are consistent with those of Garofalo et al. [63], namely in regard to progressive pneumonitis and pulmonary fibrosis, affecting all irradiated animals by four months after radiation exposure at 10 Gy. This group showed efficacy of high dose dexamethasone (1 mg/kg/day, tapered) in reducing respiratory rate, which we did not see in our study. This could be related to our choice of corticosteroid (prednisone), which has a shorter duration of activity than dexamethasone. The mean time to corticosteroid therapy was much longer in their work (116 days) relative to our median days to treatment (51 days), despite the use of a similar respiratory rate trigger of 80 breaths per minute; this may reflect the age difference in animals. Our juvenile animals had a baseline respiratory rate of around 50 breaths per minute, whereas the older animals had a lower baseline rate of around 35 breaths per minute [64]. Age could also play a role in radiation sensitivity generally; adolescent rats develop pneumonitis more rapidly than adult animals [65].

The lack of demonstrable benefit for pulmonary fibrosis is disappointing, and may indicate that an additional divergent pathogenetic pathway is involved in fibrosis. Statistical power may have been hampered by high individual variation in responses, the multifocal nature of the fibrosis, and the limited number of animals. We have shown that ongoing oxidative damage and inflammation are important in the pathogenesis of progressive pulmonary disease in rodents, and have also documented involvement of the TGF-beta pathway in radiation-induced pulmonary fibrosis in the rat model [27]. Gene expression studies of the response of primate lungs to ozone-induced oxidative injury also show not only an inflammatory response, with elevations of interleukins 6, 8 and 10, but also a matrix remodeling response, including 3- to 5-fold elevations of matrix metalloproteinase I, metallothionein, and tenascin [66]. Involvement of TGF beta and matrix remodeling pathways may provide additional preventive or therapeutic targets, in addition to oxidative damage pathways. The observation of climbing eosinophil counts in irradiated groups is another interesting finding; eosinophilia was not a prominent feature of the tissue response in the lung, but further studies of lesion progression, for example, focused on hypersensitivity responses or mast cells would be helpful.

Importantly, in this study, we saw no evidence of toxicity of the hexyl compound, at a therapeutic dose, in a NHP model more closely related to human beings than the rodents studied previously. This drug has also shown efficacy at very low doses in numerous animal models, such as the rat renal ischemia model, the rabbit cerebral palsy model, chronic morphine tolerance, stroke, subarachnoid hemorrhage and tumor radiosensitization [6–29]. The efficacy of MnTnHex-2-PyP^{5+} at a low dose (1/120th of the dose used with a hydrophilic MnTE-2-PyP^{5+} analog) is due to its highest lipophilicity within the class of water-soluble cationic *N*-alkylpyridylporphyrins [6,29]. Moreover, due to its lipophilic character and pentacationic charge, this compound crosses the blood–brain barrier, localizes in the hippocampus and other brain parts and accumulates in mitochondria (both brain and heart mitochondria) relative to the cytosol [35,36,40].

Future studies need to address the pharmacokinetics of Mn porphyrin in NHP, explore the impact of the magnitude of the dose and frequency and the duration of dosing and compare MnTnHex-2-PyP^{5+} to another similarly lipophilic and potent SOD-mimic, MnTnBuOE-2-PyP^{5+}.

5. Conclusions

Data reviewed herein show that lipophilic superoxide dismutase mimetics are effective mitigators of a range of disease processes that involve oxidative injury. New data presented here demonstrate the development of a NHP model of radiation-induced lung injury in a large animal model with high genetic and phenotypic similarity to human beings. Findings indicate potential for mitigation of radiation-induced lung injury by MnTnHex-2-PyP^{5+}. The beneficial effect on lung weight but lack of clear effect on anticipated histologic markers suggests that inflammation and fibrosis may not represent the entire picture, and that further mechanistic studies are needed.

Supplementary Materials: The following are available online at www.mdpi.com/2076-3921/7/3/40/s1.

Acknowledgments: This study was supported by National Institutes of Health, National Institute on Allergy and Infectious Disease through the Radiation Countermeasures Center of Research Excellence (U19 AI67798, PI Nelson Chao). The authors are grateful for the technical expertise of Hermina Borgerink, Russel O'Donnell, Stacey Combs, Jean Gardin, Chrystal Bragg, Matt Dwyer and Eric Steelman; and for the valuable advice of Jeff Carr, Tom MacVittie, and Jacqueline Williams.

Author Contributions: John Mark Cline designed the study, developed the monkey model of radiation, supervised the whole study and the analysis of data, and wrote the manuscript. Greg Dugan conducted the treatment of animals and analyzed the data. John Daniel Bourland designed and carried out the radiation exposure protocol and assisted in writing the manuscript. Donna L. Perry performed the histopathologic examinations of the lungs and assisted in writing the manuscript. Joel D. Stitzel and Ashley A. Weaver provided specialized Chen Jiang analytic skills and 3-D reconstruction, and assisted in writing the manuscript. Kouros Owzar and Chen Jiang carried out the statistical analyses and assisted in writing the manuscript. Artak Tovmasyan was involved in preparation of MnTnHex-2-PyP^{5+} and helped with manuscript. Ivan Spasojevic designed the SOD mimics and pharmacokinetics, including the dosing regimen for MnTnHex-2-PyP^{5+} subcutaneous injections. Ines Batinic-Haberle designed the SOD mimics, synthesized MnTnHex-2-PyP^{5+}, explored its mechanism of action and was involved in writing the manuscript. Zeljko Vujaskovic conceived and designed the experiments, participated in data analysis and preparation of the manuscript.

Conflicts of Interest: The authors report no declarations of interest.

References

1. Tsoutsou, P.G.; Koukourakis, M.I. Radiation pneumonitis and fibrosis: Mechanisms underlying its pathogenesis and implications for future research. *Int. J. Radiat. Oncol. Biol. Phys.* **2006**, *66*, 1281–1293. [CrossRef] [PubMed]
2. Van Dyk, J.; Keane, T.J.; Kan, S.; Rider, W.D.; Fryer, C.J. Radiation pneumonitis following large single dose irradiation: A re-evaluation based on absolute dose to lung. *Int. J. Radiat. Oncol. Biol. Phys.* **1981**, *7*, 461–467. [CrossRef]
3. Bradley, J.D.; Hope, A.; El Naqa, I.; Apte, A.; Lindsay, P.E.; Bosch, W.; Matthews, J.; Sause, W.; Graham, M.V.; Deasy, J.O. A nomogram to predict radiation pneumonitis, derived from a combined analysis of RTOG 9311 and institutional data. *Int. J. Radiat. Oncol. Biol. Phys.* **2007**, *69*, 985–992. [CrossRef] [PubMed]
4. Ghafoori, P.; Marks, L.B.; Vujaskovic, Z.; Kelsey, C.R. Radiation-induced lung injury. Assessment, management, and prevention. *Oncology* **2018**, *22*, 37–47.
5. Baranov, A.; Gale, R.P.; Guskova, A.; Piatkin, E.; Selidovkin, G.; Muravyova, L.; Champlin, R.E.; Danilova, N.; Yevseeva, L.; Petrosyan, L. Bone marrow transplantation after the Chernobyl nuclear accident. *N. Engl. J. Med.* **1989**, *321*, 205–212. [CrossRef] [PubMed]
6. Batinic-Haberle, I.; Tovmasyan, A.; Roberts, E.R.; Vujaskovic, Z.; Leong, K.W.; Spasojevic, I. SOD therapeutics: Latest insights into their structure-activity relationships and impact on the cellular redox-based signaling pathways. *Antioxid. Redox Signal.* **2014**, *20*, 2372–2415. [CrossRef] [PubMed]
7. Leu, D.; Spasojevic, I.; Nguyen, H.; Deng, B.; Tovmasyan, A.; Weitner, T.; Sampaio, R.S.; Batinic-Haberle, I.; Huang, T.T. CNS bioavailability and radiation protection of normal hippocampal neurogenesis by a lipophilic Mn porphyrin-based superoxide dismutase mimic, MnTnBuOE-2-PyP5. *Redox Biol.* **2017**, *12*, 864–871. [CrossRef] [PubMed]
8. Shin, S.W.; Choi, C.; Lee, G.H.; Son, A.; Kim, S.H.; Park, H.C.; Batinic-Haberle, I.; Park, W. Mechanism of the Antitumor and Radiosensitizing Effects of a Manganese Porphyrin, MnHex-2-PyP. *Antioxid. Redox Signal.* **2017**, *27*, 1067–1082. [CrossRef] [PubMed]
9. Pollard, J.M.; Reboucas, J.S.; Durazo, A.; Kos, I.; Fike, F.; Panni, M.; Gralla, E.B.; Valentine, J.S.; Batinic-Haberle, I.; Gatti, R.A. Radioprotective effects of manganese-containing superoxide dismutase mimics on ataxia-telangiectasia cells. *Free Radic. Biol. Med.* **2009**, *47*, 250–260. [CrossRef] [PubMed]

10. Tovmasyan, A.; Sheng, H.; Weitner, T.; Arulpragasam, A.; Lu, M.; Warner, D.S.; Vujaskovic, Z.; Spasojevic, I.; Batinic-Haberle, I. Design, mechanism of action, bioavailability and therapeutic effects of Mn porphyrin-based redox modulators. *Med. Princ. Pract.* **2013**, *22*, 103–130. [CrossRef] [PubMed]
11. Celic, T.; Spanjol, J.; Bobinac, M.; Tovmasyan, A.; Vukelic, I.; Reboucas, J.S.; Batinic-Haberle, I.; Bobinac, D. Mn porphyrin-based SOD mimic, MnTnHex-2-PyP^{5+}, and non-SOD mimic, $MnTBAP^{3-}$, suppressed rat spinal cord ischemia/reperfusion injury via NF-kappaB pathways. *Free Radic. Res.* **2014**, *48*, 1426–1442. [CrossRef] [PubMed]
12. Batinic-Haberle, I.; Ndengele, M.M.; Cuzzocrea, S.; Reboucas, J.S.; Spasojevic, I.; Salvemini, D. Lipophilicity is a critical parameter that dominates the efficacy of metalloporphyrins in blocking the development of morphine antinociceptive tolerance through peroxynitrite-mediated pathways. *Free Radic. Biol. Med.* **2009**, *46*, 212–219. [CrossRef] [PubMed]
13. Sheng, H.; Chaparro, R.E.; Sasaki, T.; Izutsu, M.; Pearlstein, R.D.; Tovmasyan, A.; Warner, D.S. Metalloporphyrins as therapeutic catalytic oxidoreductants in central nervous system disorders. *Antioxid. Redox Signal.* **2014**, *20*, 2437–2464. [CrossRef] [PubMed]
14. Crow, J.P. Catalytic antioxidants to treat amyotropic lateral sclerosis. *Expert Opin. Investig. Drugs* **2006**, *15*, 1383–1393. [CrossRef] [PubMed]
15. Miriyala, S.; Thippakorn, C.; Chaiswing, L.; Xu, Y.; Noel, T.; Tovmasyan, A.; Batinic-Haberle, I.; Vander Kooi, C.W.; Chi, W.; Latif, A.A.; et al. Novel role of 4-hydroxy-2-nonenal in AIFm2-mediated mitochondrial stress signaling. *Free Radic. Biol. Med.* **2016**, *91*, 68–80. [CrossRef] [PubMed]
16. Sheng, H.; Spasojevic, I.; Tse, H.M.; Jung, J.Y.; Hong, J.; Zhang, Z.; Piganelli, J.D.; Batinic-Haberle, I.; Warner, D.S. Neuroprotective efficacy from a lipophilic redox-modulating Mn(III) *N*-Hexylpyridylporphyrin, MnTnHex-2-PyP: Rodent models of ischemic stroke and subarachnoid hemorrhage. *J. Pharmacol. Exp. Ther.* **2011**, *338*, 906–916. [CrossRef] [PubMed]
17. Sheng, H.; Warner, D.S. Metalloporphyrin in CNS Injuries. In *Redox-Active Therapeutics*; Batinić-Haberle, I., Rebouças, J.S., Spasojević, I., Eds.; Springer International Publishing: Cham, Switzerland, 2016; pp. 541–561.
18. Drobyshevsky, A.; Luo, K.; Derrick, M.; Yu, L.; Du, H.; Prasad, P.V.; Vasquez-Vivar, J.; Batinic-Haberle, I.; Tan, S. Motor deficits are triggered by reperfusion-reoxygenation injury as diagnosed by MRI and by a mechanism involving oxidants. *J. Neurosci.* **2012**, *32*, 5500–5509. [CrossRef] [PubMed]
19. Fernandes, A.S.; Florido, A.; Cipriano, M.; Batinic-Haberle, I.; Miranda, J.; Saraiva, N.; Guerreiro, P.S.; Castro, M.; Oliveira, N.G. Combined effect of the SOD mimic MnTnHex-2-PyP^{5+} and doxorubicin on the migration and invasiveness of breast cancer cells. *Toxicol. Lett.* **2013**, *221S*, S59–S256. [CrossRef]
20. Costa, J.G.; Saraiva, N.; Guerreiro, P.S.; Louro, H.; Silva, M.J.; Miranda, J.P.; Castro, M.; Batinic-Haberle, I.; Fernandes, A.S.; Oliveira, N.G. Ochratoxin a-induced cytotoxicity, genotoxicity and reactive oxygen species in kidney cells: An integrative approach of complementary endpoints. *Food Chem. Toxicol.* **2016**, *87*, 65–76. [CrossRef] [PubMed]
21. Cohen, J.; Dorai, T.; Ding, C.; Batinic-Haberle, I.; Grasso, M. The administration of renoprotective agents extends warm ischemia in a rat model. *J. Endourol.* **2013**, *27*, 343–348. [CrossRef] [PubMed]
22. Dorai, T.; Fishman, A.I.; Ding, C.; Batinic-Haberle, I.; Goldfarb, D.S.; Grasso, M. Amelioration of renal ischemia-reperfusion injury with a novel protective cocktail. *J. Urol.* **2011**, *186*, 2448–2454. [CrossRef] [PubMed]
23. Saba, H.; Batinic-Haberle, I.; Munusamy, S.; Mitchell, T.; Lichti, C.; Megyesi, J.; MacMillan-Crow, L.A. Manganese porphyrin reduces renal injury and mitochondrial damage during ischemia/reperfusion. *Free Radic. Biol. Med.* **2007**, *42*, 1571–1578. [CrossRef] [PubMed]
24. Dogan, S.; Unal, M.; Ozturk, N.; Yargicoglu, P.; Cort, A.; Spasojevic, I.; Batinic-Haberle, I.; Aslan, M. Manganese porphyrin reduces retinal injury induced by ocular hypertension in rats. *Exp. Eye Res.* **2011**, *93*, 387–396. [CrossRef] [PubMed]
25. Ye, X.; Fels, D.; Tovmasyan, A.; Aird, K.M.; Dedeugd, C.; Allensworth, J.L.; Kos, I.; Park, W.; Spasojevic, I.; Devi, G.R.; et al. Cytotoxic effects of Mn(III) *N*-alkylpyridylporphyrins in the presence of cellular reductant, ascorbate. *Free Radic. Res.* **2011**, *45*, 1289–1306. [CrossRef] [PubMed]
26. Florido, A.; Saraiva, N.; Cerqueira, S.; Batinic-Haberle, I.; Miranda, J.; Castro, M.; Oliveira, N.G.; Fernandes, A.S. Impact of the SOD mimic MnTnHex-2-PyP on the adhesion and migration of doxorubicin-treated MDA-MB-231 cells. *Toxicol. Lett.* **2015**, *238S*, S241. [CrossRef]

27. Gauter-Fleckenstein, B.; Fleckenstein, K.; Owzar, K.; Jiang, C.; Batinic-Haberle, I.; Vujaskovic, Z. Comparison of two Mn porphyrin-based mimics of superoxide dismutase in pulmonary radioprotection. *Free Radic. Biol. Med.* **2008**, *44*, 982–989. [CrossRef] [PubMed]
28. Gauter-Fleckenstein, B.; Reboucas, J.S.; Fleckenstein, K.; Tovmasyan, A.; Owzar, K.; Jiang, C.; Batinic-Haberle, I.; Vujaskovic, Z. Robust rat pulmonary radioprotection by a lipophilic Mn *N*-alkylpyridylporphyrin, MnTnHex-2-PyP^{5+}. *Redox Biol.* **2014**, *2*, 400–410. [CrossRef] [PubMed]
29. Batinić-Haberle, I.; Tovmasyan, A.; Spasojević, I. Mn Porphyrin-Based Redox-Active Therapeutics. In *Redox-Active Therapeutics*; Batinić-Haberle, I., Rebouças, J.S., Spasojević, I., Eds.; Springer International Publishing: Cham, Switzerland, 2016; pp. 165–212.
30. Batinić-Haberle, I.; Spasojević, I.; Stevens, R.D.; Hambright, P.; Fridovich, I. Manganese(III) meso-tetrakis(ortho-N-alkylpyridyl)porphyrins. Synthesis, characterization, and catalysis of O_2/-dismutation. *Dalton Trans.* **2002**, *13*, 2689–2696. [CrossRef]
31. Li, A.M.; Martins, J.; Tovmasyan, A.; Valentine, J.S.; Batinic-Haberle, I.; Spasojevic, I.; Gralla, E.B. Differential localization and potency of manganese porphyrin superoxide dismutase-mimicking compounds in Saccharomyces cerevisiae. *Redox Biol.* **2014**, *3*, 1–6. [CrossRef] [PubMed]
32. Tovmasyan, A.; Reboucas, J.S.; Benov, L. Simple biological systems for assessing the activity of superoxide dismutase mimics. *Antioxid. Redox Signal.* **2014**, *20*, 2416–2436. [CrossRef] [PubMed]
33. Rajic, Z.; Tovmasyan, A.; Spasojevic, I.; Sheng, H.; Lu, M.; Li, A.M.; Gralla, E.B.; Warner, D.S.; Benov, L.; Batinic-Haberle, I. A new SOD mimic, Mn(III) ortho *N*-butoxyethylpyridylporphyrin, combines superb potency and lipophilicity with low toxicity. *Free Radic. Biol. Med.* **2012**, *52*, 1828–1834. [CrossRef] [PubMed]
34. Fernandes, A.S.; Gaspar, J.; Cabral, M.F.; Rueff, J.; Castro, M.; Batinic-Haberle, I.; Costa, J.; Oliveira, N.G. Protective role of ortho-substituted Mn(III) *N*-alkylpyridylporphyrins against the oxidative injury induced by tert-butylhydroperoxide. *Free Radic. Res.* **2010**, *44*, 430–440. [CrossRef] [PubMed]
35. Weitner, T.; Kos, I.; Sheng, H.; Tovmasyan, A.; Reboucas, J.S.; Fan, P.; Warner, D.S.; Vujaskovic, Z.; Batinic-Haberle, I.; Spasojevic, I. Comprehensive pharmacokinetic studies and oral bioavailability of two Mn porphyrin-based SOD mimics, MnTE-2-PyP(5+) and MnTnHex-2-PyP(5+). *Free Radic. Biol. Med.* **2013**, *58*, 73–80. [CrossRef] [PubMed]
36. Spasojevic, I.; Weitner, T.; Tovmasyan, A.; Sheng, H.; Miriyala, S.; Leu, D.; Rajic, Z.; Warner, D.S.; Clair, D.S.; Huang, T.-T.; et al. Pharmacokinetics, Brain Hippocampus and Cortex, and Mitochondrial Accumulation of a New Generation of Lipophilic Redox-Active Therapeutic, Mn(III) Meso Tetrakis(*N*-n-butoxyethylpyridinium-2-yl)porphyrin, MnTnBuOE-2-PyP^{5+}, in Comparison with its Ethyl and *N*-hexyl Analogs, MnTE-2-PyP^{5+} and MnTnHex-2-PyP^{5+}. *Free Radic. Biol. Med.* **2013**, *65*, S132.
37. Batinic-Haberle, I.; Reboucas, J.S.; Spasojevic, I. Superoxide dismutase mimics: Chemistry, pharmacology, and therapeutic potential. *Antioxid. Redox Signal.* **2010**, *13*, 877–918. [CrossRef] [PubMed]
38. Batinic-Haberle, I.; Tovmasyan, A. Superoxide dismutase mimics and other redox-active therapeutics. In *Oxidative Stress and Antioxidant Protection: The Science of Free Radical Biology and Disease*; Armstrong, D., Stratton, R.D., Eds.; John Wiley & Sons, Inc.: Hoboken, NJ, USA, 2016; pp. 415–470.
39. Spasojevic, I.; Chen, Y.; Noel, T.J.; Fan, P.; Zhang, L.; Reboucas, J.S.; St Clair, D.K.; Batinic-Haberle, I. Pharmacokinetics of the potent redox-modulating manganese porphyrin, MnTE-2-PyP(5+), in plasma and major organs of B6C3F1 mice. *Free Radic. Biol. Med.* **2008**, *45*, 943–949. [CrossRef] [PubMed]
40. Miriyala, S.; Spasojevic, I.; Tovmasyan, A.; Salvemini, D.; Vujaskovic, Z.; St Clair, D.; Batinic-Haberle, I. Manganese superoxide dismutase, MnSOD and its mimics. *Biochim. Biophys. Acta* **2012**, *1822*, 794–814. [CrossRef] [PubMed]
41. Bakthavatchalu, V.; Dey, S.; Xu, Y.; Noel, T.; Jungsuwadee, P.; Holley, A.K.; Dhar, S.K.; Batinic-Haberle, I.; St Clair, D.K. Manganese superoxide dismutase is a mitochondrial fidelity protein that protects Polγ against UV-induced inactivation. *Oncogene* **2012**, *31*, 2129–2139. [CrossRef] [PubMed]
42. Batinic-Haberle, I.; Rajic, Z.; Tovmasyan, A.; Reboucas, J.S.; Ye, X.; Leong, K.W.; Dewhirst, M.W.; Vujaskovic, Z.; Benov, L.; Spasojevic, I. Diverse functions of cationic Mn(III) *N*-substituted pyridylporphyrins, recognized as SOD mimics. *Free Radic. Biol. Med.* **2011**, *51*, 1035–1053. [CrossRef] [PubMed]
43. Jaramillo, M.C.; Briehl, M.M.; Batinic-Haberle, I.; Tome, M.E. Manganese (III) meso-tetrakis *N*-ethylpyridinium-2-yl porphyrin acts as a pro-oxidant to inhibit electron transport chain proteins, modulate bioenergetics, and enhance the response to chemotherapy in lymphoma cells. *Free Radic. Biol. Med.* **2015**, *83*, 89–100. [CrossRef] [PubMed]

44. Jaramillo, M.C.; Briehl, M.M.; Crapo, J.D.; Batinic-Haberle, I.; Tome, M.E. Manganese porphyrin, MnTE-2-PyP^{5+}, Acts as a pro-oxidant to potentiate glucocorticoid-induced apoptosis in lymphoma cells. *Free Radic. Biol. Med.* **2012**, *52*, 1272–1284. [CrossRef] [PubMed]
45. Tovmasyan, A.; Go, Y.-M.; Jones, D.; Spasojevic, I.; Batinic-Haberle, I. Redox Proteomics of 4T1 Breast Cancer Cell after Treatment with MnTE-2-PyP^{5+}/Ascorbate System. *Free Radic. Biol. Med.* **2016**, *100*, S112–S113. [CrossRef]
46. Zhao, Y.; Carroll, D.W.; You, Y.; Chaiswing, L.; Wen, R.; Batinic-Haberle, I.; Bondada, S.; Liang, Y.; St Clair, D.K. A novel redox regulator, MnTnBuOE-2-PyP^{5+}, enhances normal hematopoietic stem/progenitor cell function. *Redox Biol.* **2017**, *12*, 129–138. [CrossRef] [PubMed]
47. Tovmasyan, A.; Bueno-Janice, J.C.; Jaramillo, J.; Sampaio, R.S.; Reboucas, J.S.; Kyui, N.; Benov, L.; Deng, B.; Huang, T.T.; Tome, M.E.; et al. Radiation-mediated tumor growth inhibition is significantly enhanced with redox-active compounds that cycle with ascorbate. *Antioxid. Redox Signal.* **2018**. [CrossRef] [PubMed]
48. Batinic-Haberle, I.; Spasojevic, I.; Stevens, R.D.; Hambright, P.; Neta, P.; Okado-Matsumoto, A.; Fridovich, I. New class of potent catalysts of O_2•-dismutation. Mn(III) ortho-methoxyethylpyridyl- and di-ortho-methoxyethylimidazolylporphyrins. *Dalton Trans.* **2004**, 1696–1702. [CrossRef] [PubMed]
49. Singh, V.K.; Romaine, P.L.; Seed, T.M. Medical countermeasures for radiation exposure and related injuries: Characterization of medicines, FDA-approval status and inclusion into the strategic national stockpile. *Health Phys.* **2015**, *108*, 607–630. [CrossRef] [PubMed]
50. Plopper, C.G.; Hyde, D.M. The non-human primate as a model for studying COPD and asthma. *Pulm. Pharmacol. Ther.* **2008**, *21*, 755–766. [CrossRef] [PubMed]
51. Jackson, I.L.; Vujaskovic, Z.; Down, J.D. A further comparison of pathologies after thoracic irradiation among different mouse strains: Finding the best preclinical model for evaluating therapies directed against radiation-induced lung damage. *Radiat. Res.* **2011**, *175*, 510–518. [CrossRef] [PubMed]
52. Food and Drug Administration. New drug and biological drug products; evidence needed to demonstrate effectiveness of new drugs when human efficacy studies are not ethical or feasible. Final rule. *Fed. Regist.* **2002**, *67*, 37988–37998.
53. *Guide for the Care and Use of Laboratory Animals*; Committee for the Revision of the Guide for the Care and Use of Laboratory Animals: Washington, DC, USA, 2011.
54. Tovmasyan, A.; Weitner, T.; Sheng, H.; Lu, M.; Rajic, Z.; Warner, D.S.; Spasojevic, I.; Reboucas, J.S.; Benov, L.; Batinic-Haberle, I. Differential coordination demands in Fe versus Mn water-soluble cationic metalloporphyrins translate into remarkably different aqueous redox chemistry and biology. *Inorg. Chem.* **2013**, *52*, 5677–5691. [CrossRef] [PubMed]
55. Uckun, F.M.; Yanishevski, Y.; Tumer, N.; Waurzyniak, B.; Messinger, Y.; Chelstrom, L.M.; Lisowski, E.A.; Ek, O.; Zeren, T.; Wendorf, H.; et al. Pharmacokinetic features, immunogenicity, and toxicity of B43(anti-CD19)-pokeweed antiviral protein immunotoxin in cynomolgus monkeys. *Clin. Cancer Res.* **1997**, *3*, 325–337. [PubMed]
56. Becher, R.D.; Colonna, A.L.; Enniss, T.M.; Weaver, A.A.; Crane, D.K.; Martin, R.S.; Mowery, N.T.; Miller, P.R.; Stitzel, J.D.; Hoth, J.J. An innovative approach to predict the development of adult respiratory distress syndrome in patients with blunt trauma. *J. Trauma Acute Care Surg.* **2012**, *73*, 1229–1235. [CrossRef] [PubMed]
57. Daly, M.; Miller, P.R.; Carr, J.J.; Gayzik, F.S.; Hoth, J.J.; Meredith, J.W.; Stitzel, J.D. Traumatic pulmonary pathology measured with computed tomography and a semiautomated analytic method. *Clin. Imaging* **2008**, *32*, 346–354. [CrossRef] [PubMed]
58. Danelson, K.A.; Chiles, C.; Thompson, A.B.; Donadino, K.; Weaver, A.A.; Stitzel, J.D. Correlating the extent of pulmonary contusion to vehicle crash parameters in near-side impacts. *Ann. Adv. Automot. Med.* **2011**, *55*, 217–230. [PubMed]
59. Weaver, A.A.; Danelson, K.A.; Armstrong, E.G.; Hoth, J.J.; Stitzel, J.D. Investigation of pulmonary contusion extent and its correlation to crash, occupant, and injury characteristics in motor vehicle crashes. *Accid. Anal. Prev.* **2013**, *50*, 223–233. [CrossRef] [PubMed]
60. Chatterjee, A.; Kosmacek, E.A.; Oberley-Deegan, R.E. MnTE-2-PyP Treatment, or NOX4 Inhibition, Protects against Radiation-Induced Damage in Mouse Primary Prostate Fibroblasts by Inhibiting the TGF-Beta 1 Signaling Pathway. *Radiat. Res.* **2017**, *187*, 367–381. [CrossRef] [PubMed]

61. Ashcraft, K.A.; Boss, M.K.; Tovmasyan, A.; Roy Choudhury, K.; Fontanella, A.N.; Young, K.H.; Palmer, G.M.; Birer, S.R.; Landon, C.D.; Park, W.; et al. Novel Manganese-Porphyrin Superoxide Dismutase-Mimetic Widens the Therapeutic Margin in a Preclinical Head and Neck Cancer Model. *Int. J. Radiat. Oncol. Biol. Phys.* **2015**, *93*, 892–900. [CrossRef] [PubMed]
62. Weitzel, D.H.; Tovmasyan, A.; Ashcraft, K.A.; Rajic, Z.; Weitner, T.; Liu, C.; Li, W.; Buckley, A.F.; Prasad, M.R.; Young, K.H.; et al. Radioprotection of the brain white matter by Mn(III) n-Butoxyethylpyridylporphyrin-based superoxide dismutase mimic MnTnBuOE-2-PyP^{5+}. *Mol. Cancer Ther.* **2015**, *14*, 70–79. [CrossRef] [PubMed]
63. MacVittie, T.J.; Bennett, A.; Booth, C.; Garofalo, M.; Tudor, G.; Ward, A.; Shea-Donohue, T.; Gelfond, D.; McFarland, E.; Jackson, W., 3rd; et al. The prolonged gastrointestinal syndrome in rhesus macaques: The relationship between gastrointestinal, hematopoietic, and delayed multi-organ sequelae following acute, potentially lethal, partial-body irradiation. *Health Phys.* **2012**, *103*, 427–453. [CrossRef] [PubMed]
64. Garofalo, M.C.; Ward, A.A.; Farese, A.M.; Bennett, A.; Taylor-Howell, C.; Cui, W.; Gibbs, A.; Prado, K.L.; Macvittie, T.J. A pilot study in rhesus macaques to assess the treatment efficacy of a small molecular weight catalytic metalloporphyrin antioxidant (aeol 10150) in mitigating radiation-induced lung damage. *Health Phys.* **2014**, *106*, 73–83. [CrossRef] [PubMed]
65. Mahmood, J.; Jelveh, S.; Zaidi, A.; Doctrow, S.R.; Hill, R.P. Mitigation of radiation-induced lung injury with EUK-207 and genistein: Effects in adolescent rats. *Radiat. Res.* **2013**, *179*, 125–134. [CrossRef] [PubMed]
66. Hicks, A.; Kourteva, G.; Hilton, H.; Li, H.; Lin, T.A.; Liao, W.; Li, Y.; Wei, X.; March, T.; Benson, J.; et al. Cellular and molecular characterization of ozone-induced pulmonary inflammation in the Cynomolgus monkey. *Inflammation* **2010**, *33*, 144–156. [CrossRef] [PubMed]

7

Interleukin-1β Protects Neurons against Oxidant-Induced Injury via the Promotion of Astrocyte Glutathione Production

Twinkle Chowdhury, Matthew F. Allen, Trista L. Thorn, Yan He and Sandra J. Hewett *

Department of Biology, Program in Neuroscience, Syracuse University, Syracuse, NY 13210, USA; tschowdh@syr.edu (T.C.); mfallen@syr.edu (M.F.A.); tlthorn@syr.edu (T.L.T.); yhe19@syr.edu (Y.H.)
* Correspondence: shewett@syr.edu

Abstract: Interleukin-1β (IL-1β), a key cytokine that drives neuroinflammation in the Central Nervous System (CNS), is enhanced in many neurological diseases/disorders. Although IL-1β contributes to and/or sustains pathophysiological processes in the CNS, we recently demonstrated that IL-1β can protect cortical astrocytes from oxidant injury in a glutathione (GSH)-dependent manner. To test whether IL-1β could similarly protect neurons against oxidant stress, near pure neuronal cultures or mixed cortical cell cultures containing neurons and astrocytes were exposed to the organic peroxide, tert-butyl hydroperoxide (t-BOOH), following treatment with IL-1β or its vehicle. Neurons and astrocytes in mixed cultures, but not pure neurons, were significantly protected from the toxicity of t-BOOH following treatment with IL-1β in association with enhanced GSH production/release. IL-1β failed to increase the GSH levels or to provide protection against t-BOOH toxicity in chimeric mixed cultures consisting of IL-1R1$^{+/+}$ neurons plated on top of IL-1R1$^{-/-}$ astrocytes. The attenuation of GSH release via block of multidrug resistance-associated protein 1 (MRP1) transport also abrogated the protective effect of IL-1β. These protective effects were not strictly an in vitro phenomenon as we found an increased striatal vulnerability to 3-nitropropionic acid-mediated oxidative stress in IL-1R1 null mice. Overall, our data indicate that IL-1β protects neurons against oxidant injury and that this likely occurs in a non-cell-autonomous manner that relies on an increase in astrocyte GSH production and release.

Keywords: Interleukin 1β; neuroinflammation; neuroprotection; glutathione; astrocyte; neuronal injury; antioxidant; non-cell-autonomous protection

---

1. Introduction

Interleukin 1β and its signaling receptor IL-1R1 are expressed at low levels in the healthy brain, where they participate in normal brain function, including learning and memory. The inhibition of IL-1β signaling prevents the induction and/or maintenance of hippocampal long-term potentiation (LTP) [1–3] and mice null for IL-1R1 perform poorly in the Morris water maze, a hippocampus-dependent task [3]. Additionally, there is a direct indication of the role of IL-1 signaling in the regulation of sleep and sleep patterning in both rodents and humans [4–6]. An equally impressive amount of literature supports its role in Central Nervous System (CNS) pathology, although a clear cause-and-effect relationship between the presence of this neuroinflammatory factor and CNS damage does not always exist (for review see: [7]). In addition, it is becoming increasingly clear that IL-1β can protect and repair CNS tissue (for review see Reference [7]). Thus, the Janus face of IL-1β may depend heavily on the context, that is, its concentration and timing, its cellular target(s), and the presence or absence of negative feedback regulators. Work from our laboratory supports this assertion. We reported previously that

IL-1β enhances the expression and functional activity of the cystine/glutamate transporter (system x_c^-) in astrocytes, producing excitotoxic neuronal cell death in the context of energy deprivation [8–11]. However, we also find that IL-1β protects astrocytes from oxidant insults in a cell-autonomous fashion by a glutathione (GSH)-dependent mechanism [12]. Taking both in vivo and in vitro approaches herein, we investigated whether IL-1β could similarly protect neurons. We report that the loss of IL-1R1 signaling in vivo increases striatal vulnerability to 3-nitropropionic acid-mediated oxidative stress. In vitro modeling indicates that IL-1β does not protect neurons from oxidant injury directly but rather does so via stimulating the production and release of GSH from primary astrocytes.

2. Materials and Methods

2.1. Animals

This study was conducted in accordance with the National Institute of Health guidelines for the use of experimental animals and has been approved by the Institutional Animal Care and Use Committee of Syracuse University, 14-007 (approval dates: 12 September 2014–12 September 2017). CD-1 mice were obtained from Charles River Laboratories (Wilmington, MA, USA). The *il1r1* null mutant animals (Strain: B6.129S7-IL1r1^{tm1Imx}/J; stock # 003245) [13] were purchased from Jackson Laboratories (Bar Harbor, ME, USA). For in vitro experiments, *il1r1* null animals were bred in parallel with animals from the background strain (stock # 000664) whose offspring were used as wild-type controls. Experimental animals for the in vivo experiments were produced from F1 heterozygous ($^{+/-}$) breeding pairs derived from wild-type ($^{+/+}$) female and *il1r1* null ($^{-/-}$) male matings. Resulting $^{+/+}$ and $^{-/-}$ littermates from the F2 and F3 generations were used. The mice were provided food and water ad libitum. Up to five animals per cage were housed in a controlled temperature environment operating on a standard 12 h light/dark cycle. Investigator was blind to mouse's genotype at the time of experimentation.

2.2. Cell Culture

All cultures were kept at 37 °C in humidified 21% O_2; 6% CO_2-containing incubators.

Cell culture media compositions were as follows: Media stock (MS): L-glutamine-free modified Eagle's medium (Earl's salt; Cell Gro MediaTech, Inc., Manassas, VA, USA) supplemented with L-glutamine, glucose, and sodium bicarbonate to a final concentration of 2.0, 25.7, and 28.2 mM, respectively. Astrocyte plating medium: MS containing 10% fetal bovine serum (FBS; Hyclone Laboratories, Marlboro, MA, USA) and 10% calf serum (CS; Hyclone), 50 IU penicillin, and 50 µg/mL streptomycin (Gibco, Burlington, ON, Canada). Neuron plating medium: MS containing 5% bovine growth serum (BGS; Hyclone) and 5% CS, 50 IU penicillin, and 50 µg/mL streptomycin. Mixed culture maintenance medium: MS containing 10% CS and 50 IU penicillin/50 µg/mL streptomycin. Neuronal maintenance medium: Neurobasal medium (NB) containing 1×B27 supplement (Invitrogen, Carlsbad, CA, USA), 2 mM L-glutamine, 50 IU penicillin, and 50 µg/mL streptomycin.

Murine: mixed cortical cell cultures, containing neurons and astrocytes, were prepared using a two-step plating method, whereby astrocytes derived from postnatal 1–3 day pups were cultured first and grown to confluency and then purified to remove microglia [14]. Dissociated neurons from embryonic day-15 mouse fetuses (0.75–1.8 million cells/mL) were then plated on top, as described in detail previously [15]. At 5 and 9 days in vitro, 250 µL of plating medium was exchanged with a mixed culture maintenance medium. To prevent microglia cell growth and induce their death, the cultures were treated with 8 µM β-D-cytosine arabinofuranoside (Ara-C) once on day 6 or 7 in vitro, which halts cell division and induces mitotic catastrophe. Neurons and astrocytes are unaffected by this treatment as the former are post-mitotic and the latter are contact-inhibited. Two days prior to experimentation, mixed cortical cell cultures were washed into media stock (2×, 250 µL exchange). Experiments were performed at 14 days in vitro.

Near-pure neuronal cultures were derived from the cortices of embryonic day 15 CD-1 mice, as described in Reference [8]. Dissociated cortical cells were plated at a density of 1–1.4 million cells/mL on polyethyleneimine-coated plates in neuronal plating medium. Four hours later, the cell medium was exchanged fully with the neuronal maintenance medium. After two days, the neurons were treated with 1 μM of Ara-C to prevent glial cell growth. The medium was partially replenished at 4 days in vitro by exchanging 250 μL with neuronal maintenance medium made using 1×B27 supplement devoid of antioxidants (B27 minus antioxidants; Invitrogen, Carlsbad, CA, USA). Pure neuronal cultures were used at 6–7 days in vitro.

2.3. IL-1β Treatment

Cells were treated with recombinant murine IL-1β (R&D Systems, Minneapolis, MN, USA) for either 24 or 48 h in an incubation buffer of MS for mixed cultures and NB for neurons both supplemented with the vehicle, 0.1% fatty-acid-free bovine serum albumin (BSA) (Sigma, St. Louis, MO, USA). As both neurons and astrocytes have functional IL-1R1 receptors, higher concentrations for the mixed cultures were utilized to ensure optimal signaling (Birgit Fogal and Sandra J Hewett, unpublished observations).

2.4. Measurement of GSH

Total glutathione (GSH + GSSG) concentrations were determined using the GSH-Glo glutathione assay (Promega, Madison, WI, USA) per the manufacturer's instruction. The media was collected for analysis of the extracellular GSH ($[GSH]_e$) and GSH-Glo reaction buffer was directly added to the cells for analysis of the intracellular GSH ($[GSH]_i$). The samples were diluted using the reagent to keep the relative light units within the dynamic range of the standards. To determine the total GSH levels, oxidized glutathione disulfide (GSSG) within the samples was converted to GSH with the reducing agent Tris(2-carboxyethyl)phosphine hydrochloride TCEP-HCl (final concentration = 1 mM; 10 min; 25 °C; Thermo Scientific; Waltham, MA, USA). Luciferase activity was quantified using a Synergy2 microplate reader (BioTek, Winooski, VT, USA). The GSH levels were normalized to standards prepared in the GSH-Glo reagent or MS containing L-glutamine and 0.1% fatty-acid-free BSA, respectively. The intracellular GSH was normalized to cellular protein quantified using a BCA Assay Kit (Thermo Scientific, Waltham, MA, USA) as per the manufacturer's instructions.

2.5. Drug Exposure

Tert-butyl Hydroperoxide (t-BOOH) Treatment: t-BOOH is a direct-acting organic peroxide used to induce oxidative stress; its clearance requires GSH [12,16]. A stock solution of t-BOOH (1.5 M in H_2O; Acros Organics) was made and stored at 4 °C. t-BOOH was added to the cultures (final concentration: 1–4 mM) in the treatment media (MS for mixed cultures and NB for neurons). Experiments were terminated 0.5 to 3.5 h later and the tissue culture supernatant was removed for the measurement of lactate dehydrogenase (LDH) activity to quantify cell death (see below). Next, 3-(4,5-dimethylthiazol-2-yl)-2,5-diphenyltetrazolium bromide (MTT) was added and the extent of its reduction to formazan was used to quantify the cell survival (see below).

MK-571: MK-571 is a potent inhibitor of MRP1, a multi-drug resistant protein transporter used by astrocytes to export GSH [12,17]. A stock solution of MK-571 (25 mM in H_2O; Enzo Life Sciences) was made and stored at −20 °C. MK-571 was added to the mixed cultures (final concentration: 50–70 μM) in MS. After 1.5–2 h of incubation, IL-1β (final concentration = 10 ng/mL) was spiked in. Twenty-four hours later, t-BOOH was added as described in each figure's legend. The experiments were terminated 2.5 to 3.5 h later by addition of MTT to quantify cell survival.

3-Nitroproprionic Acid (3-NP) Dosing Protocol: 3-NP is a plant toxin that produces selective striatal lesions in both experimental animals and in man via mechanisms involving oxidative stress [18,19]. 3-NP (Sigma Aldrich, St. Louis, MO, USA) was dissolved in 0.9% saline to a concentration of 25 mg/mL, adjusted to pH 7.4 with 5 M NaOH, and filter sterilized (0.2 μm Nalgene). A 3-NP stock was kept at 4 °C for no more than seven days. After five days of acclimatization handling, male mice (15–18 wks) were administered 3-NP via intraperitoneal injection twice daily with an interval of 8–12 h as follows: 20 mg/kg for two days, 30 mg/kg for three days, 40 mg/kg for three days, 50 mg/kg for three days, 60 mg/kg for one day for a total cumulative dose of 920 mg/kg. Animals completing the protocol were sacrificed by cervical dislocation under isoflurane anesthesia. The brains were snap frozen in an O.C.T. compound (Sakura Finetek USA, Torrance, CA, USA). Three separate experiments were performed over two months.

2.6. Measurement of Cell Death and Viability

In vitro cell death was quantitatively determined by the spectrophotometric measurement of lactate dehydrogenase (LDH) activity, as described previously [20]. Data are expressed as a percentage of total LDH activity (defined as 100%), determined by assaying the supernatant of parallel cultures exposed to 1.5 mM t-BOOH for 20–24 h. In some mixed culture experiments, cell death was additionally assessed via propidium iodide (PI; Molecular Probes, Eugene, OR, USA) staining [20]. PI (10 μg/mL) was added to culture wells for 10 min, after which it was removed by gentle washing with PBS (3 × 750 μL). Fluorescent photos were acquired by a DP73 digital color camera (Digital Video Camera Co., Olympus, Shinjuku, Tokyo, Japan) mounted on an Olympus IX50 inverted microscope outfitted with epifluorescence controlled by CellSens Standard (Olympus, Tokyo, Japan) software. Brightness and contrast were standardized for each picture.

In vitro cell viability was quantified via colorimetric analysis of MTT (Sigma) reduction as previously described [12,21]. The percent of viable cells was quantified by normalization of experimental MTT absorbance values to values obtained from untreated control cells (i.e., highest absorbance = 100%)).

In vivo cell death was analyzed histologically. Frozen brain sections (40 μm) were collected serially from the rostrocaudal extent of each brain (+1.54 to −0.18 relative to bregma) and stained with 0.5% thionin by submersion in multiple solutions (70% EtOH, 50% EtOH, ddH_2O, thionin, ddH_2O, ddH_2O, 70% EtOH, 95% EtOH, 100% EtOH, 100% EtOH, 100% Xylene, 100% Xylene), as previously described [22]. Images were captured by scanning (Epson Perfection 3170, Epson, Long Beach, CA USA) at 2400 dpi. The lesion area, identified by the absence of thionin staining, was quantified using NIH Image J at seven levels from bregma (+1.22, +1.02, +0.72, +0.52, +0.22, +0.02, and −0.18) by three individuals blind to genotype and experimental identification. For each level, the percent striatal damage (D) was calculated as a percentage of the total striatum area (T) as (D/Tx100). Area measurements were converted to volume using Cavalieri's principle (volume = $(s_1d_1) + (s_2d_2) + (s_3d_3) + (s_4d_4) + (s_5d_5) + (s_6d_6) + (s_7d_7)$), where s = lesion surface area and d = the distance between two sections, as published in Reference [23]. The data are expressed as the percent lesion area of the striatum at all seven levels and the mean lesion volume + Standard Error of the Mean (SEM) of all seven levels derived from the mean calculated from all three individuals.

2.7. Statistical Analysis

Statistical analyses were performed using GraphPad Prism Version 6.03 or 7.03 (La Jolla, CA, USA) as described in each figure legend. Percentage data were transformed by the arcsin square root function Y = arcsin[sqrt(Y/100)], before analysis because it is, by nature, non-normally distributed. In all experiments, the data are expressed as the mean + SEM. Significance was assessed at $p < 0.05$.

3. Results

Previously, we determined that the IL-1β treatment of primary astrocytes enhanced their production and release of GSH, rendering them resistant to death induced by exposure to the organic peroxide, tert-butyl hydroperoxide (t-BOOH) [12]. Herein, we find that neurons and astrocytes in a mixed culture (Figure 1A,B)—but not neurons in isolation (Figure 2)—are also protected against t-BOOH following pretreatment with IL-1β 48 h prior to exposure. To ensure that the lack of protection in neuronal cultures was not a result of sub-optimal IL-1β concentrations, increasing concentrations of

IL-1β (5–20 ng/mL; 48 h) were tested. None protected the neurons against exposure to 2 mM t-BOOH (Supplemental Figure S1).

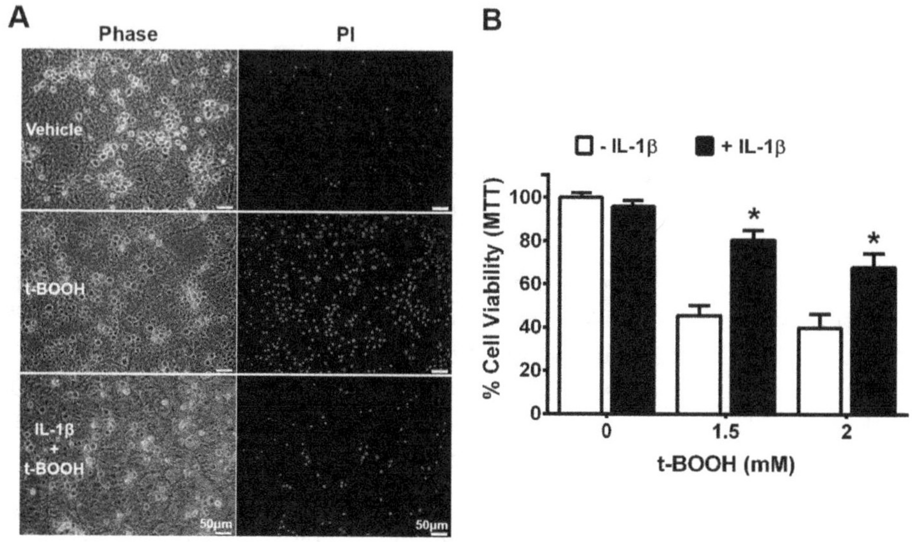

Figure 1. Interleukin-1β (IL-1β) pre-treatment protects mixed cultures against tert-butyl hydroperoxide t-BOOH toxicity. (**A**) Mixed cortical cell cultures were incubated with IL-1β (10 ng/mL) or its vehicle for 48 h after which they were treated with 1.5 mM t-BOOH for 2 h followed by the addition of propidium iodide (PI, 10 μg/mL) to assess for cell death. Phase contrast micrographs (left panel) and PI staining (right panel) of representative wells treated with vehicle, vehicle + t-BOOH, or IL-1β followed by t-BOOH; (**B**) Mixed cortical cell cultures were incubated with IL-1β (10 ng/mL) or its vehicle for 48 h after which they were treated with for 2.75–3.25 h followed by the addition of MTT to assess for cell survival. Data are expressed as % mean cell survival + SEM normalized to MTT values of non-treated control cultures (=100%). An asterisk (*) denotes a significant between-group difference (+ IL-1β vs. −IL-1β at each t-BOOH concentration) as determined via two-way analysis of variance (ANOVA) followed by Bonferroni's test for multiple comparisons (n = 7–16 from three separate dissections; $p < 0.001$).

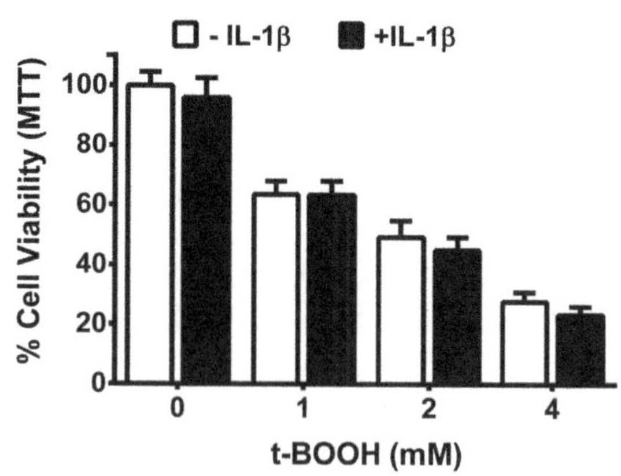

Figure 2. IL-1β pre-treatment does not protect pure neurons against t-BOOH-toxicity. Cortical neurons cultured in isolation were washed twice with the treatment media and incubated with IL-1β (5 ng/mL) or its vehicle for 48 h. Next, the cells were treated with t-BOOH at the indicated concentrations for 1.25–4.5 h. Cell viability was determined using the MTT assay. Data are expressed as % neuronal cell viability (mean + SEM) normalized to MTT values of the untreated group (=100%). No significant between-group differences (+IL-1β vs. −IL-1β at each t-BOOH concentration) were observed as assessed by two-way ANOVA followed by Bonferroni's test for multiple comparisons (n = 6–9 from two separate dissections).

In the mixed cultures, the protective effect of IL-1β was associated with a significant increase and decrease in the supernatant and cellular GSH levels, respectively (Figure 3A). IL-1β produced no alterations in either intracellular or extracellular GSH concentrations from pure neurons (Figure 3B).

This IL-1β-mediated increase in extracellular GSH levels in mixed cultures was absent in chimeric mixed cultures grown with *il1r1*$^{-/-}$ astrocytes, that is, astrocytes derived from mice lacking the IL-1β signaling receptor (Figure 4). Neurons and astrocytes in chimeric cultures containing *il1r1*$^{-/-}$ astrocytes were also no longer protected against t-BOOH toxicity (1.5 mM t-BOOH; 2 h) by prior IL-1β treatment (10 ng/mL, 48 h), whereas those containing *il1r1*$^{+/+}$ astrocytes were still rescued (Figure 5). These results suggest that extracellular GSH produced by astrocytes is essential for the neuroprotective effects of IL-1β. To examine this idea directly, the ability of IL-1β to protect against t-BOOH exposure following the abrogation of GSH release with MK-571 was tested. The GSH release was significantly reduced by the inclusion of MK-571 (50 μM and 70 μM) in both control and IL-1β-treated cultures, as expected (Figure 6A). The MK-571 treatment also rendered mixed cultures more vulnerable to the toxicity of t-BOOH exposure (1.5 mM, 2.45 h) and significantly attenuated the ability of IL-1β to protect them from this oxidant (Figure 6B). Thus, the neuroprotective, antioxidant potential of IL-1β rests on its ability to increase GSH production and release from astrocytes in the mixed culture.

Finally and importantly, these protective effects were not strictly an in vitro phenomenon as we found an increased striatal vulnerability to 3-nitropropionic acid in mice lacking the signaling receptor for IL-1β (IL-1R1 null mice) when compared to their wild-type littermate controls. Lesion size was significantly greater in IL-1R1 null mice (Figure 7). Secondly, lesion incidence—defined as the proportion of total mice from each genotype treated with 3-NP with a lesion of any size—was also greater in IL-1R1 null mice. While only 3/8 (37.5%) of *il1r1*$^{+/+}$ mice showed histological evidence of 3-NP-induced striatal neurodegeneration, 7/11 (64%) of *il1r1*$^{-/-}$ did ($p = 0.13$, Chi-square test). The total striatal volume was not different between the *il1r1*$^{+/+}$ and *il1r1*$^{-/-}$ mice (10.6 ± 0.5 and 11.8 ± 0.4 mm^3, respectively). This increased vulnerability could not be explained by the differential metabolism of 3-NP as the striatal succinate dehydrogenase activity was inhibited to the same extent in both genotypes (data not shown). The present results indicate that loss of IL-1β signaling is detrimental to the striatum in the setting of chronic, systemic 3-NP exposure.

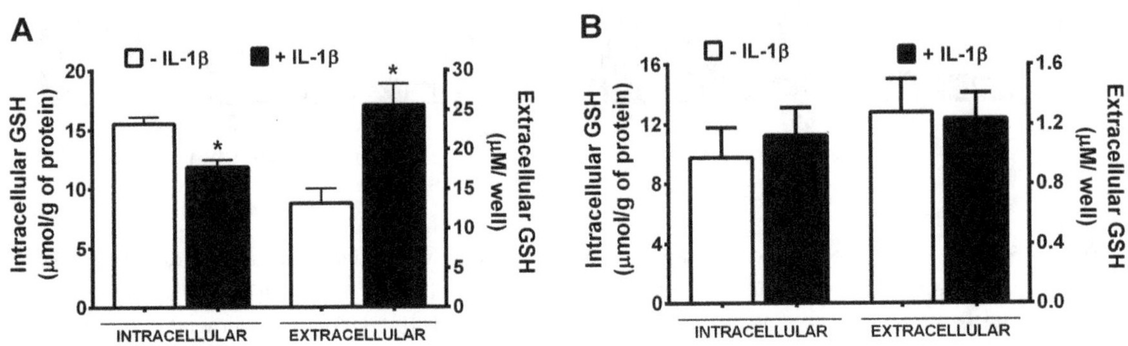

Figure 3. Mixed cultures, but not pure neurons, produce and release glutathione (GSH) upon stimulation with IL-1β. (**A**) Mixed cortical cultures were treated with media containing vehicle (−IL-1β; white bars) or 10 ng/mL IL-1β (+ IL-1β; black bars) (n = 22–24 from three to five separate dissections; well volume = 400 μL); (**B**) Neurons were treated with its vehicle or 5 ng/mL IL-1β (n = 9 from three separate dissections; 0.36 ± 0.024 mg protein/well). Forty-eight hours later, the total intracellular or supernatant GSH levels were measured as described in the methods. Data are expressed as mean + SEM. An asterisk (*) denotes a significant between-group difference (−IL-1β vs. +IL-1β) as determined by two-way ANOVA followed by Bonferroni's test for multiple comparisons.

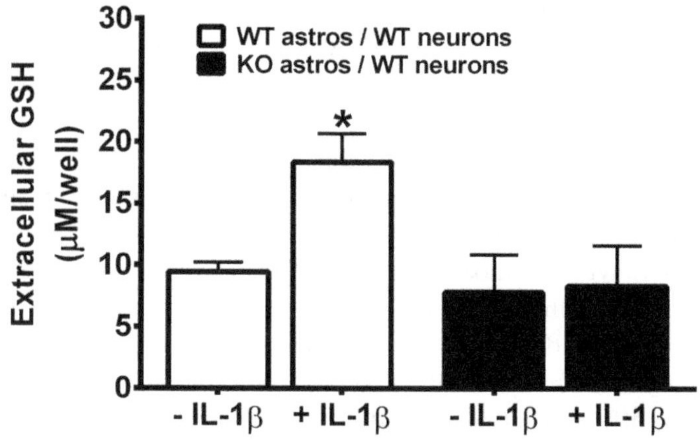

Figure 4. IL-1β-mediated increase in extracellular GSH in mixed cultures is dependent on astrocyte activation. Wild-type neurons plated on astrocytes cultured from *il1r1*$^{+/+}$ or *il1r1*$^{-/-}$ mice were treated with vehicle (−IL-1β) or 10 ng/mL IL-1β (+ IL-1β) for 48 h after which the total supernatant GSH levels were measured. The data are expressed as the mean μM GSH/well + SEM. An asterisk (*) denotes significant between-group difference (+ and −IL-1β within the same combination of chimeric culture) as assessed by two-way ANOVA followed by Bonferroni's test for multiple comparisons (n = 8 each from two separate dissections; p = 0.001). WT: *il1r1*$^{+/+}$; KO: *il1r1*$^{-/-}$.

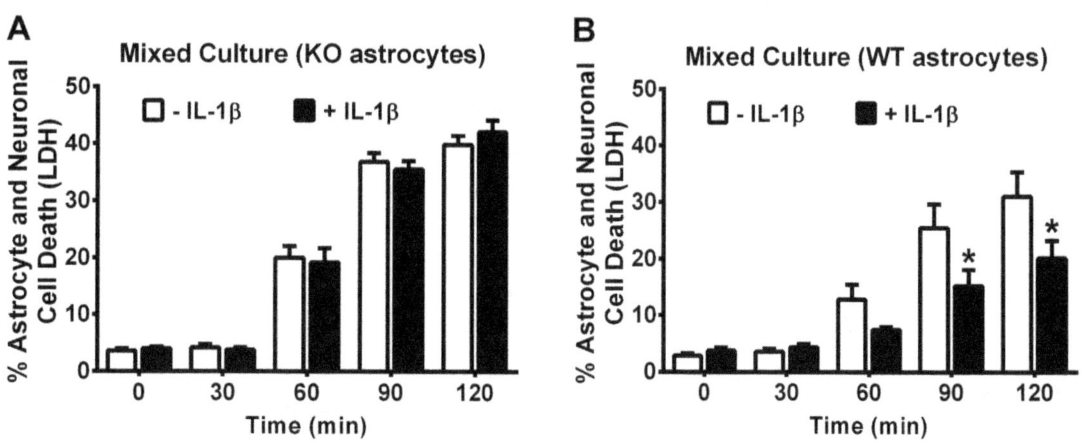

Figure 5. IL-1β-mediated protection against t-BOOH-toxicity in mixed cultures is dependent on astrocyte activation. Wild-type neurons plated on astrocytes cultured from (**A**) *il1r1*$^{-/-}$ or (**B**) *il1r1*$^{+/+}$ mice were treated with its vehicle (−IL-1β) or 10 ng/mL IL-1β (+IL-1β) for 48 h followed by treatment with 1.5 mM t-BOOH. Supernatants were collected for measurement of lactate dehydrogenase LDH at each time point, as indicated. Cultures were then washed free of t-BOOH, and medium collected again at 165 min (total time of exposure plus post-wash incubation) from each well. Values were summed and normalized to LDH released from cultures treated with 1.5 mM t-BOOH for 20–24 h (=100% cell death). Data are mean % cell death + SEM (**A**) There were no statistically significant group effects as determined by two-way ANOVA (n = 16 from 4 separate dissections); (**B**) p values were equal to 0.0035 for the IL-1β treatment effect, <0.0001 for the effect of time of t-BOOH exposure, and 0.0149 for the treatment × time interaction. An asterisk (*) depicts significant between-group difference ($p < 0.05$). Two-way ANOVA followed by Bonferroni's test for multiple comparisons (n = 16 from 4 separate dissections). WT: *il1r1*$^{+/+}$; KO: *il1r1*$^{-/-}$.

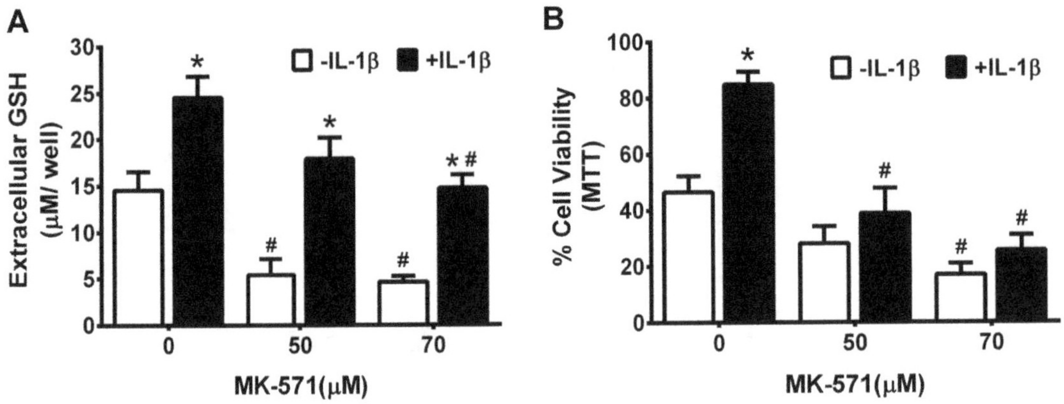

Figure 6. Attenuation of astrocytic GSH release abrogates the protective effect of IL-1β against t-BOOH-induced toxicity. Mixed cortical cell cultures (n = 8 from three separate dissections) were treated with MK-571 at the indicated concentrations for 2 h, after which IL-1β (10 ng/mL) or its vehicle was spiked in for an additional 24 h. (**A**) The supernatant was removed for measurement of the total GSH expressed as the mean μM/well + SEM, as described in the methods; (**B**) The same cells were treated with 1.5 mM t-BOOH (2.45 h) and the experiment was terminated by the addition of MTT. The results are expressed as mean % cell survival normalized to the MTT values of the non-treated control cultures (not shown = 100%). An asterisk (*) denotes significant between-group difference (−IL-1β vs +IL-1β) and a pound (#) denotes significant within-group difference (MK-571 treated with or without IL-1β) as assessed by two-way ANOVA followed by Bonferroni's test for multiple comparisons. Significance was set at $p < 0.05$.

4. Discussion

The present results demonstrate that IL-1β protects neurons against oxidant injury both in vitro and in vivo and that this likely occurs in a non-cell-autonomous manner that relies on an increase in astrocyte GSH production and release. These data fit in with a larger literature reporting the ability of IL-1β to mount protective responses in the CNS. For instance, enhanced neuronal sprouting and/or regeneration in various in vitro and in vivo model systems follow IL-1β treatment [24–26]. IL-1β—either endogenously produced or administered exogenously—has been shown to mediate ischemic tolerance in gerbil [27]. Treatment with IL-1β, at the same concentration as used herein in mixed cultures (10 ng/mL), protected organotypic hippocampal cultures from simulated ischemia, although hypoxic neuronal damage was enhanced [28]. IL-1β has been reported to protect against excitotoxic neuronal injury in neuronal cell cultures [29,30] and organotypic hippocampal cultures [28]. Interestingly, APP/PS1 Alzheimer's disease mice whose astrocytes chronically overexpress IL-1β have reduced hippocampal amyloid load [31], although contextual and spatial memory impairments in control animals were evident [32,33]. Additionally, loss of IL-1β signaling exacerbated motor deficits and increased the levels of mutant huntingtin in the striatum of the N171-82Q Huntington's disease (HD) mouse. Of note, repeated systemic administration of 3-NP—a phyto/fungal toxin that irreversibly inhibits the electron transport enzyme succinate dehydrogenase (SDH) preferentially in neurons in vivo [34]—as used herein, is often used as a chemical model of HD [18,35]. Striatal lesions subsequent to 3-NP-mediated metabolic inhibition [36–38] result from oxidative stress that occurs via multiple mechanisms [19,39,40]. Thus, the more numerous and larger striatal lesions in IL-1R1 null mice (Figure 7) as compared to wild-type littermate controls seen in this study, suggests that endogenous IL1-β signaling protects against 3-NP-mediated oxidative stress in vivo.

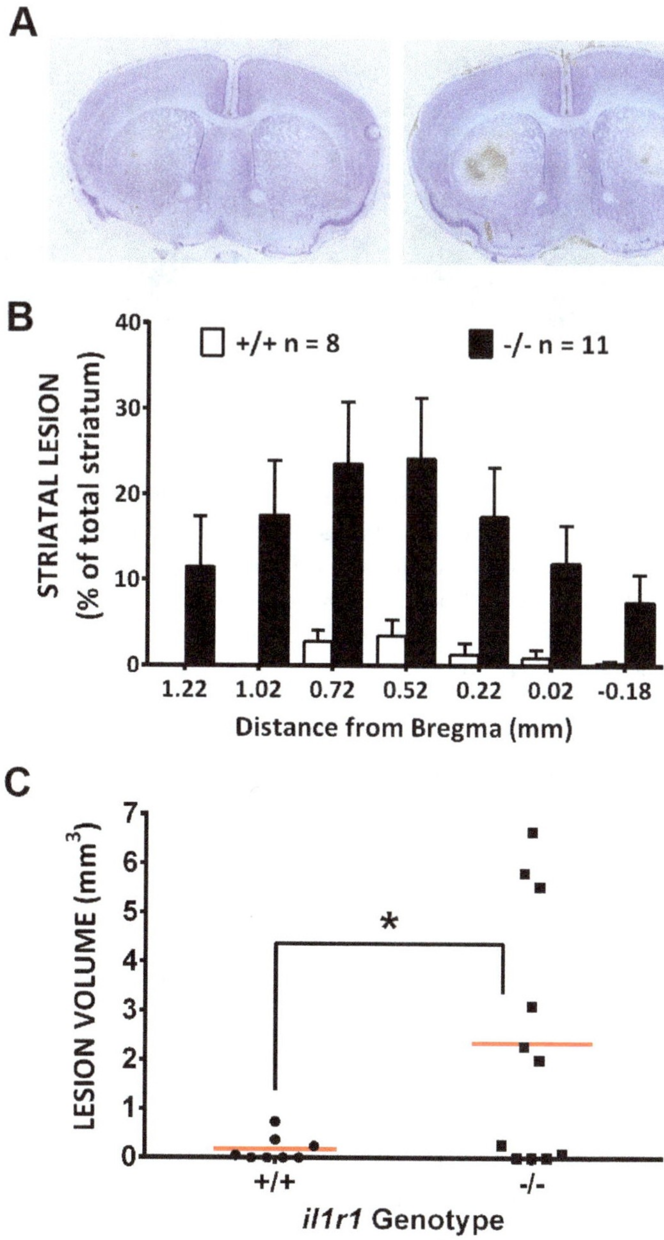

Figure 7. Mice deficient in IL-1R1 signaling (*il1r1*$^{-/-}$) have larger striatal lesions following systemic 3-NP treatment as compared to their wild-type littermate (*il1r1*$^{+/+}$) controls. Male *il1r1*$^{-/-}$ ($n = 11$) and *il1r1*$^{+/+}$ ($n = 8$) were injected twice daily with 3-NP as described in the methods. (**A**) Representative photomicrographs of thionin-stained sections (+0.52 from bregma) taken from 3-NP-treated *il1r1*$^{+/+}$ (left) and *il1r1*$^{-/-}$ mice (right); (**B**) Comparison of lesion area between *il1r1*$^{+/+}$ and *il1r1*$^{-/-}$ mice expressed as a percentage of total striatal area. A significant difference between genotypes occurs at every level of bregma as determined by repeated measures two-way ANOVA ($p = 0.0163$), followed by Sidaks post-hoc *t*-tests for multiple comparisons ($p < 0.0001$ at all levels); (**C**) Comparison of lesion volume between *il1r1*$^{+/+}$ and *il1r1*$^{-/-}$ mice determined using the Cavalieri's method. Data points represent the lesion volume (mm^3) for each individual mouse, while a horizontal line represents the mean mm^3 for each group. A one-tailed *t*-test with Welch's correction revealed a significant difference (*) between genotypes at $p = 0.01$.

Consistent with our in vivo results, we find that neurons and astrocytes in mixed culture treated with IL-1β also enjoy protection against oxidant injury resulting from the direct addition of the organic peroxide, t-BOOH (Figure 1). Despite the fact that both neurons and astrocytes have been shown to express IL-1R1 [41–45], this IL-1β-mediated protection did not extend to neurons cultured in isolation (Figure 2), indicating the need for astrocyte involvement. The importance of astrocyte signaling to the protective effects of IL-1β was directly confirmed using chimeric cultures consisting of wild-type neurons plated on astrocytes cultured from IL-1RI$^{-/-}$ mice (Figure 5). Cell-type-specific effects of IL-1β have been reported previously. For instance, nuclear translocation of the p65 NF-κB subunit in response to IL-1β treatment of mixed hippocampal neuron-astrocyte co-cultures also occurs in astrocytes, but not neurons [46]. Interestingly, treatment of mouse primary astrocytes with IL-1β results in an NF-κB-dependent increase in the production and release of the antioxidant GSH, which subsequently rendered treated astrocytes less susceptible to oxidant injury [12]. In this study, the protective effect of IL-1β, or lack thereof, also correlated remarkably with its ability to stimulate GSH production and release from the cultures (Figures 3 and 4), with again astrocytes taking center stage (Figure 4). This may not be surprising given the numerous studies demonstrating that astrocytes possess higher concentrations of GSH than neurons [47–51], that astrocytes protect neurons against oxidative insults [49,52–55], and that the depletion of astrocyte GSH renders neurons more susceptible to oxidative insults [49,56–58]. Interestingly, the release of GSH into the mixed culture medium was accompanied by a small but significant loss of intracellular GSH (Figure 3A). Since we see no change in intracellular GSH in IL-1β-treated neurons (Figure 3B), we interpret this to mean that the release from astrocytes in mixed culture is not completely matched by the synthesis, as it is when astrocytes cultures are treated with IL-1β in isolation [12]. This suggests that the dynamics of astrocyte GSH synthesis and/or release are altered by the presence of neurons. In support of this assertion, the GSH release from mixed cultures—confirmed to be astrocyte-derived in Figure 4—is 4–5 fold higher (Figure 3A) than from astrocytes cultured alone [12,59].

The cycling of GSH and/or its metabolites between astrocytes and neurons appears necessary for the maintenance of neuronal GSH levels [60–62]. Astrocytes reportedly facilitate neuronal GSH synthesis [47,48,63] by releasing GSH into the extracellular space [17,50,64,65] where it is cleaved to cysteinylglycine by γ-glutamyltranspeptidase [66] and hydrolyzed by a neuronal ectopeptidase to its constituent amino acids for uptake [67,68]. Our data demonstrating that the attenuation of GSH release via a block of MRP1 transport abrogates the protective effect of IL-1β in mixed culture also supports this notion of astrocyte to neuron GSH cycling. With respect to the GSH site of action, it should be noted that peroxides are certainly generated intracellularly but also in the extracellular space in vivo by infiltrating inflammatory cells [69–71] and/or resident microglia [72,73]; this latter process is what extracellular t-BOOH exposure to mixed cultures likely models. Additionally, hydrogen peroxide readily crosses cell membranes and this has been shown to occur through aquaporins [74], which are expressed by astrocytes and some neurons [75,76]. Finally, we previously demonstrated the increase in the intracellular reactive oxygen species in astrocytes follow extracellular t-BOOH exposure [12]. Thus, it seems likely that GSH exerts both intracellular and extracellular effects.

How does IL-1β facilitate astrocyte production of GSH? We previously demonstrated that IL-1β enhanced system x_c^- expression and thus, activity in the primary astrocytes (but not neurons [8]) in isolation [8,59] or in mixed culture [9] (also see Supplemental Figure S2). System x_c^- operates as an obligate exchanger, which links the export of L-glutamate to the import of L-cystine. Rapid reduction of intracellular cystine to cysteine allows for its incorporation into proteins as well as into GSH [77–79]. One of the major determinates of the rate of GSH synthesis is the availability of its substrate cyst(e)ine [47,63,80]. In fact, we found that enhanced GSH export that followed IL-1β treatment is abolished in astrocytes derived from mice null for xCT, the substrate-specific light chain for the antiporter, system x_c^- [59]. Unlike with xCT, we did not find a change in the steady-state mRNA levels of the regulatory enzyme of GSH synthesis, glutamate cysteine ligase (either the catalytic and modifier domain), or of MRP1 following IL-1β exposure of cultured astrocytes (Supplemental Figure S2). However, this does not rule out the possibility that IL-1β facilitates post-translational modifications leading to changes in enzymatic activity or in the trafficking of MRP1 to the plasma membrane, the latter of which has been previously shown for bilirubin-treated astrocytes [81]. If the latter is true, this could explain why MK-571 was less effective in reducing GSH efflux under IL-1β-treated conditions (Figure 6A). Moreover, various other pathways for GSH release from astrocytes have been described in the literature including gap junction hemichannels [64,65,82] and the Organic Anion-transporting Polypeptide-1, (Oatp) [83]. Whether any of these pathways are modified by IL-1β exposure was not determined.

5. Conclusions

IL-1β is traditionally thought of as a classic pro-inflammatory cytokine that participates in processes leading to neurodegeneration (see References [7,84]). Contrary to this notion, we describe data demonstrating the ability of IL-1β signaling to protect neurons against oxidant injury both in vitro and in vivo. The totality of our results are consistent with the conclusion that this likely occurs in a non-cell-autonomous manner that relies on an increase in astrocyte GSH production and release. This pleiotropic nature of IL-1β in the CNS (see References [7,84]) indicates that a detailed understanding of the both the physiological, pathophysiological, and protective potential of its signaling in the brain under different contexts and conditions is necessary so that we can devise strategies to exploit its benefits while simultaneously reducing its unfavorable effects.

Supplementary Materials: The following are available online at http://www.mdpi.com/2076-3921/7/8/100/s1, Figure S1: IL-1β does not protect neurons cultured in isolation against t-BOOH-mediated toxicity at any concentration tested, Figure S2: Effect of IL-1β on molecules involved in GSH synthesis and export.

Author Contributions: T.C., M.F.A., Y.H. and S.J.H. conceived and designed the experiments; T.C., T.L.T. and Y.H. performed in vitro experiments, while M.F.A. performed the in vivo experiments. T.C., M.F.A., Y.H. and S.J.H. analyzed the data; Y.H. finalized/standardized the figures. T.C. and S.J.H. wrote the paper with input from M.F.A., T.L.T. and Y.H.

Funding: This work was supported by NIH/NINDS R01NS051445-08, which also covered the funds to publish open access. An American Heart Post-doctoral Fellowship supported Y.H.

Conflicts of Interest: The authors declare no conflict of interest. Additionally, the funding sponsors had no role in the design of the study; in the collection, analyses, or interpretation of data; in the writing of the manuscript, and in the decision to publish the results. T.C. is currently at Amgen, Cambridge, MA, USA.

References

1. Ross, F.M.; Allan, S.M.; Rothwell, N.J.; Verkhratsky, A. A dual role for interleukin-1 in LTP in mouse hippocampal slices. *J. Neuroimmunol.* **2003**, *144*, 61–67. [CrossRef] [PubMed]
2. Schneider, H.; Pitossi, F.; Balschun, D.; Wagner, A.; del Rey, A.; Besedovsky, H.O. A neuromodulatory role of interleukin-1β in the hippocampus. *Proc. Natl. Acad. Sci. USA* **1998**, *95*, 7778–7783. [CrossRef] [PubMed]
3. Avital, A.; Goshen, I.; Kamsler, A.; Segal, M.; Iverfeldt, K.; Richter-Levin, G.; Yirmiya, R. Impaired interleukin-1 signaling is associated with deficits in hippocampal memory processes and neural plasticity. *Hippocampus* **2003**, *13*, 826–834. [CrossRef] [PubMed]
4. Fang, J.; Wang, Y.; Krueger, J.M. Effects of interleukin-1 beta on sleep are mediated by the type I receptor. *Am. J. Physiol.* **1998**, *274*, R655–R660. [PubMed]
5. Krueger, J.M.; Fang, J.; Taishi, P.; Chen, Z.; Kushikata, T.; Gardi, J. Sleep. A physiologic role for IL-1 beta and TNF-alpha. *Ann. N. Y. Acad. Sci.* **1998**, *856*, 148–159. [CrossRef] [PubMed]
6. Schmidt, E.M.; Linz, B.; Diekelmann, S.; Besedovsky, L.; Lange, T.; Born, J. Effects of an interleukin-1 receptor antagonist on human sleep, sleep-associated memory consolidation, and blood monocytes. *Brain Behav. Immun.* **2015**, *47*, 178–185. [CrossRef] [PubMed]
7. Hewett, S.J.; Jackman, N.A.; Claycomb, R.J. Interleukin-1β in central nervous system injury and repair. *Eur. J. Neurodegener. Dis.* **2012**, *1*, 195–211. [PubMed]
8. Jackman, N.A.; Uliasz, T.F.; Hewett, J.A.; Hewett, S.J. Regulation of system x_c^- activity and expression in astrocytes by interleukin-1beta: Implications for hypoxic neuronal injury. *Glia* **2010**, *58*, 1806–1815. [CrossRef] [PubMed]

9. Fogal, B.; Li, J.; Lobner, D.; McCullough, L.D.; Hewett, S.J. System x_c^- activity and astrocytes are necessary for interleukin-1beta-mediated hypoxic neuronal injury. *J. Neurosci.* **2007**, *27*, 10094–10105. [CrossRef] [PubMed]
10. Fogal, B.; Hewett, J.A.; Hewett, S.J. Interleukin-1beta potentiates neuronal injury in a variety of injury models involving energy deprivation. *J. Neuroimmunol.* **2005**, *161*, 93–100. [CrossRef] [PubMed]
11. Jackman, N.A.; Melchior, S.E.; Hewett, J.A.; Hewett, S.J. Non-cell autonomous influence of the astrocyte system x_c^- on hypoglycaemic neuronal cell death. *ASN Neuro* **2012**, *4*, e00074. [CrossRef] [PubMed]
12. He, Y.; Jackman, N.A.; Thorn, T.L.; Vought, V.E.; Hewett, S.J. Interleukin-1beta protects astrocytes against oxidant-induced injury via an nf-kappab-dependent upregulation of glutathione synthesis. *Glia* **2015**, *63*, 1568–1580. [CrossRef] [PubMed]
13. Glaccum, M.B.; Stocking, K.L.; Charrier, K.; Smith, J.L.; Willis, C.R.; Maliszewski, C.; Livingston, D.J.; Peschon, J.J.; Morrissey, P.J. Phenotypic and functional characterization of mice that lack the type I receptor for IL-1. *J. Immunol.* **1997**, *159*, 3364–3371. [PubMed]
14. Hamby, M.E.; Uliasz, T.F.; Hewett, S.J.; Hewett, J.A. Characterization of an improved procedure for the removal of microglia from confluent monolayers of primary astrocytes. *J. Neurosci. Methods* **2006**, *150*, 128–137. [CrossRef] [PubMed]
15. Trackey, J.L.; Uliasz, T.F.; Hewett, S.J. Sin-1-induced cytotoxicity in mixed cortical cell culture: Peroxynitrite-dependent and -independent induction of excitotoxic cell death. *J. Neurochem.* **2001**, *79*, 445–455. [CrossRef] [PubMed]
16. Dringen, R.; Kussmaul, L.; Hamprecht, B. Rapid clearance of tertiary butyl hydroperoxide by cultured astroglial cells via oxidation of glutathione. *Glia* **1998**, *23*, 139–145. [CrossRef]
17. Hirrlinger, J.; Schulz, J.B.; Dringen, R. Glutathione release from cultured brain cells: Multidrug resistance protein 1 mediates the release of GSH from rat astroglial cells. *J. Neurosci. Res.* **2002**, *69*, 318–326. [CrossRef] [PubMed]
18. Borlongan, C.V.; Koutouzis, T.K.; Freeman, T.B.; Cahill, D.W.; Sanberg, P.R. Behavioral pathology induced by repeated systemic injections of 3-nitropropionic acid mimics the motoric symptoms of huntington's disease. *Brain Res.* **1995**, *697*, 254–257. [CrossRef]
19. Schulz, J.B.; Henshaw, D.R.; MacGarvey, U.; Beal, M.F. Involvement of oxidative stress in 3-nitropropionic acid neurotoxicity. *Neurochem. Int.* **1996**, *29*, 167–171. [CrossRef]
20. Uliasz, T.F.; Hewett, S.J. A microtiter trypan blue absorbance assay for the quantitative determination of excitotoxic neuronal injury in cell culture. *J. Neurosci. Methods* **2000**, *100*, 157–163. [CrossRef]
21. Lobner, D. Comparison of the LDH and mtt assays for quantifying cell death: Validity for neuronal apoptosis? *J. Neurosci. Methods* **2000**, *96*, 147–152. [CrossRef]
22. He, Y.; Akumuo, R.C.; Yang, Y.; Hewett, S.J. Mice deficient in l-12/15 lipoxygenase show increased vulnerability to 3-nitropropionic acid neurotoxicity. *Neurosci. Lett.* **2017**, *643*, 65–69. [CrossRef] [PubMed]
23. Shih, A.Y.; Imbeault, S.; Barakauskas, V.; Erb, H.; Jiang, L.; Li, P.; Murphy, T.H. Induction of the Nrf2-driven antioxidant response confers neuroprotection during mitochondrial stress in vivo. *J. Biol. Chem.* **2005**, *280*, 22925–22936. [CrossRef] [PubMed]
24. Wang, J.; Bankiewicz, K.S.; Plunkett, R.J.; Oldfield, E.H. Intrastriatal implantation of interleukin-1. Reduction of parkinsonism in rats by enhancing neuronal sprouting from residual dopaminergic neurons in the ventral tegmental area of the midbrain. *J. Neurosurg.* **1994**, *80*, 484–490. [CrossRef] [PubMed]
25. Fagan, A.M.; Gage, F.H. Cholinergic sprouting in the hippocampus: A proposed role for IL-1. *Exp. Neurol.* **1990**, *110*, 105–120. [CrossRef]
26. Temporin, K.; Tanaka, H.; Kuroda, Y.; Okada, K.; Yachi, K.; Moritomo, H.; Murase, T.; Yoshikawa, H. IL-1beta promotes neurite outgrowth by deactivating RhoA via p38 mapk pathway. *Biochem. Biophys. Res. Commun.* **2008**, *365*, 375–380. [CrossRef] [PubMed]
27. Ohtsuki, T.; Ruetzler, C.A.; Tasaki, K.; Hallenbeck, J.M. Interleukin-1 mediates induction of tolerance to global ischemia in gerbil hippocampal CA1 neurons. *J. Cereb. Blood Flow Metab.* **1996**, *16*, 1137–1142. [CrossRef] [PubMed]
28. Pringle, A.K.; Niyadurupola, N.; Johns, P.; Anthony, D.C.; Iannotti, F. Interleukin-1beta exacerbates hypoxia-induced neuronal damage, but attenuates toxicity produced by simulated ischaemia and excitotoxicity in rat organotypic hippocampal slice cultures. *Neurosci. Lett.* **2001**, *305*, 29–32. [CrossRef]

29. Carlson, N.G.; Wieggel, W.A.; Chen, J.; Bacchi, A.; Rogers, S.W.; Gahring, L.C. Inflammatory cytokines IL-1 alpha, IL-1 beta, IL-6, and TNF-alpha impart neuroprotection to an excitotoxin through distinct pathways. *J. Immunol.* **1999**, *163*, 3963–3968. [PubMed]
30. Strijbos, P.J.; Rothwell, N.J. Interleukin-1 beta attenuates excitatory amino acid-induced neurodegeneration in vitro: Involvement of nerve growth factor. *J. Neurosci.* **1995**, *15*, 3468–3474. [CrossRef] [PubMed]
31. Shaftel, S.S.; Kyrkanides, S.; Olschowka, J.A.; Miller, J.N.; Johnson, R.E.; O'Banion, M.K. Sustained hippocampal IL-1 beta overexpression mediates chronic neuroinflammation and ameliorates alzheimer plaque pathology. *J. Clin. Investig.* **2007**, *117*, 1595–1604. [CrossRef] [PubMed]
32. Moore, A.H.; Wu, M.; Shaftel, S.S.; Graham, K.A.; O'Banion, M.K. Sustained expression of interleukin-1beta in mouse hippocampus impairs spatial memory. *Neuroscience* **2009**, *164*, 1484–1495. [CrossRef] [PubMed]
33. Matousek, S.B.; Hein, A.M.; Shaftel, S.S.; Olschowka, J.A.; Kyrkanides, S.; O'Banion, M.K. Cyclooxygenase-1 mediates prostaglandin E_2 elevation and contextual memory impairment in a model of sustained hippocampal interleukin-1beta expression. *J. Neurochem.* **2010**, *114*, 247–258. [PubMed]
34. Hassel, B.; Sonnewald, U. Selective inhibition of the tricarboxylic acid cycle of gabaergic neurons with 3-nitropropionic acid in vivo. *J. Neurochem.* **1995**, *65*, 1184–1191. [CrossRef] [PubMed]
35. Brouillet, E.; Conde, F.; Beal, M.F.; Hantraye, P. Replicating huntington's disease phenotype in experimental animals. *Prog. Neurobiol.* **1999**, *59*, 427–468. [CrossRef]
36. Beal, M.F.; Brouillet, E.; Jenkins, B.G.; Ferrante, R.J.; Kowall, N.W.; Miller, J.M.; Storey, E.; Srivastava, R.; Rosen, B.R.; Hyman, B.T. Neurochemical and histologic characterization of striatal excitotoxic lesions produced by the mitochondrial toxin 3-nitropropionic acid. *J. Neurosci.* **1993**, *13*, 4181–4192. [CrossRef] [PubMed]
37. Brouillet, E.; Jacquard, C.; Bizat, N.; Blum, D. 3-nitropropionic acid: A mitochondrial toxin to uncover physiopathological mechanisms underlying striatal degeneration in huntington's disease. *J. Neurochem.* **2005**, *95*, 1521–1540. [CrossRef] [PubMed]
38. Palfi, S.; Ferrante, R.J.; Brouillet, E.; Beal, M.F.; Dolan, R.; Guyot, M.C.; Peschanski, M.; Hantraye, P. Chronic 3-nitropropionic acid treatment in baboons replicates the cognitive and motor deficits of huntington's disease. *J. Neurosci.* **1996**, *16*, 3019–3025. [CrossRef] [PubMed]
39. Reynolds, D.S.; Carter, R.J.; Morton, A.J. Dopamine modulates the susceptibility of striatal neurons to 3-nitropropionic acid in the rat model of huntington's disease. *J. Neurosci.* **1998**, *18*, 10116–10127. [CrossRef] [PubMed]
40. Beal, M.F. Aging, energy, and oxidative stress in neurodegenerative diseases. *Ann. Neurol.* **1995**, *38*, 357–366. [CrossRef] [PubMed]
41. Ban, E.M. Interleukin-1 receptors in the brain: Characterization by quantitative in situ autoradiography. *Immunomethods* **1994**, *5*, 31–40. [CrossRef] [PubMed]
42. Ban, E.M.; Sarlieve, L.L.; Haour, F.G. Interleukin-1 binding sites on astrocytes. *Neuroscience* **1993**, *52*, 725–733. [CrossRef]
43. Choi, S.; Friedman, W.J. Inflammatory cytokines IL-1beta and TNF-alpha regulate $p75^{NTR}$ expression in CNS neurons and astrocytes by distinct cell-type-specific signalling mechanisms. *ASN Neuro* **2009**, *1*, e00010. [CrossRef] [PubMed]
44. Friedman, W.J. Cytokines regulate expression of the type 1 interleukin-1 receptor in rat hippocampal neurons and glia. *Exp. Neurol.* **2001**, *168*, 23–31. [CrossRef] [PubMed]
45. Tomozawa, Y.; Inoue, T.; Satoh, M. Expression of type I interleukin-1 receptor mrna and its regulation in cultured astrocytes. *Neurosci. Lett.* **1995**, *195*, 57–60. [CrossRef]
46. Srinivasan, D.; Yen, J.H.; Joseph, D.J.; Friedman, W. Cell type-specific interleukin-1beta signaling in the CNS. *J. Neurosci.* **2004**, *24*, 6482–6488. [CrossRef] [PubMed]
47. Sagara, J.I.; Miura, K.; Bannai, S. Maintenance of neuronal glutathione by glial cells. *J. Neurochem.* **1993**, *61*, 1672–1676. [CrossRef] [PubMed]
48. Sun, X.; Shih, A.Y.; Johannssen, H.C.; Erb, H.; Li, P.; Murphy, T.H. Two-photon imaging of glutathione levels in intact brain indicates enhanced redox buffering in developing neurons and cells at the cerebrospinal fluid and blood-brain interface. *J. Biol. Chem.* **2006**, *281*, 17420–17431. [CrossRef] [PubMed]
49. Shih, A.Y.; Johnson, D.A.; Wong, G.; Kraft, A.D.; Jiang, L.; Erb, H.; Johnson, J.A.; Murphy, T.H. Coordinate regulation of glutathione biosynthesis and release by Nrf2-expressing glia potently protects neurons from oxidative stress. *J. Neurosci.* **2003**, *23*, 3394–3406. [CrossRef] [PubMed]

50. Keelan, J.; Allen, N.J.; Antcliffe, D.; Pal, S.; Duchen, M.R. Quantitative imaging of glutathione in hippocampal neurons and glia in culture using monochlorobimane. *J. Neurosci. Res.* **2001**, *66*, 873–884. [CrossRef] [PubMed]
51. Raps, S.P.; Lai, J.C.; Hertz, L.; Cooper, A.J. Glutathione is present in high concentrations in cultured astrocytes but not in cultured neurons. *Brain Res.* **1989**, *493*, 398–401. [CrossRef]
52. Jakel, R.J.; Townsend, J.A.; Kraft, A.D.; Johnson, J.A. Nrf2-mediated protection against 6-hydroxydopamine. *Brain Res.* **2007**, *1144*, 192–201. [CrossRef] [PubMed]
53. Tanaka, J.; Toku, K.; Zhang, B.; Ishihara, K.; Sakanaka, M.; Maeda, N. Astrocytes protect neuronal death induced by reactive oxygen and nitrogen species. *Glia* **1999**, *28*, 85–96. [CrossRef]
54. Desagher, S.; Glowinski, J.; Premont, J. Astrocytes protect neurons from hydrogen peroxide toxicity. *J. Neurosci.* **1996**, *16*, 2553–2562. [CrossRef] [PubMed]
55. Makar, T.K.; Nedergaard, M.; Preuss, A.; Gelbard, A.S.; Perumal, A.S.; Cooper, A.J. Vitamin E, ascorbate, glutathione, glutathione disulfide, and enzymes of glutathione metabolism in cultures of chick astrocytes and neurons: Evidence that astrocytes play an important role in antioxidative processes in the brain. *J. Neurochem.* **1994**, *62*, 45–53. [CrossRef] [PubMed]
56. Gegg, M.E.; Clark, J.B.; Heales, S.J.R. Co-culture of neurones with glutathione deficient astrocytes leads to increased neuronal susceptibility to nitric oxide and increased glutamate-cysteine ligase activity. *Brain Res.* **2005**, *1036*, 1–6. [CrossRef] [PubMed]
57. Drukarch, B.; Schepens, E.; Jongenelen, C.A.M.; Stoof, J.C.; Langeveld, C.H. Astrocyte-mediated enhancement of neuronal survival is abolished by glutathione deficiency. *Brain Res.* **1997**, *770*, 123–130. [CrossRef]
58. Abramov, A.Y.; Canevari, L.; Duchen, M.R. Changes in intracellular calcium and glutathione in astrocytes as the primary mechanism of amyloid neurotoxicity. *J. Neurosci.* **2003**, *23*, 5088–5095. [CrossRef] [PubMed]
59. Shi, J.; He, Y.; Hewett, S.J.; Hewett, J.A. Interleukin 1beta regulation of the system x_c^- substrate-specific subunit, xCT, in primary mouse astrocytes involves the RNA-binding protein HuR. *J. Biol. Chem.* **2016**, *291*, 1643–1651. [CrossRef] [PubMed]
60. Dringen, R.; Gutterer, J.M.; Hirrlinger, J. Glutathione metabolism in brain. Metabolic interaction between astrocytes and neurons in the defense against reactive oxygen species. *Eur. J. Biochem.* **2000**, *267*, 4912–4916. [CrossRef] [PubMed]
61. Dringen, R.; Pfeiffer, B.; Hamprecht, B. Synthesis of the antioxidant glutathione in neurons: Supply by astrocytes of CysGly as precursor for neuronal glutathione. *J. Neurosci.* **1999**, *19*, 562–569. [CrossRef] [PubMed]
62. Schulz, J.B.; Lindenau, J.; Seyfried, J.; Dichgans, J. Glutathione, oxidative stress and neurodegeneration. *Eur. J. Biochem.* **2000**, *267*, 4904–4911. [CrossRef] [PubMed]
63. Kranich, O.; Hamprecht, B.; Dringen, R. Different preferences in the utilization of amino acids for glutathione synthesis in cultured neurons and astroglial cells derived from rat brain. *Neurosci. Lett.* **1996**, *219*, 211–214. [CrossRef]
64. Stridh, M.H.; Tranberg, M.; Weber, S.G.; Blomstrand, F.; Sandberg, M. Stimulated efflux of amino acids and glutathione from cultured hippocampal slices by omission of extracellular calcium: Likely involvement of connexin hemichannels. *J. Biol. Chem.* **2008**, *283*, 10347–10356. [CrossRef] [PubMed]
65. Rana, S.; Dringen, R. Gap junction hemichannel-mediated release of glutathione from cultured rat astrocytes. *Neurosci. Lett.* **2007**, *415*, 45–48. [CrossRef] [PubMed]
66. Hanigan, M.H.; Ricketts, W.A. Extracellular glutathione is a source of cysteine for cells that express gamma-glutamyl transpeptidase. *Biochemistry* **1993**, *32*, 6302–6306. [CrossRef] [PubMed]
67. Olson, C.K.; Binkley, F. Metabolism of glutathione. III. Enzymatic hydrolysis of cysteinylglycine. *J. Biol. Chem.* **1950**, *186*, 731–735. [PubMed]
68. Dringen, R.; Gutterer, J.M.; Gros, C.; Hirrlinger, J. Aminopeptidase n mediates the utilization of the GSH precursor CysGly by cultured neurons. *J. Neurosci. Res.* **2001**, *66*, 1003–1008. [CrossRef] [PubMed]
69. Babior, B.M. Oxygen-dependent microbial killing by phagocytes (second of two parts). *N. Engl. J. Med.* **1978**, *298*, 721–725. [CrossRef] [PubMed]
70. Babior, B.M. Oxygen-dependent microbial killing by phagocytes (first of two parts). *N. Engl. J. Med.* **1978**, *298*, 659–668. [CrossRef] [PubMed]

71. Carreras, M.C.; Pargament, G.A.; Catz, S.D.; Poderoso, J.J.; Boveris, A. Kinetics of nitric oxide and hydrogen peroxide production and formation of peroxynitrite during the respiratory burst of human neutrophils. *FEBS Lett.* **1994**, *341*, 65–68. [CrossRef]
72. Zhang, P.; Hatter, A.; Liu, B. Manganese chloride stimulates rat microglia to release hydrogen peroxide. *Toxicol. Lett.* **2007**, *173*, 88–100. [CrossRef] [PubMed]
73. Banati, R.B.; Gehrmann, J.; Schubert, P.; Kreutzberg, G.W. Cytotoxicity of microglia. *Glia* **1993**, *7*, 111–118. [CrossRef] [PubMed]
74. Henzler, T.; Steudle, E. Transport and metabolic degradation of hydrogen peroxide in chara corallina: Model calculations and measurements with the pressure probe suggest transport of H_2O_2 across water channels. *J. Exp. Bot.* **2000**, *51*, 2053–2066. [CrossRef] [PubMed]
75. Badaut, J.; Lasbennes, F.; Magistretti, P.J.; Regli, L. Aquaporins in brain: Distribution, physiology, and pathophysiology. *J. Cereb. Blood Flow Metab.* **2002**, *22*, 367–378. [CrossRef] [PubMed]
76. Badaut, J.; Fukuda, A.M.; Jullienne, A.; Petry, K.G. Aquaporin and brain diseases. *Biochim. Biophys. Acta* **2014**, *1840*, 1554–1565. [CrossRef] [PubMed]
77. Sato, H.; Tamba, M.; Ishii, T.; Bannai, S. Cloning and expression of a plasma membrane cystine/glutamate exchange transporter composed of two distinct proteins. *J. Biol. Chem.* **1999**, *274*, 11455–11458. [CrossRef] [PubMed]
78. Bassi, M.T.; Gasol, E.; Manzoni, M.; Pineda, M.; Riboni, M.; Martin, R.; Zorzano, A.; Borsani, G.; Palacin, M. Identification and characterisation of human xCT that co-expresses, with 4F2 heavy chain, the amino acid transport activity system xc. *Pflugers Archiv Eur. J. Physiol.* **2001**, *442*, 286–296. [CrossRef]
79. Bridges, C.C.; Kekuda, R.; Wang, H.; Prasad, P.D.; Mehta, P.; Huang, W.; Smith, S.B.; Ganapathy, V. Structure, function, and regulation of human cystine/glutamate transporter in retinal pigment epithelial cells. *Investig. Ophthalmol. Vis. Sci.* **2001**, *42*, 47–54.
80. Deneke, S.M.; Fanburg, B.L. Regulation of cellular glutathione. *Am. J. Physiol.* **1989**, *257*, L163–L173. [CrossRef] [PubMed]
81. Gennuso, F.; Fernetti, C.; Tirolo, C.; Testa, N.; L'Episcopo, F.; Caniglia, S.; Morale, M.C.; Ostrow, J.D.; Pascolo, L.; Tiribelli, C.; et al. Bilirubin protects astrocytes from its own toxicity by inducing up-regulation and translocation of multidrug resistance-associated protein 1 (Mrp1). *Proc. Natl. Acad. Sci. USA* **2004**, *101*, 2470–2475. [CrossRef] [PubMed]
82. Ye, B.; Shen, H.; Zhang, J.; Zhu, Y.G.; Ransom, B.R.; Chen, X.C.; Ye, Z.C. Dual pathways mediate beta-amyloid stimulated glutathione release from astrocytes. *Glia* **2015**, *63*, 2208–2219. [CrossRef] [PubMed]
83. Ballatori, N.; Hammond, C.L.; Cunningham, J.B.; Krance, S.M.; Marchan, R. Molecular mechanisms of reduced glutathione transport: Role of the MRP/CFTR/ABCC and OATP/SLC21A families of membrane proteins. *Toxicol. Appl. Pharmacol.* **2005**, *204*, 238–255. [CrossRef] [PubMed]
84. Becher, B.; Spath, S.; Goverman, J. Cytokine networks in neuroinflammation. *Nat. Rev. Immunol.* **2017**, *17*, 49–59. [CrossRef] [PubMed]

8

Comparing Palm Oil, Tocotrienol-Rich Fraction and α-Tocopherol Supplementation on the Antioxidant Levels of Older Adults

Nor Helwa Ezzah Nor Azman [1], Jo Aan Goon [1,*], Siti Madiani Abdul Ghani [1], Zalina Hamid [2] and Wan Zurinah Wan Ngah [1]

1 Department of Biochemistry, Faculty of Medicine, Universiti Kebangsaan Malaysia, Jalan Yaacob Latif, Kuala Lumpur 56000, Malaysia; ezzahafezzi@gmail.com (N.H.E.N.A.); ctiemadiani@gmail.com (S.M.A.G.); wwanzurinah@yahoo.com (W.Z.W.N.)

2 Sime Darby Foods and Beverages Marketing Sdn. Bhd, Petaling Jaya 47301, Selangor, Malaysia; zalina.hamid@simedarby.com

* Correspondence: joaan@ukm.edu.my

Abstract: Background: Tocotrienol and tocopherol are known to prevent numerous degenerative diseases. The aim of this study is to compare the effects of tocotrienol-rich fraction (TRF) with α-tocopherol (α-TF) on the antioxidant status of healthy individuals aged between 50 and 55 years. Methods: Volunteers were divided into groups receiving placebo (n = 23), α-TF (n = 24) and TRF (n = 24). Fasting venous blood samples were taken at baseline (0 month), 3 months and 6 months of supplementation for the determination of superoxide dismutase (SOD), catalase (CAT), and glutathione peroxidase (GPx) activities as well as for reduced glutathione (GSH) and oxidized glutathione (GSSG) concentrations. Results: CAT and GPx were unaffected by TRF and α-TF supplementations. SOD activity increased significantly after six months of TRF supplementation. Analysis by gender showed that only female subjects had significant increases in SOD and GPx activities after six months of TRF supplementation. GPx activity was also significantly higher in females compared to males after six months of TRF supplementation. The GSH/GSSG ratio increased significantly after six months of TRF and α-TF supplementation in only the female subjects. Conclusion: TRF and α-TF supplementation exhibited similar effects to the antioxidant levels of older adults with TRF having more significant effects in females.

Keywords: aging; oxidative stress; vitamin E; oxidative status; enzyme

---

1. Introduction

Vitamin E is a potent chain-breaking antioxidant that has been shown to reduce oxidative stress and prevent the propagation of free radical reactions. There are eight naturally occurring forms of vitamin E that are distinguished by the methylation pattern on the chromanol ring. These are further divided into four isomers designated as alpha (α), beta (β), delta (δ), and gamma (γ) tocopherols and tocotrienols [1]. Tocopherols and tocotrienols have the same basic chemical structure characterized by a long chain attached at the second position of a chromanol ring. Tocotrienols differ from tocopherols because they possess a farnesyl rather than a saturated isoprenoid C_{16} side chain [2]. All tocopherols and tocotrienols are potent antioxidants with lipoperoxyl radical-scavenging activities [3]. Based on a recent review, tocotrienol is not considered a part of the vitamin E family because it has distinct biological activities, cellular targets and molecular mechanism of action that is different from α-tocopherol [4]. In tabulating the Dietary Reference Intakes for vitamin E, the United States Pharmacopoeia also standardizes the units definition of different vitamin E analogues according to the efficiency of α-tocopherol because β-, γ- and δ-tocopherol and the tocotrienols are considered to be less active [5].

Most research on vitamin E has primarily focused on α-tocopherol (α-TF) [6] because α-TF is the predominant form of vitamin E in tissues and human plasma. However, varying outcomes have been obtained regarding its protective role in the prevention or treatment of chronic diseases such as cancer and cardiovascular diseases [7,8]. Tocotrienol has been reported to be more effective in the prevention of disease progression compared to tocopherol [9–15]. However, most studies were done using animals and in vitro models. To date, very limited data is available from human interventional studies using tocotrienol.

We previously reported that tocotrienol-rich fraction (TRF) supplementation restored the redox balance of individuals over 50 years of age after six months of supplementation [16,17]. Increases of plasma α-TF and tocotrienol with supplementation have been associated with a reduction in DNA damage, and improvements in lipid profile and oxidative status in older adults [17,18]. To the best of our knowledge, studies comparing the efficacy between tocopherols and tocotrienols supplementation in humans are still scarce and gender response disparities to the supplements is yet to be determined.

Humans are equipped with an extremely sophisticated and complex antioxidant protection system to protect the cells and organ systems of the body against free radicals [19,20]. The enzymatic components of the antioxidative defense system comprises several antioxidant enzymes such as superoxide dismutase (SOD), catalase (CAT), glutathione peroxidase (GPx), enzymes of ascorbate-glutathione (AsA-GSH) cycle, ascorbate peroxidase (APX), monodehydroascorbate reductase (MDHAR), dehydroascorbate reductase (DHAR), and glutathione reductase (GR) [21] as well as non-enzymatic antioxidant systems such as bilirubin, glutathione (GSH), carotenoids, and vitamins C and E. The antioxidant enzymes operate in different subcellular compartments and respond in concert when cells are exposed to oxidative stress [22]. However, the effectiveness of the natural antioxidant network has been reported to decline with aging [23–25]. Thus, the purpose of this study is to compare the effects of TRF and α-TF supplementation, respectively, on the antioxidant levels of healthy individuals aged between 50 and 55 years.

2. Materials and Methods

2.1. Study Subjects

The protocol of this study was approved by the Research and Ethics Committee of the Faculty of Medicine, Universiti Kebangsaan Malaysia (UKM 1.5.3.5/244/FF-434-2011). A total of 237 volunteers aged 50 to 55 years were approached for general health screening. Volunteers with a positive history of cardiovascular disease, stroke, chronic inflammatory diseases, hematological diseases or surgery within 6 months; serious medical illness such as cancer, malignant hypertension, uncontrolled diabetes or cardiopulmonary insufficiency; and consumption of supplements or pharmaceutical products with antioxidant properties were excluded. Physical activity of volunteers was not documented. However, volunteers were advised to be persistent with their daily physical activities when enrolled into the study to prevent modifications of oxidative status in the body by sudden onset of any exercise regime. A total of 86 healthy, non-smoking and non-alcoholic volunteers were enrolled into the study after obtaining written informed consent. Among this number, 71 subjects completed the supplementation study, while 15 subjects dropped out due to personal reasons and health problems.

2.2. Experimental Design

Recruited subjects were randomly divided into three groups and supplemented accordingly for 6 months with placebo (n = 23), α-TF (400 IU/day) (n = 24) and TRF (150 mg/day) (n = 24). The doses of supplementation used were based on positive results of previous human studies [26–29]. All subjects were requested to consume the supplements after dinner to ensure proper absorption [30,31] and encouraged to maintain their usual diet and lifestyle throughout the study period. The supplements including placebo were supplied by Sime Darby Food and Beverages Marketing Sdn. Bhd (previously known as Sime Darby Bioganic). Each TRF capsule contained 70.4 mg α-tocotrienol, 4.8 mg β-tocotrienol, 33.6 mg δ-tocotrienol, 57.6 mg γ-tocotrienol, and 48 mg α-tocopherol. α-TF capsules contained only tocopherol, while the placebo contained olive oil. The treatment was double-blinded throughout the study period until all data were collected, after which the randomization code was broken. Compliance of subjects was verified by the determination of plasma TRF and α-TF levels by high-performance liquid chromatography. The data of increased TRF and α-TF plasma levels after supplementation was reported earlier in a separate publication [23].

2.3. Sample Collection

Blood sampling was performed at baseline (0 months), 3 months and 6 months of supplementation. Venous blood samples (15 mL) were drawn into heparin tubes between 08:00 a.m. and 10:00 a.m. and processed within 1 to 2 h. Plasma was separated by centrifugation at 1800 rpm for 30 min at 4 °C. The obtained erythrocytes were washed two times with 0.9% sodium chloride solution. The mixture was then separated again by centrifugation at 3000 *g* for 10 min at 4 °C. Washed erythrocytes were used for the determination of antioxidant activities (SOD, CAT and GPx) and non-enzymatic antioxidant (reduced GSH and oxidized glutathione (GSSG)). Samples were then stored at −80 °C until further analysis.

2.4. Determination of Erythrocyte Antioxidant Enzymes (SOD, CAT, GPx)

Blood antioxidant enzymes activity (SOD, CAT and GPx) were measured via Cayman Chemical assay kit (Cayman Chemical Company, Ann Arbor, MI, USA). The SOD assay kit utilizes a tetrazolium salt for detection of the superoxide radicals generated by xanthine oxidase and hypoxanthine. The amount of enzyme required to exhibit 50% dismutation of superoxide radical is defined as one unit of SOD. This assay kit can measure three types of SOD: Cu/Zn, Mn, and FeSOD. SOD activity was expressed as U/mL.

The CAT assay kit is based on the reaction of the enzyme with methanol in the presence of an optimal concentration of hydrogen peroxide (H_2O_2). The formaldehyde produced was measured colorimetrically with Purpald, a chromogen that specifically forms a bicyclic heterocycle with aldehydes, which upon oxidation changes from colorless to a purple color and quantified at an absorbance of 540 nm. CAT activity was expressed as nmol/min/mL.

GPx activity was determined via the coupled reaction with GR and measured by a decreased absorbance at 340 nm. GPx produces GSSG upon reduction of hydroperoxide while GR returns GSSG to its reduced state. GPx activity was expressed as nmol/min/mL.

2.5. Determination of Erythrocyte GSH and GSSG Concentration

Reduced GSH and GSSG were measured by Cayman Chemical Glutathione assay kit (Cayman Chemical Company, Ann Arbor, MI, USA). The assay kit used glutathione reductase through the enzymatic recycling method for the quantification of GSH. The sulfhydryl group of GSH reacts with 5,5′-dithio-bis-2-nitrobenzoic acid (DTNB) to form a yellow-colored 5-thio-2-nitrobenzoic acid (TNB). The rate of TNB production was directly proportional to the concentration of GSH in all samples. The erythrocyte lysate was deproteinated using metaphosphoric acid (Sigma-Aldrich, St. Louis, MO, USA), 2-vinylpyridine (Merck, Jerman, Kenilworth, NJ, USA) and triethanolamine (Sigma-Aldrich, St. Louis, MO, USA) to avoid interferences from particulates and sulfhydryl group in proteins. GSH concentration in the samples was measured at 405–414 nm absorbance and expressed as μM.

2.6. Statistical Analysis

Statistical analysis was performed using the Statistical Package for Social Sciences (SPSS) Version 22.0 (IBM Corp., Chicago, IL, USA). The Shapiro–Wilk test was used to check the normality of the variables. Statistical evaluation was measured using two-way analysis of variance (ANOVA) test to compare changes from baseline to 3 and 6 months for all variables to verify the effects of treatment. A post hoc Least Significant Difference (LSD) multiple comparison test was performed to compare the average of the treatment group to the average of the control group and the impact of gender. Statistical tests with $p < 0.05$ were considered as significant. All the results are presented in mean ± S.E.M.

3. Results

3.1. Demography of Subjects

The mean ± SEM age for the subjects were 52.2 ± 2.1 for placebo, 52.5 ± 2.5 for α-TF, and 53.4 ± 1.5 for TRF. The number of subjects from each gender was comparable for the placebo, α-TF, and TRF groups (Table 1). The mean age of supplemented groups was not significantly different compared to placebo.

Table 1. Baseline and intervention characteristics of the subjects.

	Group								
	Placebo			α-Tocopherol			(Tocotrienol-Rich Fraction) TRF		
	Male	Female	Total	Male	Female	Total	Male	Female	Total
Subjects (n)	8	15	23	9	15	24	9	15	24
Age (years)	52.7 ± 1.6	52.1 ± 1.7	52.2 ± 2.1	53.5 ± 1.5	52.7 ± 1.2	52.5 ± 2.5	53.1 ± 1.3	52.7 ± 1.9	53.4 ± 1.5
p value	-	-	-	0.335	0.49	0.845	0.609	0.678	0.935

3.2. Antioxidant Enzymes Activities (SOD, CAT and GPx)

A significant effect was observed in SOD activity with supplementation of TRF. TRF supplementation significantly increased SOD activity after 6 months of treatment compared to baseline (0 month) (Figure 1). Further analysis by grouping of gender showed that SOD activity increased in female subjects after 6 months of TRF supplementation compared to baseline (0 month) (Figure 2).

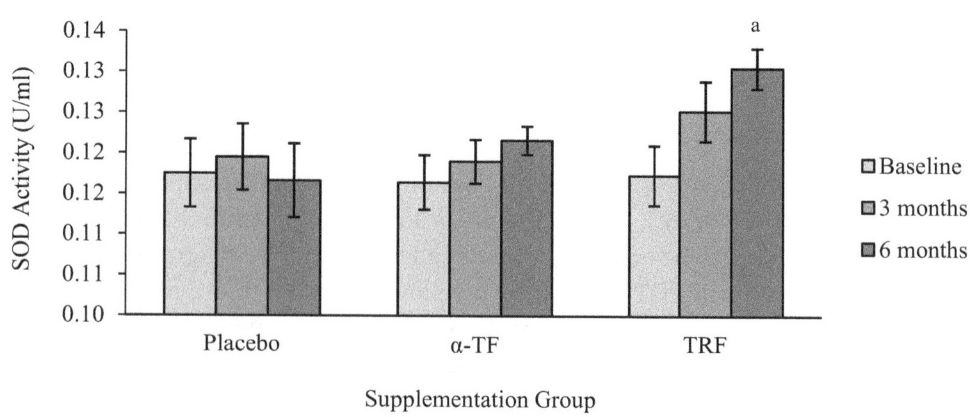

Figure 1. Effect of α-tocopherol (α-TF) and tocotrienol-rich fraction (TRF) supplementation on superoxide dismutase (SOD) activity for 6 months. a = statistically significant compared to 0-month TRF group, $p < 0.05$.

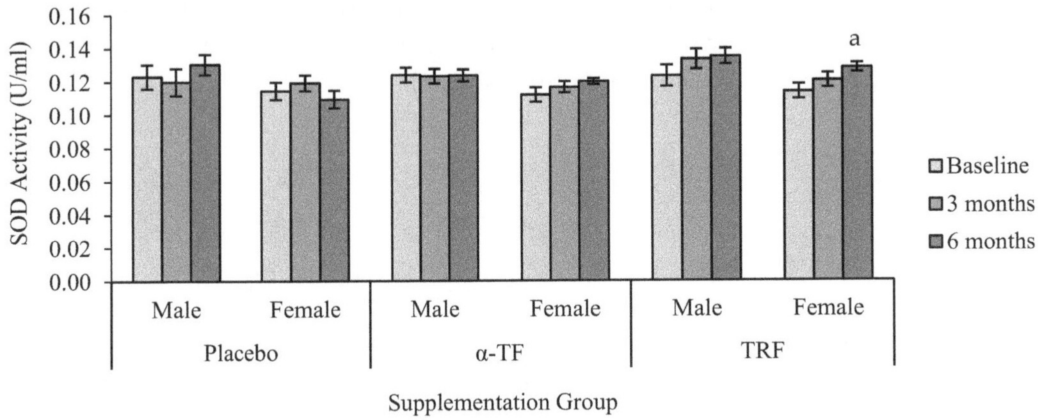

Figure 2. Effect of α-TF and TRF supplementation between males and females on SOD activity for 6 months. a = statistically significant compared to 0-month TRF group (female), $p < 0.05$.

CAT activity remained unchanged in TRF and α-TF supplemented groups (Figure 3). By contrast, CAT activity decreased after 6 months in the placebo group, particularly among the female subjects when compared to the baseline (0 month) (Figure 4).

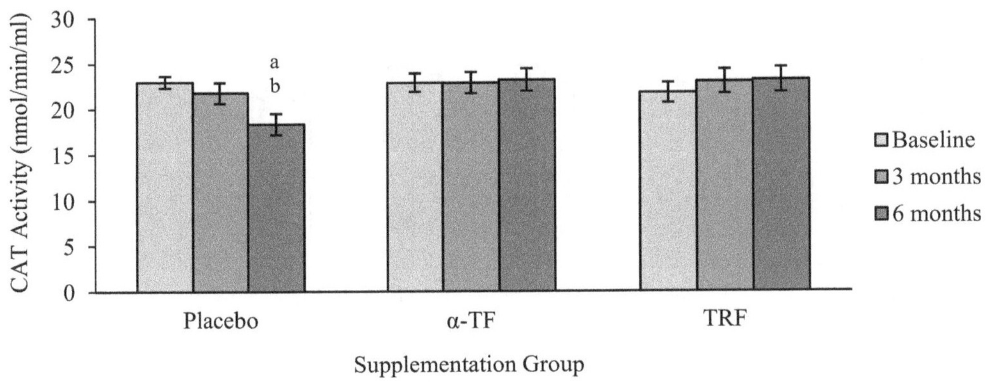

Figure 3. Effect of α-TF and TRF supplementation on catalase (CAT) activity for 6 months. a = statistically significant compared to 0-month placebo group, b = statistically significant compared to 3 months placebo group, $p < 0.05$.

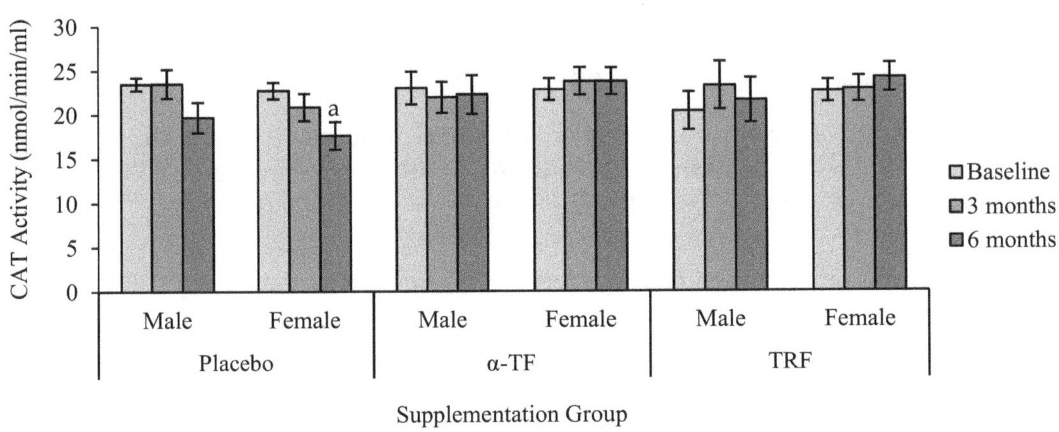

Figure 4. Effect of α-TF and TRF supplementation between males and females on CAT activity for 6 months. a = statistically significant compared to 0-month placebo group (female), $p < 0.05$.

However, no significant differences were found in the activity of GPx between all groups (Figure 5). Similar to the results of SOD, only female subjects had increased GPx activity after 6 months of TRF supplementation compared to baseline (0 month) (Figure 6).

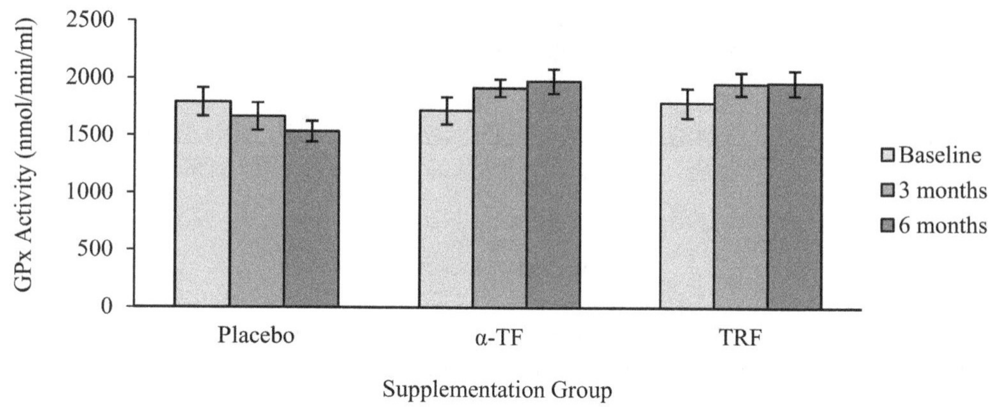

Figure 5. Effect of α-TF and TRF supplementation on glutathione peroxidase (GPx) activity for 6 months. GPx activity remained unchanged throughout the study with both supplements.

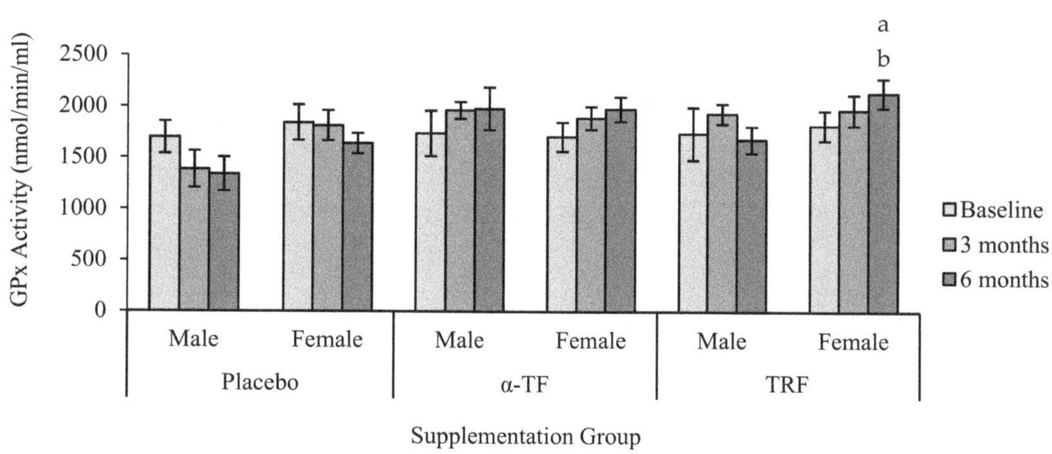

Figure 6. Effect of α-TF and TRF supplementation between males and females on GPx activity for 6 months. a = statistically significant compared to 0-month TRF group (female), b = statistically significant compared to 6 months TRF group (male), $p < 0.05$.

3.3. *Non-Enzymatic Antioxidant (GSH and GSSG)*

No significant differences were found in the concentration of GSH with TRF and α-TF supplementations (Figure 7). In addition, there were no apparent differences in GSH concentration between male and female subjects after TRF and α-TF supplementation (Figure 8).

GSSG concentration was significantly decreased after 6 months of α-TF supplementation compared to baseline (month 0) and 3 months (Figure 9). Similarly, TRF supplementation also decreased the concentration of GSSG after 6 months of supplementation. Analysis by gender revealed a marked reduction of GSSG in the male subjects after 6 months of α-TF supplementation (Figure 10). No differences were observed between the two genders in the TRF and placebo groups.

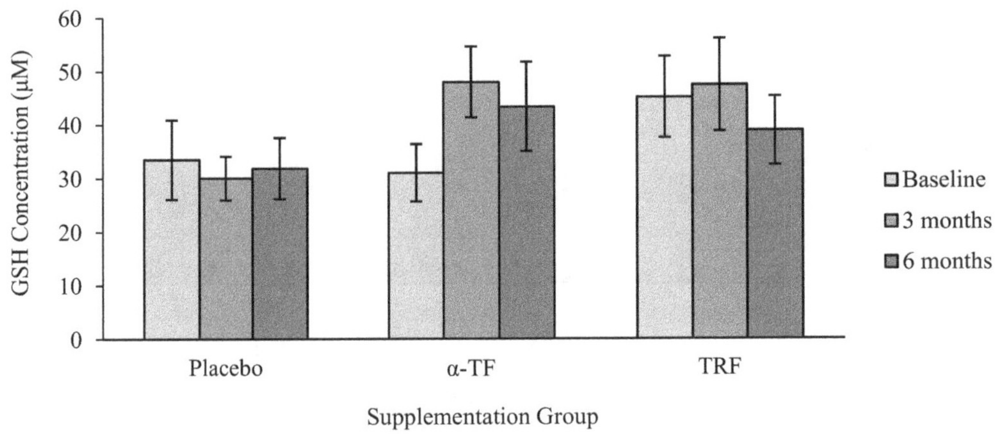

Figure 7. Effect of α-TF and TRF supplementation on glutathione (GSH) concentration for 6 months. The level of GSH remained unchanged throughout the supplementation period in both groups of vitamins.

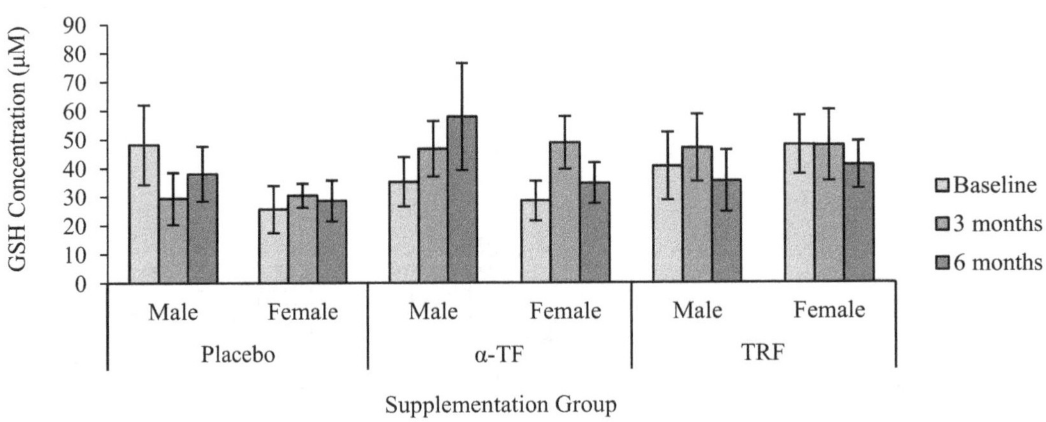

Figure 8. Effect of α-TF and TRF supplementation between males and females on GSH concentration for 6 months. No differences in the level of GSH were found between genders in all supplemented groups.

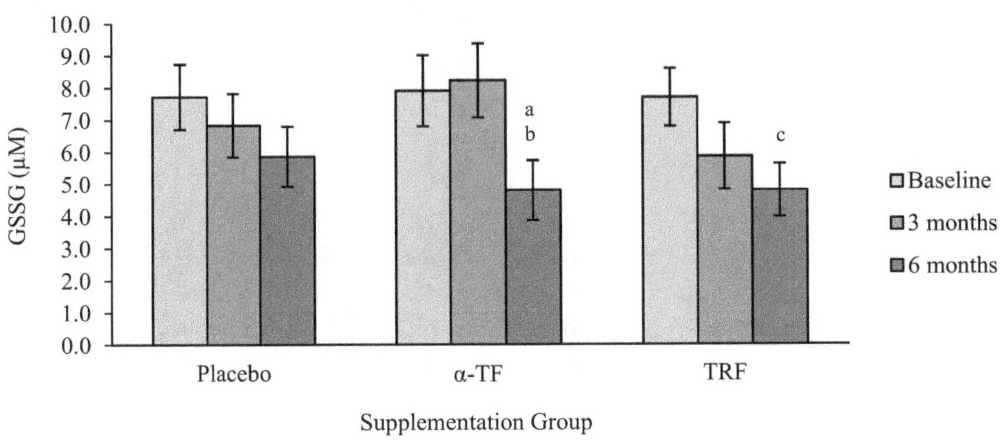

Figure 9. Effect of α-TF and TRF supplementation on oxidized glutathione (GSSG) concentration for 6 months. a = significantly different compared to 0-month α-TF, b = significantly different compared to 3 months α-TF, c = significantly different compared to 0 month TRF, $p < 0.05$.

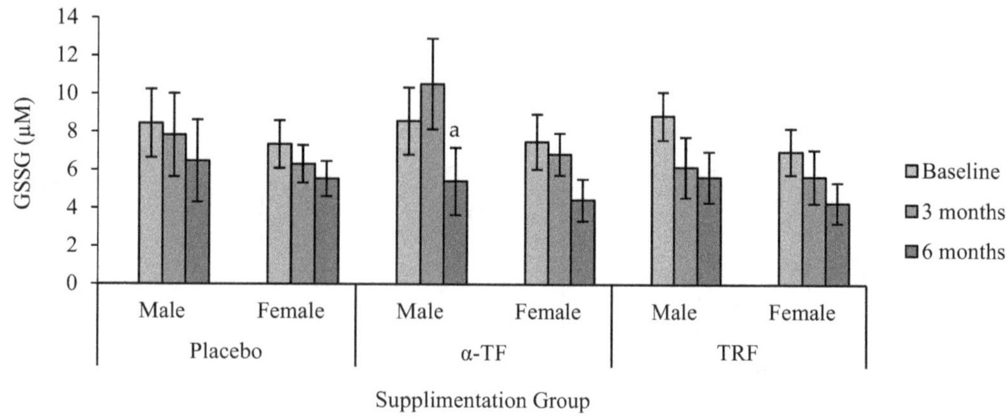

Figure 10. Effect of α-TF and TRF supplementation between males and females on GSSG concentration for 6 months. a = significantly different compared to 3-month α-TF (male), $p < 0.05$.

The ratio of GSH/GSSG increased after 6 months of TRF and α-TF supplementation (Figure 11). These effects were seen only in female subjects with both supplementations (Figure 12).

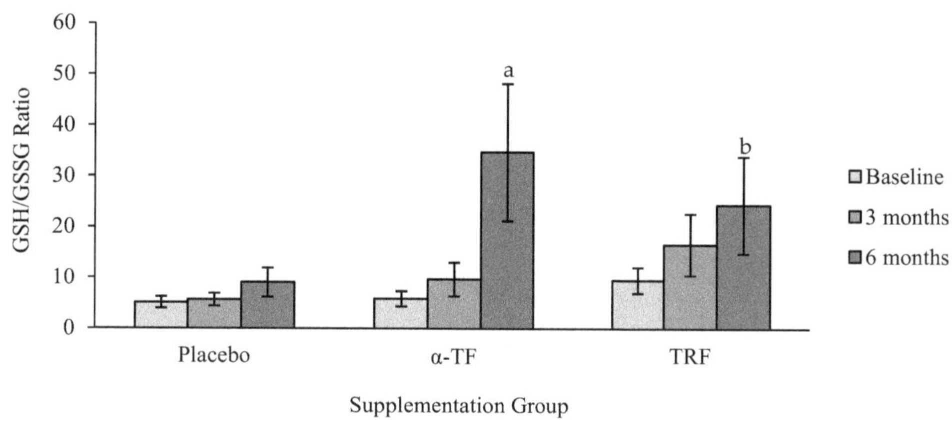

Figure 11. Effect of α-TF and TRF supplementation on GSH/GSSG ratio for 6 months. a = significantly different compared to 0-month α-TF, b = significantly different compared to 0-month TRF, $p < 0.05$.

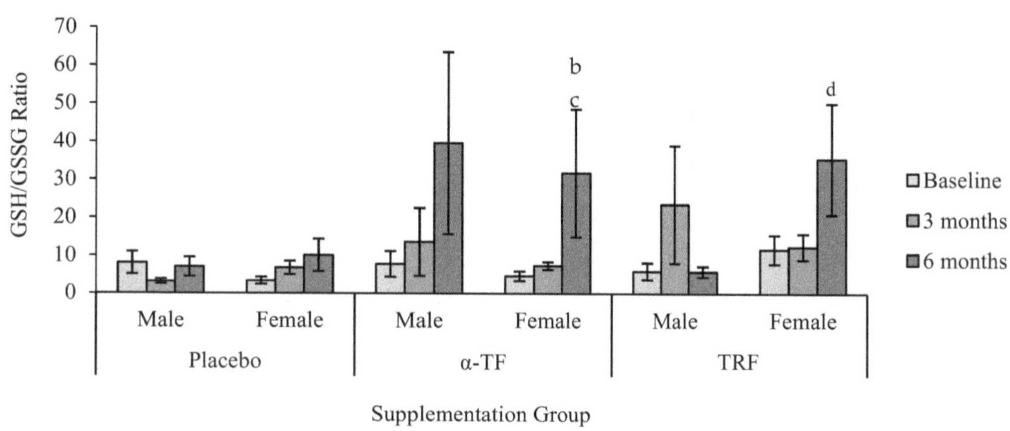

Figure 12. Effect of α-TF and TRF supplementation between male and female on GSH/GSSG ratio for 6 months. b = significantly different compared to 0-month α-TF (female), c = significantly different compared to 3-month α-TF (female), d = significantly different compared to 0-month TRF (female), $p < 0.05$.

4. Discussion

Oxidative stress is known to increase with age. Many studies have highlighted the benefits of vitamin E as an antioxidant to prevent damages to macromolecules in aging [27,32]. Results of this comparative study between TRF and α-TF further elucidate the role of these vitamin E isomers in preventing oxidative damages as reported previously.

SOD is an intracellular enzymatic antioxidant that catalyzes the conversion of superoxide anions to molecular oxygen and H_2O_2, whereas CAT and GPx promote the conversion of H_2O_2 into water and oxygen [33]. In this study, the activities of SOD and GPx were found to increase after 6 months of TRF supplementation. These outcomes are seen to be beneficial as SOD and GPx help neutralize reactive oxygen species that are generated extensively with age.

The activity of CAT remained unchanged throughout the study period regardless of supplementation with TRF or α-TF. However, its activity decreased after six months in the placebo group. Given the fact that both CAT and GPx remove H_2O_2 in the antioxidant network, the reduction of CAT activity suggests that the removal of H_2O_2 was predominantly accomplished by GPx in the placebo group. In line with the current results, TRF supplementation was also found to increase the activity of GPx without altering the activity of CAT in our previous study [16].

The unaltered activity of CAT with TRF and α-TF observed in this study is seen as a positive effect because the placebo group had decreased CAT activity after six months of study. Both supplements may have helped to maintain the oxidative status of the older adults through upregulation of other antioxidants as reported earlier.

According to a previous finding, premenopausal women aged 53.2 ± 5.7 years have been found to have increased oxidative stress manifested by elevated total antioxidant status [34]. The development of oxidative stress was suggested to be a consequence of reduced levels of circulating estrogens and increased abdominal and total body fat in women. Although it was not ascertained whether the female subjects in the present study were premenopausal, TRF supplementation effectively increased SOD and GPx activities in females of similar age.

The discrepancy between the response to antioxidant supplementation seen between men and women in this study could be due to the difference in the level of estrogen. This hormone has been implicated as a phenolic antioxidant due to the presence of phenolic A-ring in its structure [35]. Previous researches have shown that estrogen can upregulate the expression of antioxidant enzymes and protect against the release of cytochrome c by mitochondria [36,37]. This hormone is known to decrease in aged women but not in aged men [38]. We postulate that the level of estrogen in the female subjects of this study could have been lower compared to men, hence their antioxidant status was more receptive and responsive to antioxidant therapy. However, further research is needed to determine the extent of the role of estrogen in the oxidative status of women compared to men in aging.

Glutathione is an important constituent in the endogenous antioxidant defense system. Reduced GSH is a biological antioxidant that helps to protect the cells from reactive oxygen species such as free radicals, heavy metals, lipid peroxides and peroxides. It is the major endogenous antioxidant produced by the cells, participating directly in the neutralization of free radicals and reactive oxygen compounds, as well as maintaining exogenous antioxidants [39,40]. GSH is synthesized in the liver and GSH deficiency is associated with aging, cardiovascular disease, and cancer [41–44].

GSSG is usually reduced into reduced GSH via GSSG reductase, an enzyme that uses nicotine adenine dinucleotide phosphate (NADPH) as a cofactor [45]. The increase in GSSG levels is associated with oxidative stress [46,47] and may contribute to many chronic degenerative diseases. High level of GSSG is also found to promote the formation of extensive disulfide mixture and deactivation of SH-dependent enzyme.

The ratio of reduced GSH to GSSG levels in the blood is an indicator of cellular health. The GSH/GSSG ratio is considered very important as an index of oxidative status and guidance to a range of chronic risk to humans [48,49]. Decreased ratio of GSH/GSSG was proposed as a major contributing factor to some chronic diseases such as pneumonia, amyotrophic lateral sclerosis, kidney failure, malignant disorders, diabetes, high blood pressure, Parkinson's disease, Alzheimer's disease, and cataract formation [50–54].

In this study, supplementation of TRF and α-TF significantly increased the ratio of GSH/GSSG after 6 months. Tocotrienol and tocopherol are known to result in noncompetitive inhibition toward the substrates (GSH and 1-chloro-2,4-dinitrobenzene) of glutathione S-transferase (GST). Conformational changes of the enzyme lead to marked reduction of GST activity [55]. The mechanistic action of TRF and α-TF towards GST together with an improved redox balance could have led to the increase of GSH and reduction of GSSG concentrations as measured in this study after six months of supplementation. Interestingly, α-TF and TRF supplementations increased the ratio of GSH/GSSG only in the female subjects. Since not many studies have compared the levels of GSH and GSSG between genders in humans, further research engaging a larger number of subjects is needed to elucidate gender-associated differences in oxidative status.

5. Conclusions

TRF supplementation showed comparable effects to α-TF in modulating the activities of antioxidant enzymes and increasing the ratio of GSH/GSSG in healthy older adults. TRF seemed to improve the antioxidant levels of females more significantly compared to males. Nevertheless, a study with a bigger sample size is necessary to conclude this gender-associated disparity as this study is limited to an unequal number of males and females in every supplemented group.

Author Contributions: N.H.E.N.A. was conducted the study, analysis and interpretation of data in addition to drafting the manuscript. J.A.G. contributed to the content of the manuscript. S.M.A.G. was involved in subject screening, assessed the physical activity questionnaire and interpretation of data. Z.H. contributed to supply the supplementation of placebo, a-TF and TRF capsules. W.Z.W.N. was instrumental in the study's inception, design the study, obtained approval while providing critical analysis of data interpretation and manuscript review. The final manuscript has been read and approved by all authors.

Funding: Financial support for this study was provided by UKM Economic Transformation Programme grant (ETP-2013-007).

Acknowledgments: The authors thank Zalina Hamid from Sime Darby Foods and Beverages Marketing Sdn. Bhd (previously known as Sime Darby Bioganic) for supplying the TRF, α-TF and placebo capsules used in the study.

Conflicts of Interest: The authors declare that they have no competing interests.

References

1. Ulatowski, L.M.; Manor, D. Vitamin E and neurodegeneration. *Neurobiol. Dis.* **2015**, *84*, 78–83. [CrossRef] [PubMed]
2. Rizvi, S.; Raza, S.T.; Ahmed, F.; Ahmad, A.; Abbas, S.; Mahdi, F. The role of vitamin E in human health and some diseases. *Sultan Qaboos Univ. Med. J.* **2014**, *14*, e157–e165. [PubMed]
3. Jiang, Q. Natural forms of vitamin E: Metabolism, antioxidant and anti-inflammatory activities and the role in disease prevention and therapy. *Free Radic. Biol. Med.* **2014**, *72*, 76–90. [CrossRef] [PubMed]
4. Comitato, R.; Ambra, R.; Virgili, F. Tocotrienols: A Family of Molecules with Specific Biological Activities. *Antioxidants* **2017**, *6*, 93. [CrossRef] [PubMed]
5. Board, F.A.N.; Medicine, I.O. *Dietary Reference Intakes for Vitamin C, Vitamin E, Selenium, and Carotenoids*; The National Academies Press: Washington, DC, USA, 2000.
6. Jiang, Q.; Christen, S.; Shigenaga, M.K.; Ames, B.N. Gamma-tocopherol, the major form of vitamin E in the US diet, deserves more attention. *Am. J. Clin. Nutr.* **2001**, *74*, 714–722. [CrossRef] [PubMed]
7. Moya-Camarena, S.; Jiang, Q. The Role of Vitamin E Forms in Cancer Prevention and Therapy—Studies in Human Intervention Trials and Animal Models. In *Nutraceuticals and Cancer*; Sarkar, F.H., Ed.; Springer: Dordrecht, The Netherlands, 2012; pp. 323–354.
8. Myung, S.-K.; Ju, W.; Cho, B.; Oh, S.-W.; Park, S.M.; Koo, B.-K.; Park, B.J.; Korean Meta-Analysis (KORMA) Study Group. Efficacy of vitamin and antioxidant supplements in prevention of cardiovascular disease: Systematic review and meta-analysis of randomised controlled trials. *BMJ* **2013**, *346*, f10. [CrossRef] [PubMed]

9. Inokuchi, H.; Hirokane, H.; Tsuzuki, T.; Nakagawa, K.; Igarashi, M.; Miyazawa, T. Anti-angiogenic activity of tocotrienol. *Biosci. Biotechnol. Biochem.* **2003**, *67*, 1623–1627. [CrossRef] [PubMed]
10. Mizushina, Y.; Nakagawa, K.; Shibata, A.; Awata, Y.; Kuriyama, I.; Shimazaki, N.; Koiwai, O.; Uchiyama, Y.; Sakaguchi, K.; Miyazawa, T.; et al. Inhibitory effect of tocotrienol on eukaryotic DNA polymerase λ and angiogenesis. *Biochem. Biophys. Res. Commun.* **2006**, *339*, 949–955. [CrossRef] [PubMed]
11. Nesaretnam, K.; Dorasamy, S.; Darbre, P.D. Tocotrienols inhibit growth of ZR-75-1 breast cancer cells. *Int. J. Food Sci. Nutr.* **2000**, *51*, 95–103. [CrossRef]
12. Qureshi, A.A.; Qureshi, N.; Wright, J.; Shen, Z.; Kramer, G.; Gapor, A.; Chong, Y.H.; DeWitt, G.; Ong, A.; Peterson, D.M. Lowering of serum cholesterol in hypercholesterolemic humans by tocotrienols (palmvitee). *Am. J. Clin. Nutr.* **1991**, *53*, 1021S–1026S. [CrossRef] [PubMed]
13. Qureshi, A.A.; Sami, S.A.; Salser, W.A.; Khan, F.A. Dose-dependent suppression of serum cholesterol by tocotrienol-rich fraction (TRF 25) of rice bran in hypercholesterolemic humans. *Atherosclerosis* **2002**, *161*, 199–207. [CrossRef]
14. Sen, C.K.; Khanna, S.; Roy, S.; Packer, L. Molecular basis of vitamin E action tocotrienol potently inhibits glutamate-induced pp60(c-Src) kinase activation and death of Ht4 neuronal cells. *J. Biol. Chem.* **2000**, *275*, 13049–13055. [CrossRef] [PubMed]
15. Thor, H.; Ng, T. Effects of administration of α-tocopherol and tocotrienols on serum lipids and liver HMG CoA reductase activity. *Int. J. Food Sci. Nutr.* **2000**, *51*, S3–S11. [CrossRef]
16. Chin, S.F.; Ibahim, J.; Makpol, S.; Abdul Hamid, N.A.; Abdul Latiff, A.; Zakaria, Z.; Mazlan, M.; Mohd Yusof, Y.A.; Abdul Karim, A.; Wan Ngah, W.Z. Tocotrienol rich fraction supplementation improved lipid profile and oxidative status in healthy older adults: A randomized controlled study. *Nutr. Metab.* **2011**, *8*, 42. [CrossRef] [PubMed]
17. Heng, E.; Karsani, S.; Abdul Rahman, M.; Abdul Hamid, N.; Hamid, Z.; Wan Ngah, W. Supplementation with tocotrienol-rich fraction alters the plasma levels of Apolipoprotein A-I precursor, Apolipoprotein E precursor, and C-reactive protein precursor from young and old individuals. *Eur. J. Nutr.* **2013**, *52*, 1811–1820. [CrossRef] [PubMed]
18. Jeno, P.; Mini, T.; Moes, S.; Hintermann, E.; Horst, M. Internal sequences from proteins digested in polyacrylamide gels. *Anal. Biochem.* **1995**, *224*, 75–82. [CrossRef] [PubMed]
19. Andreescu, S.; Hepel, M. *Oxidative Stress: Diagnostics, Prevention, and Therapy*; ACS Symposium Series; ACS Publication: Washington, DC, USA, 2011; Volume 1083.
20. Sen, S.; Chakraborty, R. The Role of Antioxidants in Human Health. In *Oxidative Stress: Diagnostics, Prevention, and Therapy*; ACS Publication: Washington, DC, USA, 2011; Volume 1083, pp. 1–37.
21. Noctor, G.; Foyer, C.H. Ascorbate and glutathione: Keeping active oxygen under control. *Annu. Rev. Plant Biol.* **1998**, *49*, 249–279. [CrossRef] [PubMed]
22. Sharma, P.; Jha, A.B.; Dubey, R.S.; Pessarakli, M. Reactive oxygen species, oxidative damage, and antioxidative defense mechanism in plants under stressful conditions. *J. Bot.* **2012**, *2012*, 217037. [CrossRef]
23. Goon, J.A.; Azman, N.H.E.N.; Ghani, S.M.A.; Hamid, Z.; Ngah, W.Z.W. Comparing palm oil tocotrienol rich fraction with a-tocopherol supplementation on oxidative stress in healthy older adults. *Clin. Nutr. ESPEN* **2017**, *21*, 1–12. [CrossRef]
24. Khor, S.C.; Ngah, W.Z.W.; Yusof, Y.A.M.; Karim, N.A.; Makpol, S. Tocotrienol-Rich Fraction Ameliorates Antioxidant Defense Mechanisms and Improves Replicative Senescence-Associated Oxidative Stress in Human Myoblasts. *Oxid. Med. Cell. Longev.* **2017**, *2017*, 3868305. [CrossRef] [PubMed]
25. Aliahmat, N.S.; Noor, M.R.M.; Yusof, W.J.W.; Makpol, S.; Ngah, W.Z.W.; Yusof, Y.A.M. Antioxidant enzyme activity and malondialdehyde levels can be modulated by *Piper betle*, tocotrienol rich fraction and *Chlorella vulgaris* in aging C57BL/6 mice. *Clinics* **2012**, *67*, 1447–1454. [CrossRef]
26. Ford, E.S.; Ajani, U.A.; Mokdad, A.H. Brief communication: The prevalence of high intake of vitamin E from the use of supplements among US adults. *Ann. Intern. Med.* **2005**, *143*, 116–120. [CrossRef] [PubMed]
27. Sun, Y.; Ma, A.; Li, Y.; Han, X.; Wang, Q.; Liang, H. Vitamin E supplementation protects erythrocyte membranes from oxidative stress in healthy Chinese middle-aged and elderly people. *Nutr. Res.* **2012**, *32*, 328–334. [CrossRef] [PubMed]
28. Werninghaus, K.; Meydani, M.; Bhawan, J.; Margolis, R.; Blumberg, J.B.; Gilchrest, B.A. Evaluation of the photoprotective effect of oral vitamin E supplementation. *Arch. Dermatol.* **1994**, *130*, 1257–1261. [CrossRef] [PubMed]

29. Chin, S.-F.; Hamid, N.A.A.; Latiff, A.A.; Zakaria, Z.; Mazlan, M.; Yusof, Y.A.; Karim, A.A.; Ibahim, J.; Hamid, Z.; Ngah, W.Z.; et al. Reduction of DNA damage in older healthy adults by Tri E® Tocotrienol supplementation. *Nutrition* **2008**, *24*, 1–10. [CrossRef] [PubMed]
30. Mastaloudis, A.; Leonard, S.W.; Traber, M.G. Oxidative stress in athletes during extreme endurance exercise. *Free Radic. Biol. Med.* **2001**, *31*, 911–922. [CrossRef]
31. O'Byrne, D.; Grundy, S.; Packer, L.; Devaraj, S.; Baldenius, K.; Hoppe, P.P.; Kraemer, K.; Jialal, I.; Traber, M.G. Studies of LDL oxidation following α-, γ-, or δ-tocotrienyl acetate supplementation of hypercholesterolemic humans. *Free Radic. Biol. Med.* **2000**, *29*, 834–845. [CrossRef]
32. Andriollo-Sanchez, M.; Hininger-Favier, I.; Meunier, N.; Venneria, E.; O'Connor, J.M.; Maiani, G.; Coudray, C.; Roussel, A.M. Age-related oxidative stress and antioxidant parameters in middle-aged and older European subjects: The ZENITH study. *Eur. J. Clin. Nutr.* **2005**, *59*, S58–S62. [CrossRef] [PubMed]
33. Guemouri, L.; Artur, Y.; Herbeth, B.; Jeandel, C.; Cuny, G.; Siest, G. Biological variability of superoxide dismutase, glutathione peroxidase, and catalase in blood. *Clin. Chem.* **1991**, *37*, 1932–1937. [PubMed]
34. Žitňanová, I.; Rakovan, M.; Paduchová, Z.; Dvořáková, M.; Andrezálová, L.; Muchová, J.; Šimko, M.; Waczulíková, I.; Ďuračková, Z. Oxidative stress in women with perimenopausal symptoms. *Menopause* **2011**, *18*, 1249–1255. [CrossRef] [PubMed]
35. Prokai, L.; Prokai-Tatrai, K.; Perjési, P.; Simpkins, J.W. Mechanistic insights into the direct antioxidant effects of estrogens. *Drug Dev. Res.* **2005**, *66*, 118–125. [CrossRef]
36. Borras, C.; Sastre, J.; Garcia-Sala, D.; Lloret, A.; Pallardo, F.V.; Vina, J. Mitochondria from females exhibit higher antioxidant gene expression and lower oxidative damage than males. *Free Radic. Biol. Med.* **2003**, *34*, 546–552. [CrossRef]
37. Borrás, C.; Gambini, J.; López-Grueso, R.; Pallardó, F.V.; Viña, J. Direct antioxidant and protective effect of estradiol on isolated mitochondria. *Biochem. Biophys. Acta* **2010**, *1802*, 205–211. [CrossRef] [PubMed]
38. Greenblatt, R.B.; Oettinger, M.; Bohler, C.S. Estrogen-Androgen Levels in Aging Men and Women: Therapeutic Considerations. *J. Am. Geriatr. Soc.* **1976**, *24*, 173–178. [CrossRef] [PubMed]
39. Scholz, R.W.; Graham, K.S.; Gumpricht, E.; Reddy, C.C. Mechanism of Interaction of Vitamin E and Glutathione in the Protection against Membrane Lipid Peroxidation. *Ann. N. Y. Acad. Sci.* **1989**, *570*, 514–517. [CrossRef]
40. Halprin, K.M.; Ohkawara, A. The Measurement of Glutathione in Human Epidermis Using Glutathione Reductase. *J. Investig. Dermatol.* **1967**, *48*, 149–152. [CrossRef] [PubMed]
41. Codoñer-Franch, P.; Pons-Morales, S.; Boix-García, L.; Valls-Bellés, V. Oxidant/antioxidant status in obese children compared to pediatric patients with type 1 diabetes mellitus. *Pediatr. Diabetes* **2010**, *11*, 251–257. [CrossRef] [PubMed]
42. Moskaug, J.Ø.; Carlsen, H.; Myhrstad, M.C.; Blomhoff, R. Polyphenols and glutathione synthesis regulation. *Am. J. Clin. Nutr.* **2005**, *81*, 277S–283S. [CrossRef] [PubMed]
43. Papp, L.V.; Holmgren, A.; Khanna, K.K. Selenium and selenoproteins in health and disease. *Antioxid. Redox Signal.* **2010**, *12*, 793–795. [CrossRef] [PubMed]
44. Valko, M.; Leibfritz, D.; Moncol, J.; Cronin, M.T.; Mazur, M.; Telser, J. Free radicals and antioxidants in normal physiological functions and human disease. *Int. J. Biochem. Cell Biol.* **2007**, *39*, 44–84. [CrossRef] [PubMed]
45. Orlowski, M.; Karkowsky, A. Glutathione metabolism and some possible functions of glutathione in the nervous system. *Int. Rev. Neurobiol.* **1976**, *19*, 75–121. [PubMed]
46. Sies, H. Hydroperoxides and Thiol Oxidants in the Study of Oxidative Stress in Intact Cells and Organs. In *Oxidative Stress*; Academic Press: London, UK, 1985; pp. 73–90.
47. White, C.W.; Mimmack, R.E.; Repine, J.E. Accumulation of lung tissue oxidized glutathione (GSSG) as a marker of oxidant induced lung injury. *Chest* **1986**, *89*, 111S–113S. [CrossRef] [PubMed]
48. Dalle-Donne, I.; Rossi, R.; Colombo, R.; Giustarini, D.; Milzani, A. Biomarkers of oxidative damage in human disease. *Clin. Chem.* **2006**, *52*, 601–623. [CrossRef] [PubMed]
49. Owen, J.B.; Butterfield, D.A. Measurement of oxidized/reduced glutathione ratio. *Methods Mol. Biol.* **2010**, *648*, 269–277. [PubMed]
50. Bonnefont-Rousselot, D.; Lacomblez, L.; Jaudon, M.-C.; Lepage, S.; Salachas, F.; Bensimon, G.; Bizard, C.; Doppler, V.; Delattre, J.; Meininger, V. Blood oxidative stress in amyotrophic lateral sclerosis. *J. Neurol. Sci.* **2000**, *178*, 57–62. [CrossRef]

51. Cecchi, C.; Latorraca, S.; Sorbi, S.; Iantomasi, T.; Favilli, F.; Vincenzini, M.T.; Liguri, G. Gluthatione level is altered in lymphoblasts from patients with familial Alzheimer's disease. *Neurosci. Lett.* **1999**, *275*, 152–154. [CrossRef]
52. Lang, C.A.; Mills, B.J.; Mastropaolo, W.; Liu, M.C. Blood glutathione decreases in chronic diseases. *J. Lab. Clin. Med.* **2000**, *135*, 402–405. [CrossRef] [PubMed]
53. Mills, B.J.; Weiss, M.M.; Lang, C.A.; Liu, M.C.; Ziegler, C. Blood glutathione and cysteine changes in cardiovascular disease. *J. Lab. Clin. Med.* **2000**, *135*, 396–401. [CrossRef] [PubMed]
54. Samiec, P.S.; Drews-Botsch, C.; Flagg, E.W.; Kurtz, J.C.; Sternberg, P., Jr.; Reed, R.L.; Jones, D.P. Glutathione in human plasma: Decline in association with aging, age-related macular degeneration, and diabetes. *Free Radic. Biol. Med.* **1998**, *24*, 699–704. [CrossRef]
55. Van Haaften, R.I.M.; Haenen, G.R.M.M.; Evelo, C.T.A.; Bast, A. Tocotrienols Inhibit Human Glutathione S-Transferase P1-1. *IUBMB Life* **2002**, *54*, 81–84. [CrossRef] [PubMed]

9

Mechanisms of LPS-Induced Acute Kidney Injury in Neonatal and Adult Rats

Egor Y. Plotnikov [1,2,3,*], Anna A. Brezgunova [4], Irina B. Pevzner [1,2], Ljubava D. Zorova [1,2], Vasily N. Manskikh [1], Vasily A. Popkov [1,2,5], Denis N. Silachev [1,2] and Dmitry B. Zorov [1,2,*]

1 A.N. Belozersky Institute of Physico-Chemical Biology, Lomonosov Moscow State University, 119992 Moscow, Russia; irinapevzner@mail.ru (I.B.P.); lju_2003@list.ru (L.D.Z.); manskikh@mail.ru (V.N.M.); popkov.vas@gmail.com (V.A.P.); silachevdn@belozersky.msu.ru (D.N.S.)
2 V.I. Kulakov National Medical Research Center of Obstetrics, Gynecology and Perinatology, 117997 Moscow, Russia
3 Institute of Molecular Medicine, Sechenov First Moscow State Medical University, 119991 Moscow, Russia
4 Biological Faculty, Lomonosov Moscow State University, 119992 Moscow, Russia; elqu7@yandex.ru
5 Faculty of Bioengineering and Bioinformatics, Lomonosov Moscow State University, 119992 Moscow, Russia
* Correspondence: plotnikov@belozersky.msu.ru (E.Y.P.); zorov@belozersky.msu.ru (D.B.Z.)

Abstract: Neonatal sepsis is one of the major causes of mortality and morbidity in newborns, greatly associated with severe acute kidney injury (AKI) and failure. Handling of newborns with kidney damage can be significantly different compared to adults, and it is necessary to consider the individuality of an organism's response to systemic inflammation. In this study, we used lipopolysaccharide (LPS)-mediated acute kidney injury model to study mechanisms of kidney cells damage in neonatal and adult rats. We found LPS-associated oxidative stress was more severe in adults compared to neonates, as judged by levels of carbonylated proteins and products of lipids peroxidation. In both models, LPS-mediated septic simulation caused apoptosis of kidney cells, albeit to a different degree. Elevated levels of proliferating cell nuclear antigen (PCNA) in the kidney dropped after LPS administration in neonates but increased in adults. Renal fibrosis, as estimated by smooth muscle actin levels, was significantly higher in adult kidneys, whereas these changes were less profound in LPS-treated neonatal kidneys. We concluded that in LPS-mediated AKI model, renal cells of neonatal rats were more tolerant to oxidative stress and suffered less from long-term pathological consequences, such as fibrosis. In addition, we assume that by some features LPS administration simulates the conditions of accelerated aging.

Keywords: kidney injury; renal failure; endotoxin; sepsis; age; oxidative stress; fibrosis; regeneration

1. Introduction

Neonatal sepsis, when it occurs at up to 28 days of age, is one of the major causes of mortality and morbidity in newborns. According to the World Health Organization, in 2010, more than 1.3 million newborns in the United States died before reaching 28 days of age because of infections [1,2]. Sepsis is commonly considered a complex clinical syndrome, which is mostly defined by severe systemic inflammation leading to multiple pathologies and organs dysfunction and failure [3,4]. The immune system is considered to be a key player in sepsis development due to its association with infection (bacterial or fungal). However, the immune system of newborns is known to mature only at 24 weeks [5], being underdeveloped before this term. This fact heavily affects sepsis onset and propagation in neonates, thus making diagnostics and treatment of sepsis and SIRS (systemic inflammatory response syndrome) in neonates quite different from adults [6].

The immature immune system of infants is poorly studied and understood, and it is extremely difficult for clinicians to predict responses to both inflammation-inducing agents and treatment [7]. For example, term newborns usually react to sepsis by elevated temperature (more than 37.8 °C), but preterm newborns more often react by hypothermia due to their underdeveloped temperature control system [8]. It is also known that neutrophils activity [9] and concentrations of IgG [9,10] are low in neonates. Monocytes and macrophages of neonates contain less toll-like receptor 4 (TLR4) [11–14], and their response to antigens and endotoxin is retarded, thus yielding low production of proinflammatory cytokines. The complement system in neonates is under-regulated as well [15]. In concert, these factors lead to newborns being more susceptible to infections, which increases both the chance of sepsis development and its severity [16]. On the other hand, these features can be beneficial against the inflammatory aspect of sepsis pathogenesis, which is the leading damaging factor.

Lastly, the mother's health should also be considered. It is common for neonates to receive infection from their mothers, and the mother's inflammatory response could strongly affect the fetus, with further complications occurring after birth [17].

The kidney is one of the main organs that suffer from sepsis. Sepsis triggers 50% of all acute kidney injury (AKI) cases in critically ill patients, and its mortality rate reaches 60% [18–20]. Moreover, in neonates, due to their immature immune system, the situation is usually complicated by administered antibiotics, which are required to fight infection but more likely to causing damage to the kidneys. Antibiotic therapy can complicate the dysfunction of many organs, but the kidney becomes the most vulnerable organ because of the well-known nephrotoxicity of antibiotics [21–23]. Since kidney damage in systemic inflammatory response can arise both from infectious and noninfectious causes and can include hyperactive or hypoactive inflammation phases, this leads to a new view on sepsis management that is based on consideration of key points of the process, including mitochondria dysfunction and changes in redox homeostasis. This is not only a new approach for therapy but the only one which is considered to be ubiquitous to all sepsis patients as it addresses the mechanism of cellular damage directly. Recently, the existence of the "sepsis redox cycle" was postulated by researchers [24]. According to this cycle, interleukins (IL6, IL8) activate NF-κB (nuclear factor κB), which upregulates inducible nitric oxide (NO) synthase (iNOS). This leads to elevated NO levels, which inhibit cytochrome oxidase and thus decelerate mitochondrial electron transport, resulting in increased production of superoxide anion radical and hydrogen peroxide in mitochondria [25]. Hydrogen peroxide further activates NF-κB, which closes this positive self-amplifying loop, ultimately yielding mitochondria, cell, and organ dysfunction. This is highly applicable to the kidney, where damage during sepsis is associated with mitochondria dysfunction, and where reactive oxygen species (ROS) generation [26]—with ROS generation as a self-promoting loop [27]—might be terminated on initial stages by right approaches.

The possibility of treating ROS-associated kidney pathologies through addressed maintenance of redox homeostasis reached by different agents, like antioxidants, looks very promising. We have also demonstrated the efficiency of this approach on adult kidney damage models in our earlier work [28,29]. However, for neonatal kidneys, the method requires careful study of oxidative stress development under septic conditions with a proper comparison to those in adult kidneys. In this study, we have chosen lipopolysaccharide (LPS)-mediated acute kidney injury as a model for our studies because it triggers the same mechanisms as natural sepsis does and ultimately results in the same mitochondria-mediated damage. At the same time, it is much more controllable and reproducible than bacterial models. This study aims to compare AKI, particularly the associated oxidative damage in neonatal and adult rats during LPS-mediated sepsis simulation, and to identify mechanisms of kidney cells damage following AKI that is common to both groups.

2. Materials and Methods

2.1. Animal Experiments

The animal protocols used in this work were evaluated and approved by the institutional animal ethics committee (Protocol 9/17 from 28 April 2017) in accordance with Federation for Laboratory Animal Science Associations (FELASA) guidelines. The experiments were performed on outbred white rats. Dams and their pups were kept in cages with a temperature-controlled environment (23 ± 2 °C) with light on from 9 a.m. to 9 p.m. Dams had ad libitum access to food and water, and pups were checked daily for health. The number of pups in a litter was 9–12. Endotoxin-mediated AKI was performed on 3-days-old neonatal and adult rats by intraperitoneal administration of LPS from *E. coli* (0127:B8 strain, Sigma Aldrich, St. Louis, MO, USA) in concentration 4 mg/kg; the control group was administrated with saline infusion. The total number of animals in each group was 6 (from different litters). The experimental design is presented in Figure 1. Briefly, 24 h after LPS administration, blood, urine and kidneys were taken from animals. Urine samples were diluted 1:1 with 2× sample buffer and boiled for 5 min and then centrifuged at 12,000× *g* for 3 min. Blood samples were taken to determine blood urea nitrogen (BUN) using AU480 Chemistry System (Beckman Coulter, Brea, CA, USA).

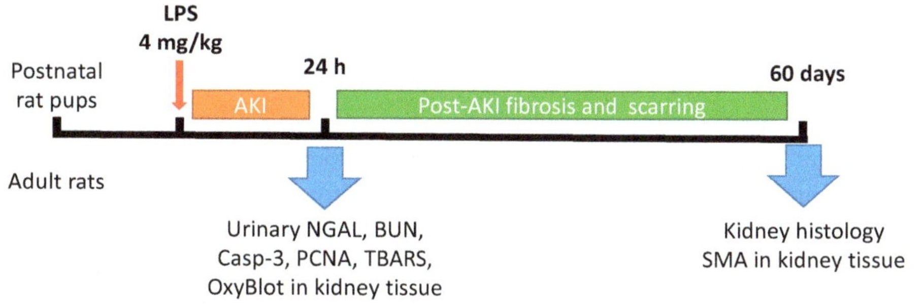

Figure 1. Design of experiments with lipopolysaccharide (LPS)-mediated acute kidney injury (AKI) in adult and newborn rats. NGAL: neutrophil gelatinase-associated lipocalin 2; BUN: blood urea nitrogen; PCNA: proliferating cell nuclear antigen; TBARS: thiobarbituric acid-reactive substances; SMA: α-smooth muscle actin.

2.2. Western Blotting

Kidneys were homogenized in 1 mL of phosphate buffered saline (PBS) with 1 mM of protease inhibitor phenylmethylsulfonyl fluoride (PMSF), then centrifuged at 1000× *g* for 3 min. Five microliters of the supernatant were used to measure protein concentration using the bicinchoninic acid kit (Sigma Aldrich, St. Louis, MO, USA); the rest was taken for blotting analysis to evaluate the proliferative potential, protein oxidation, and apoptotic activity. Samples were loaded onto 15% Tris-glycine polyacrylamide gels (10 μg protein per lane). After electrophoresis, gels were blotted onto polyvinylidene difluoride (PVDF) membranes (Amersham Pharmacia Biotech, Amersham, UK). Membranes were blocked with 5% non-fat milk in PBS/0.1% Tween-20 and subsequently incubated with primary rabbit antibodies to neutrophil gelatinase-associated lipocalin 2 (NGAL) 1:1000 (Abcam, Cambridge, UK), proliferating cell nuclear antigen (PCNA) 1:1000 (13110, Cell Signaling Technology, Danvers, MA, USA), and to caspase-3 1:500 (9661, Cell Signaling Technology, Danvers, MA, USA). Fibrosis formation was examined two months after a single LPS administration using rabbit antibodies for α-smooth muscle actin (SMA) 1:500 (14968, Cell Signaling Technology, Danvers, MA, USA). Carbonylated proteins (protein oxidation marker) were measured using OxyBlot kit (S7150 OxyBlot Protein Oxidation DetectionKit, Millipore, Burlington, MA, USA). Membranes were processed with secondary antibodies conjugated with horseradish peroxidase 1:10,000 (IMTEK, Moscow, Russia). Detection was performed by ChemiDoc™ MP imaging system (BioRad, Hercules, CA, USA) with WesternBright™ Enhanced Chemiluminescence kit (Advansta, Menlo Park, CA, USA).

2.3. Renal Histology

After sacrificing the animal, the kidneys were immediately taken, fixed in a 10% neutral buffered formalin solution, embedded in paraffin, and used for histopathological examination. Five-micrometer-thick sections were cut, deparaffinized, hydrated, and stained with Masson trichrome [30]. The renal sections were examined for fibrosis in an automated fashion by quantification of a specific color in the kidney tissue using ImageJ (National Institutes of Health, Bethesda, MD, USA) color threshold plugin. Color threshold settings were adjusted manually for each image. Percentage of the field of view with positive staining was considered to be fibrosis ratio. A minimum of seven fields of view for each kidney slice was examined.

2.4. Measurement Thiobarbituric Acid-Reactive Substances (TBARS)

TBARS in kidney tissue homogenates were explored by a conventional colorimetric method with the use of malondialdehyde–thiobarbituric acid reaction according to Mihara and Uchiyama [31]. Briefly, each sample was mixed with 0.8% thiobarbituric acid and 1% H_3PO_4 in the ratio by volume 0.9:1.0:3.0. The mixture was boiled for 45 min, cooled to room temperature, and then centrifuged at $15{,}000\times\ g$ for 10 min. The absorbance of the resulting supernatant at 532 nm was measured using a Hitachi 557 spectrophotometer. 1,3,3-tetraetoxipropan (Sigma Aldrich, St. Louis, MO, USA) was used as a calibration standard. The content of thiobarbituric acid (TBA)-reactive products was finally normalized by total protein content.

2.5. Statistics

Statistical analyses were performed using STATISTICA 7.0 for Windows (StatSoft, Inc., Palo Alto, CA, USA). Values are given as mean ± standard error of the mean (SEM). Variance homogeneity was assessed with Levene's test. Statistical differences were analyzed using the Kruskal–Wallis test with the Mann–Whitney u-test (the Bonferroni post hoc correction was applied). Differences were considered significant at $p \leq 0.05$.

3. Results

3.1. Oxidative Stress in Kidneys of Neonatal and Adult Rats

We analyzed the development of oxidative stress and accumulation of oxidative modified (carbonylated) proteins and lipids (TBARS) in 3-days-old neonates and adult rats (Figure 2). After 24 h of LPS administration, we observed much higher levels of carbonylated proteins in both adult and neonatal rats compared to the relevant control. However, in neonatal AKI kidneys this increase was smaller compared to the adult AKI group. While in adult kidneys, the signal of OxyBlot was about 20 times higher after LPS treatment, the same signal rose only about two times in neonatal kidneys (Figure 2C). Note that while adult rats demonstrated a higher increase in carbonylated proteins level, the intact neonatal kidneys initially had a slightly higher Oxyblot signal than the intact adult kidneys. Our results indicate that oxidative stress during LPS-induced, sepsis-like kidney injury is more severe in adults than in neonates.

TBA-reactive products reporting on the content of the main product of lipid oxidation—malondialdehyde (MDA)—as well as some other lipid peroxides are other markers of oxidative damage in kidney cells. We found (Figure 2D) that similar to carbonylated proteins, TBARS levels in kidney tissue were much higher after LPS injection, both in adult and neonatal rats compared to intact controls. However, in neonatal AKI kidneys, this increase was less than in adult AKI group. Thus, our results indicate that LPS-mediated sepsis indeed leads to oxidative stress and that oxidative kidney tissue damage is less severe in neonates.

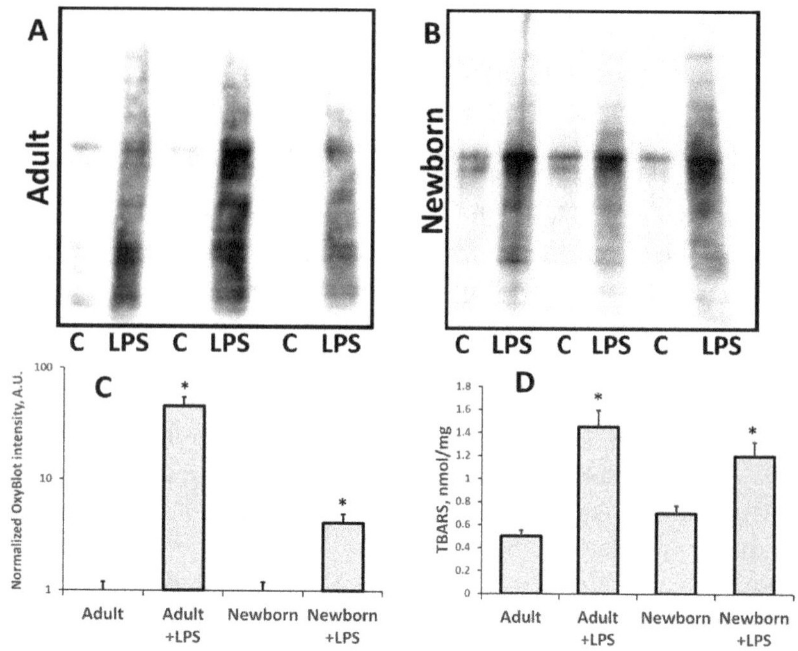

Figure 2. Oxidative stress in neonatal and adult kidneys 24 h after LPS treatment. Estimation of carbonylated proteins in kidney tissue of (**A**) adult rats and (**B**) newborn rats. (**C**) Densitometry of OxyBlot® plots. (**D**) Analysis of lipid peroxidation in kidneys as measured by thiobarbituric acid-reactive substances (TBARS) accumulation. Number of animals for Oxyblot densitometry and TBARS analysis: Adult ($n = 6$), Newborn ($n = 6$), Adult + LPS ($n = 5$), Newborn + LPS ($n = 5$). *: $p < 0.05$.

3.2. Changes Associated with LPS-Mediated Oxidative Stress

It is well known that oxidative stress can induce cell death of different nature, including apoptosis. To evaluate apoptosis activation in kidney cells in response to LPS administration, we measured levels of active caspase-3 using western blotting. Twenty-four hours after LPS injection, levels of cleaved (active) caspase-3 in both adult and neonatal rats were increased two times vs. relevant intact groups (Figure 3). There was no significant difference in apoptosis activation in response to LPS-mediated injury between adults and neonates.

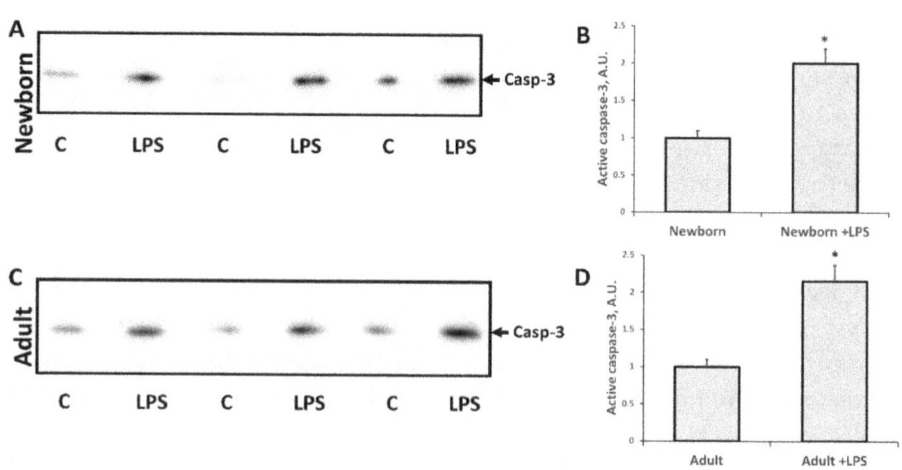

Figure 3. Induction of apoptosis in neonatal and adult kidneys 24 h after LPS treatment. Immunoblots for cleaved procaspase-3 (caspase-3, i.e., mature, active form) levels in kidneys of (**A**,**B**) neonatal rats and (**C**,**D**) adult rats. Densitometry analysis of bands in newborn and adults are presented in (**B**) and (**D**), respectively. Number of animals for western blot densitometry: Adult ($n = 6$), Newborn ($n = 6$), Adults + LPS ($n = 5$), Newborn + LPS ($n = 5$). *: $p < 0.05$.

We demonstrated that LPS injection led to acute kidney damage. Twenty-four hours after administration of LPS, a significant increase in NGAL (highly sensitive biomarker of AKI) was observed in the urine of neonatal and adult rats (Figure 4). In addition, there was a trend of increasing BUN in both experimental groups (Figure 4E,F) indicating some renal failure. While only slight renal failure was observed by this indicator after exposure to LPS, the AKI marker NGAL in urine demonstrated the presence of severe AKI in neonatal and adult rats in the first 24 h.

Another marker associated with kidney injury and regeneration after damage is the level of proliferation marker PCNA. Since cell proliferation is almost absent in adult kidneys, it is believed that injury activates PCNA expression as part of a signal for regeneration. Indeed, in our study, PCNA levels in adult kidneys were significantly increased 24 h after LPS administration (Figure 5A,B). However, in neonates, the response was opposite (Figure 5C,D), possibly due to the fact that until the seventh day after birth, the kidney is still developing with proper proliferative activity. PCNA level in intact neonates kidneys was already much higher compared to the adult ones (compare Figure 4A,C) as described earlier [32]. LPS-mediated injury caused a drop of PCNA levels in neonatal rats, which was the opposite of the adult kidneys' response.

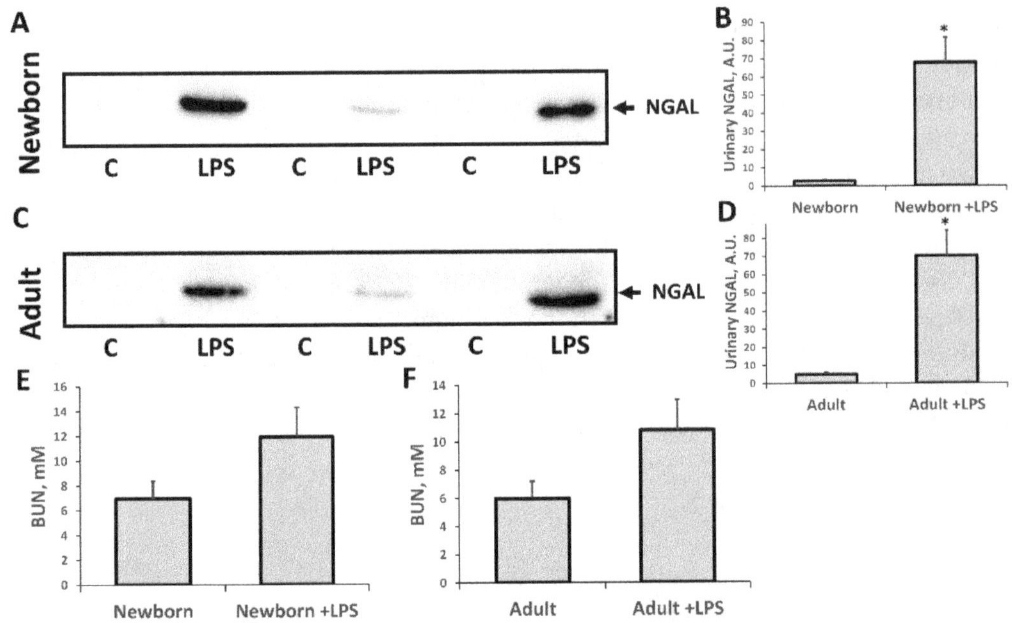

Figure 4. Acute kidney injury in (**A**,**B**,**E**) neonatal rats and (**C**,**D**,**F**) adult rats 24 h after LPS treatment. Significant increase in urinary neutrophil gelatinase-associated lipocalin 2 (NGAL) content and some rise of blood urea nitrogen (BUN) was observed. Diagrams on B, D represent densitometry analysis of corresponding bands on the blots. Number of animals for western blot densitometry: Adult (n = 4), Newborn (n = 4), Adult + LPS (n = 4), Newborn + LPS (n = 4). *: $p < 0.05$.

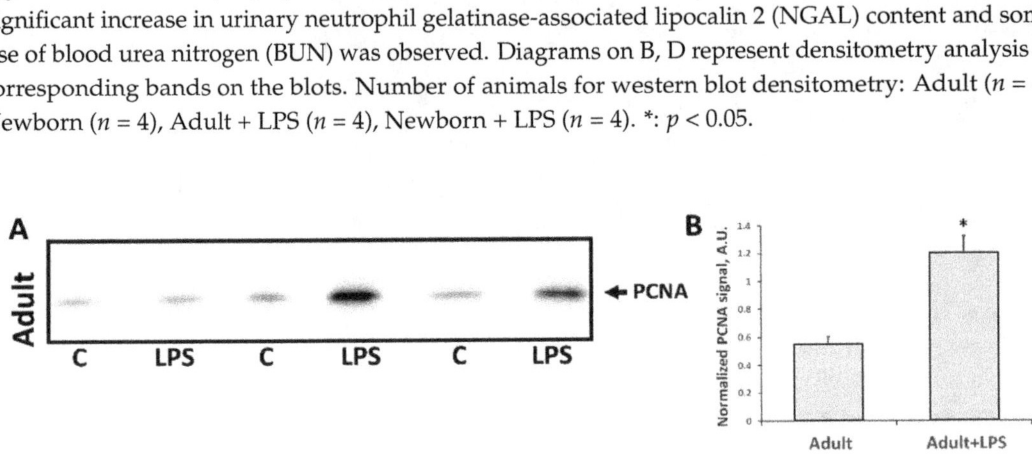

Figure 5. *Cont.*

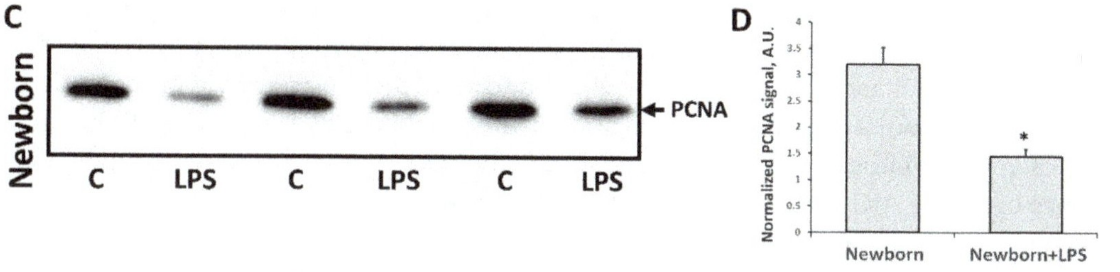

Figure 5. Proliferative activity of kidney cells of newborn and adult rats 24 h after LPS treatment. Immunoblots for proliferating cell nuclear antigen (PCNA) levels in (**A**) adult kidneys and (**C**) neonatal kidneys and their densitometry analysis in (**B**,**D**), respectively. Number of animals for western blot densitometry: Adult (n = 6), Newborn (n = 6), Adult + LPS (n = 5), Newborn + LPS (n = 5). *: $p < 0.05$.

3.3. Fibrosis Formation after Acute Kidney Injury

One of the most severe consequences of any AKI is a fibrosis formation, i.e., replacement of functional kidney tissue by fibroblasts and connective tissue scarring. We evaluated fibrosis formation two months after LPS administration using classical histological approach (Figure 6). Connective tissue (collagen formations) was found in both LPS-treated groups (those that received LPS in infancy or adult age) after two months, indicating that fibrosis formation had taken place. We found more pronounced renal fibrotic scaring in the adult group compared to neonatal kidneys, as shown in the digital image analysis (Figure 6C). Moreover, α-smooth muscle actin (SMA) levels—one of the well-established markers for fibrosis formation in kidneys—demonstrated significant differences (Figure 7). SMA levels in adult kidneys two months after LPS injection were significantly higher compared to intact animals. In kidneys of rats treated with LPS in neonatal age, SMA levels were higher as well but not as much as in adult kidneys. Overall, these results indicate that fibrosis formation took place two months after LPS-induced AKI and that SMA accumulation was less in neonatal kidneys than in the adult one.

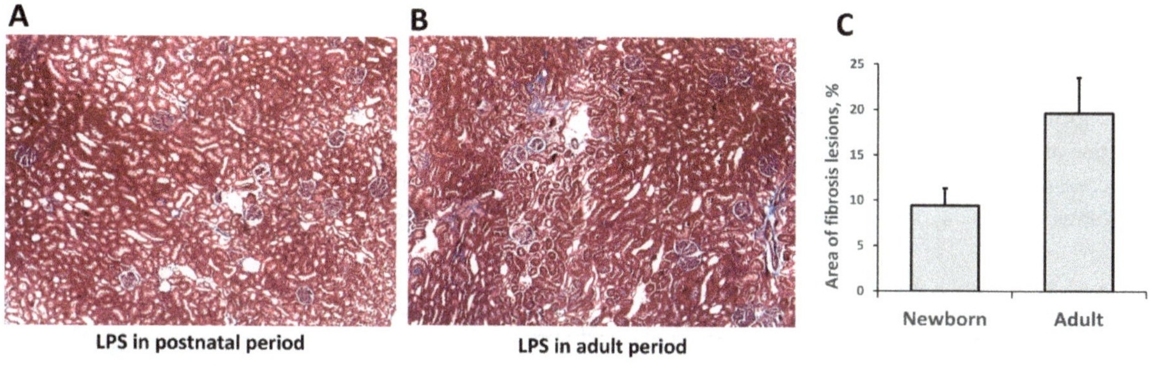

Figure 6. Histological evaluation of fibrotic changes in neonatal and adult kidneys two months after LPS treatment. (**A**) Kidneys of rats that received LPS in neonatal age and (**B**) kidney of rats treated with LPS in adult age. (**C**) Evaluation of fibrotic lesions revealed increased fibrosis in adult group. Number of animals: Adult (n = 3), Newborn (n = 3).

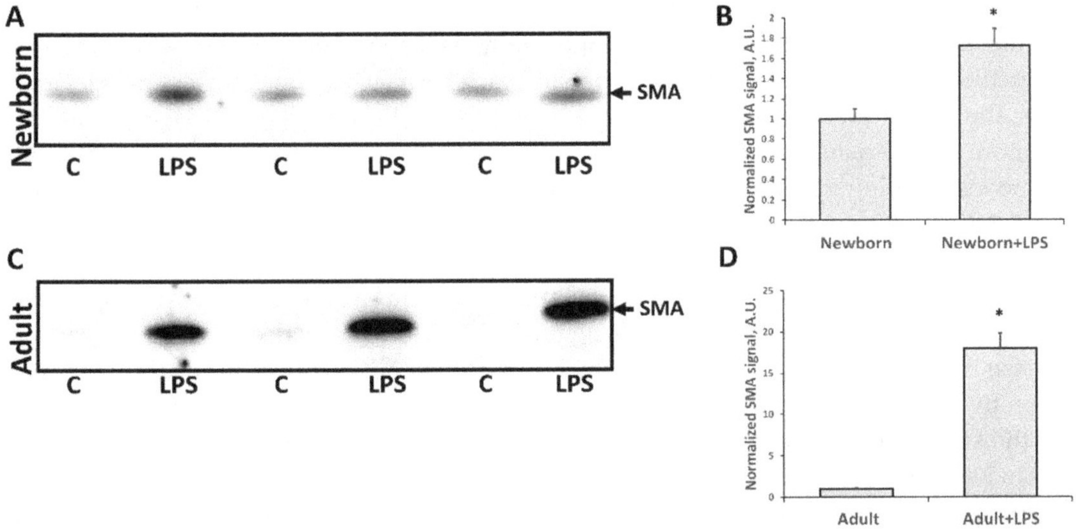

Figure 7. Kidney fibrosis, estimated by α-smooth muscle actin (SMA) levels in kidney tissue two months after LPS treatment. (**A**,**B**) Immunoblots of kidneys of rats that received LPS in neonatal age and (**C**,**D**) rats treated with LPS in adult age. (**B**,**D**) Densitometry analysis of bands in neonates and adults, respectively. Number of animals for Western blot densitometry: Adult (n = 6), Newborn (n = 6), Adults + LPS (n = 5), Newborn + LPS (n = 5). *: $p < 0.05$.

4. Discussion

Most biological studies of sepsis and AKI were carried out on adult animals. However, translating experimental results from bench to bedside is difficult because for a wide spectrum of diseases, adults are the least presented patients in clinics and hospital beds, while children and old people are the most often presented group. Sepsis is one such pathology that affects neonates more often [2] and has pathogenesis that is quite different in neonates compared to adults or elders. Sepsis is a complex condition, which includes heterogeneous interconnected processes—bacterial invasion, inflammation, and oxidative stress—that are all highly affected by neonatal status. An immature immune system compromises an organism's ability to fight a disease in case of bacterial sepsis. On the other hand, it is not clear how underdeveloped immune system affects inflammatory component of sepsis, i.e., whether it relieves or burdens the pathology. Finally, neonates are believed to have deficient antioxidant systems [33–36], possibly due to the fact that intrauterine fetuses are exposed to three times lower O_2 concentration than after birth (pO_2 30 and 90 mm Hg, respectively) [37]. Levels and activity of antioxidant enzymes superoxide dismutase and glutathione peroxidase and other antioxidants are low in neonate plasma, making neonates potentially more vulnerable to pathologies associated with oxidative stress [33,38,39]. Therefore, the antioxidant system in the first few days after birth does not correspond to the environmental oxygen challenge. However, neonates also have lower capacities to produce ROS [40], and this feature could affect oxidative stress-associated pathologies outcomes as well. Weaker antioxidant system could complicate the course of septic damage in newborns, whereas weaker ROS production may have a beneficial effect.

In our study, we found the last assumption to be true for AKI—both carbonylated proteins levels and TBARS after LPS-mediated kidney injury were higher in adults than in neonates. This indicates that oxidative stress in septic kidneys is lower in neonates. A possible explanation of decreased oxidative damage is the underdeveloped immune response of newborns, i.e., underexpression of TLR4 interacting with LPS. Thus, the immature immune system in neonates might afford some protection by preventing the initiating steps of "sepsis redox cycle", which triggers oxidative damage in adults.

Considering the mechanisms of kidney injury in sepsis, we should mention three main approaches for modeling sepsis: LPS injection, bacteria injection, and caecal ligation and puncture (CLP) [41]. All of them have their specificity and disadvantages and address different aspects of sepsis pathogenesis. LPS injection is the most reproducible and simple model as it allows exploring of basic processes such as inflammation and oxidative damage by bypassing bacteria-related factors, such as toxins production. Moreover, the LPS model is more relevant for sepsis-like conditions like SIRS. Bacteria injection and CLP are more appropriate models for clinical sepsis pathogenesis but are less reproducible and more heterogeneous, making it harder to study molecular mechanisms in these models. Also, bacterial toxins and antibiotics administration could dramatically affect the flow and outcome of the pathology. Since the aim of our work was to address oxidative damage and antioxidant capacities in neonates, we studied LPS-mediated AKI and revealed that oxidative damage per se was less severe in neonates.

Regarding the mechanisms of development of AKI in LPS-simulated sepsis, it is worth noting the increase in the cleaved procaspase-3, which is a marker of apoptosis induction. The observed increase in the level of this protein in the kidney indicates that the endotoxin action causes apoptotic death of the kidney cells. Note that at the same time, the AKI marker NGAL in the urine is increased. Thus, it can be assumed that kidney damage is associated with apoptosis of the tubular cells. However, between the groups of newborns and adult rats, there was no difference in the manifestation of these two parameters when exposed to LPS.

We also observed an increase in PCNA levels in adult kidney tissues and a reduction in neonatal kidneys after AKI. PCNA elevation is commonly associated with activation of tubular regeneration, and it has been well described that AKI activates regeneration in the adult kidney [42]. However, basal levels of PCNA in kidneys of intact newborn rats is essentially higher compared to adults. We believe that even after an LPS-induced drop of PCNA in neonates, the proliferation remains will be higher or equal to AKI-induced increased level of PCNA in adults. We speculate that this is due to the ongoing development of kidney in neonates, which is associated with tubular cells proliferation that keeps the basal level of PCNA elevated. Thus, LPS exposure affects these proliferating cells and causes a drop in their number because of cell death. However, we could give an alternative explanation of different reaction of PCNA level in adult and newborn kidney. PCNA is a marker of proliferation, and fibroblasts proliferation during fibrosis development could also lead to an increase of this protein. In our study, we demonstrated fibrotic scaring after LPS-mediated kidney injury as indicated by collagen appearing in kidney tissue two months after AKI. Moreover, SMA levels were much higher in adults after AKI compared to neonates, which reflects progressing fibroblasts proliferation and transformation to myofibroblasts [43]. Thus, the possibility exists that PCNA increase in adult kidney tissue can be associated to some extent with fibroblast proliferation and that it is a part of fibrosis formation rather than just being a sign of regeneration.

5. Conclusions

Our data suggest that in the model of LPS-mediated AKI, neonatal rats kidney are more tolerant to oxidative stress, with less oxidative damage to renal cell and less long-term pathological consequences like fibrosis. We propose that it could be partially due to the immature immune system of newborns, which is the main player contributing to oxidative stress associated with sepsis in adults. We emphasize that the key component of sepsis development—oxidative stress—is still poorly described in neonates, at least in relation to the kidney. We need a comprehensive understanding of sepsis impact on susceptible organs of neonates, such as the kidney, to create specific approaches for treating this dangerous pathology in newborns and infants.

Author Contributions: Investigation, A.A.B., I.B.P., L.D.Z., V.N.M.; Conceptualization, E.Y.P.; Methodology, E.Y.P.; Software, V.A.P.; Validation, E.Y.P., D.N.S., D.B.Z.; Formal Analysis, V.A.P.; Writing-Original Draft Preparation, V.A.P.; Writing-Review; Editing, V.A.P., E.Y.P., D.N.S., D.B.Z.; Visualization, E.Y.P.; Supervision, E.Y.P., D.B.Z.

Funding: The study was supported by Russian science foundation grant 18-15-00058.

Conflicts of Interest: The authors declare no conflict of interest.

References

1. Edmond, K.M.; Kortsalioudaki, C.; Scott, S.; Schrag, S.J.; Zaidi, A.K.; Cousens, S.; Heath, P.T. Group B streptococcal disease in infants aged younger than 3 months: Systematic review and meta-analysis. *Lancet* **2012**, *379*, 547–556. [CrossRef]
2. Watson, R.S.; Carcillo, J.A.; Linde-Zwirble, W.T.; Clermont, G.; Lidicker, J.; Angus, D.C. The epidemiology of severe sepsis in children in the United States. *Am. J. Respir. Crit. Care Med.* **2003**, *167*, 695–701. [CrossRef] [PubMed]
3. Bone, R.C.; Balk, R.A.; Cerra, F.B.; Dellinger, R.P.; Fein, A.M.; Knaus, W.A.; Schein, R.M.H.; Sibbald, W.J. Definitions for sepsis and organ failure and guidelines for the use of innovative therapies in sepsis. *Chest* **1992**, *101*, 1644–1655. [CrossRef] [PubMed]
4. Celes, M.R.N.; Prado, C.M.; Rossi, M.A. Sepsis: Going to the heart of the matter. *Pathobiology* **2012**, *80*, 70–86. [CrossRef] [PubMed]
5. Tissières, P.; Ochoda, A.; Dunn-Siegrist, I.; Drifte, G.; Morales, M.; Pfister, R.; Berner, M.; Pugin, J. Innate immune deficiency of extremely premature neonates can be reversed by interferon-γ. *PLoS ONE* **2012**, *7*. [CrossRef] [PubMed]
6. Aneja, R.K.; Carcillo, J.A. Differences between adult and pediatric septic shock. *Minerva Anestesiol.* **2011**, *77*, 986–992. [PubMed]
7. Basha, S.; Surendran, N.; Pichichero, M. Immune responses in neonates. *Expert Rev. Clin. Immunol.* **2014**, *10*, 1171–1184. [CrossRef] [PubMed]
8. Hofer, N.; Müller, W.; Resch, B. Neonates presenting with temperature symptoms: Role in the diagnosis of early onset sepsis. *Pediatr. Int.* **2012**, *54*, 486–490. [CrossRef] [PubMed]
9. Nussbaum, C.; Gloning, A.; Pruenster, M.; Frommhold, D.; Bierschenk, S.; Genzel-Boroviczeny, O.; von Andrian, U.H.; Quackenbush, E.; Sperandio, M. Neutrophil and endothelial adhesive function during human fetal ontogeny. *J. Leukoc. Biol.* **2013**, *93*, 175–184. [CrossRef] [PubMed]
10. Filias, A.; Theodorou, G.L.; Mouzopoulou, S.; Varvarigou, A.A.; Mantagos, S.; Karakantza, M. Phagocytic ability of neutrophils and monocytes in neonates. *BMC Pediatr.* **2011**, *11*. [CrossRef] [PubMed]
11. Yan, S.R.; Qing, G.; Byers, D.M.; Stadnyk, A.W.; Al-Hertani, W.; Bortolussi, R. Role of MyD88 in Diminished Tumor Necrosis Factor Alpha Production by Newborn Mononuclear Cells in Response to Lipopolysaccharide. *Infect. Immun.* **2004**, *72*, 1223–1229. [CrossRef] [PubMed]
12. Förster-Waldl, E.; Sadeghi, K.; Tamandl, D.; Gerhold, B.; Hallwirth, U.; Rohrmeister, K.; Hayde, M.; Prusa, A.R.; Herkner, K.; Boltz-Nitulescu, G.; et al. Monocyte toll-like receptor 4 expression and LPS-induced cytokine production increase during gestational aging. *Pediatr. Res.* **2005**, *58*, 121–124. [CrossRef] [PubMed]
13. Al-Hertani, W.; Sen, R.Y.; Byers, D.M.; Bortolussi, R. Human newborn polymorphonuclear neutrophils exhibit decreased levels of MyD88 and attenuated p38 phosphorylation in response to lipopolysaccharide. *Clin. Investig. Med.* **2007**, *30*, 44–53. [CrossRef]
14. Sadeghi, K.; Berger, A.; Langgartner, M.; Prusa, A.; Hayde, M.; Herkner, K.; Pollak, A.; Spittler, A.; Förster-Waldl, E. Immaturity of Infection Control in Preterm and Term Newborns Is Associated with Impaired Toll-Like Receptor Signaling. *J. Infect. Dis.* **2007**, *195*, 296–302. [CrossRef] [PubMed]
15. McGreal, E.P.; Hearne, K.; Spiller, O.B. Off to a slow start: Under-development of the complement system in term newborns is more substantial following premature birth. *Immunobiology* **2012**, *217*, 176–186. [CrossRef] [PubMed]
16. Wynn, J.L.; Levy, O. Role of innate host defenses in susceptibility to early-onset neonatal sepsis. *Clin. Perinatol.* **2010**, *37*, 307–337. [CrossRef] [PubMed]
17. Buhimschi, C.S.; Baumbusch, M.A.; Dulay, A.T.; Oliver, E.A.; Lee, S.; Zhao, G.; Bhandari, V.; Ehrenkranz, R.A.; Weiner, C.P.; Madri, J.A.; et al. Characterization of RAGE, HMGB1, and S100β in inflammation-induced preterm birth and fetal tissue injury. *Am. J. Pathol.* **2009**, *175*, 958–975. [CrossRef] [PubMed]
18. Uchino, S.; Kellum, J.A.; Bellomo, R.; Doig, G.S.; Morimatsu, H.; Morgera, S.; Schetz, M.; Tan, I.; Bouman, C.; Macedo, E.; et al. Acute renal failure in critically ill patients: A multinational, multicenter study. *J. Am. Med. Assoc.* **2005**, *294*, 813–818. [CrossRef] [PubMed]
19. Murugan, R.; Karajala-Subramanyam, V.; Lee, M.; Yende, S.; Kong, L.; Carter, M.; Angus, D.C.; Kellum, J.A. Acute kidney injury in non-severe pneumonia is associated with an increased immune response and lower survival. *Kidney Int.* **2010**, *77*, 527–535. [CrossRef] [PubMed]

20. Bagshaw, S.M.; Uchino, S.; Bellomo, R.; Morimatsu, H.; Morgera, S.; Schetz, M.; Tan, I.; Bouman, C.; Macedo, E.; Gibney, N.; et al. Septic acute kidney injury in critically ill patients: Clinical characteristics and outcomes. *Clin. J. Am. Soc. Nephrol.* **2007**, *2*, 431–439. [CrossRef] [PubMed]
21. Eliopoulos, G.M.; Drusano, G.L.; Ambrose, P.G.; Bhavnani, S.M.; Bertino, J.S.; Nafziger, A.N.; Louie, A. Back to the Future: Using Aminoglycosides Again and How to Dose Them Optimally. *Clin. Infect. Dis.* **2007**, *45*, 753–760. [CrossRef] [PubMed]
22. Ordooei Javan, A.; Shokouhi, S.; Sahraei, Z. A review on colistin nephrotoxicity. *Eur. J. Clin. Pharmacol.* **2015**, *71*, 801–810. [CrossRef] [PubMed]
23. Mergenhagen, K.A.; Borton, A.R. Vancomycin nephrotoxicity: A review. *J. Pharm. Pract.* **2014**, *27*, 545–553. [CrossRef] [PubMed]
24. Bajčetić, M.; Spasić, S.; Spasojević, I. Redox therapy in neonatal sepsis: Reasons, targets, strategy, and agents. *Shock* **2014**, *42*, 179–184. [CrossRef] [PubMed]
25. Romeo, C.; Eaton, S.; Spitz, L.; Pierro, A. Nitric oxide inhibits neonatal hepatocyte oxidative metabolism. *J. Pediatr. Surg.* **2000**, *35*, 44–48. [CrossRef]
26. Plotnikov, E.Y.; Pavlenko, T.A.; Pevzner, I.B.; Zorova, L.D.; Manskikh, V.N.; Silachev, D.N.; Sukhikh, G.T.; Zorov, D.B. The role of oxidative stress in acute renal injury of newborn rats exposed to hypoxia and endotoxin. *FEBS J.* **2017**, *284*, 3069–3078. [CrossRef] [PubMed]
27. Zorov, D.B.; Juhaszova, M.; Sollott, S.J. Mitochondrial reactive oxygen species (ROS) and ROS-induced ROS release. *Physiol. Rev.* **2014**, *94*, 909–950. [CrossRef] [PubMed]
28. Plotnikov, E.Y.; Morosanova, M.; Pevzner, I.B.; Zorova, L.D.; Manskikh, V.N.; Pulkova, N.V.; Galkina, S.I.; Skulachev, V.P.; Zorov, D.B. Protective effect of mitochondria-targeted antioxidants in an acute bacterial infection. *Proc. Natl. Acad. Sci. USA* **2013**, *110*, 3100–3108. [CrossRef] [PubMed]
29. Plotnikov, E.Y.; Chupyrkina, A.A.; Jankauskas, S.S.; Pevzner, I.B.; Silachev, D.N.; Skulachev, V.P.; Zorov, D.B. Mechanisms of nephroprotective effect of mitochondria-targeted antioxidants under rhabdomyolysis and ischemia/reperfusion. *Biochim. Biophys. Acta* **2011**, *1812*, 77–86. [CrossRef] [PubMed]
30. Kiernan, J.A. *Histological and Histochemical Methods: Theory and Practice*, 3rd ed.; Butterworth-Heinemann: Boston, MA, USA; Oxford, UK, 1999.
31. Mihara, M.; Uchiyama, M. Determination of malonaldehyde precursor in tissues by thiobarbituric acid test. *Anal. Biochem.* **1978**, *86*, 271–278. [PubMed]
32. Balbi, A.P.C.; Costa, R.S.; Coimbra, T.M. Postnatal renal development of rats from mothers that received increased sodium intake. *Pediatr. Nephrol.* **2004**, *19*, 1212–1218. [CrossRef] [PubMed]
33. Asikainen, T.M.; Raivio, K.O.; Saksela, M.; Kinnula, V.L. Expression and developmental profile of antioxidant enzymes in human lung and liver. *Am. J. Respir. Cell Mol. Biol.* **1998**, *19*, 942–949. [CrossRef] [PubMed]
34. Hayashibe, H.; Asayama, K.; Dobashi, K.; Kato, K. Prenatal development of antioxidant enzymes in rat lung, kidney, and heart: Marked increase in immunoreactive superoxide dismutases, glutathione peroxidase, and catalase in the kidney. *Pediatr. Res.* **1990**, *27*, 472–475. [CrossRef] [PubMed]
35. Gopinathan, V.; Miller, N.J.; Milner, A.D.; Rice-Evans, C.A. Bilirubin and ascorbate antioxidant activity in neonatal plasma. *FEBS Lett.* **1994**, *349*, 197–200. [CrossRef]
36. Nassi, N.; Ponziani, V.; Becatti, M.; Galvan, P.; Donzelli, G. Anti-oxidant enzymes and related elements in term and preterm newborns. *Pediatr. Int.* **2009**, *51*, 183–187. [CrossRef] [PubMed]
37. Longo, L.D. Respiratory Gas Exchange in the Placenta. In *Comprehensive Physiology*; John Wiley & Sons Inc.: Hoboken, NJ, USA, 2011; pp. 351–401, ISBN 9780470650714.
38. Saugstad, O.D. Mechanisms of tissue injury by oxygen radicals: Implications for neonatal disease. *Acta Paediatr. Int. J. Paediatr.* **1996**, *85*, 1–4. [CrossRef]
39. Buonocore, G.; Groenendaal, F. Anti-oxidant strategies. *Semin. Fetal Neonatal Med.* **2007**, *12*, 287–295. [CrossRef] [PubMed]
40. Komatsu, H.; Tsukimori, K.; Hata, K.; Satoh, S.; Nakano, H. The characterization of superoxide production of human neonatal neutrophil. *Early Hum. Dev.* **2001**, *65*, 11–19. [CrossRef]
41. Doi, K.; Leelahavanichkul, A.; Yuen, P.S.T.; Star, R.A. Animal models of sepsis and sepsis-induced kidney injury. *J. Clin. Investig.* **2009**, *119*, 2868–2878. [CrossRef] [PubMed]

42. Park, S.K.; Kang, M.J.; Kim, W.; Koh, G.Y. Renal tubule regeneration after ischemic injury is coupled to the up-regulation and activation of cyclins and cyclin dependent kinases. *Kidney Int.* **1997**, *52*, 706–714. [CrossRef] [PubMed]
43. Meran, S.; Steadman, R. Fibroblasts and myofibroblasts in renal fibrosis. *Int. J. Exp. Pathol.* **2011**, *92*, 158–167. [CrossRef] [PubMed]

10

Iron and the Breastfed Infant

James Friel [1,*], Wafaa Qasem [2] and Chenxi Cai [1]

1 Department of Food and Human Nutritional Sciences, University of Manitoba, Winnipeg, MB R3T 2N2, Canada; caic3@myumanitoba.ca
2 Food and Nutrition Administration, Ministry of Health, P.O. Box 4078, Safat 13041, Kuwait; qasemw@myumanitoba.ca
* Correspondence: James.Friel@umanitoba.ca

Abstract: The first 6 months of life is a crucial time in meeting iron needs. The purpose of this review is to examine iron in mother's milk and whether or not it meets the physiological needs of the growing infant. Key issues include iron content and iron transport from the mammary gland as well as when and what foods should be added to the solely breastfed infant. We examine these topics in light of new molecular biology findings in the mammary gland.

Keywords: iron; infant; mother's milk

---

1. Introduction

Iron (Fe) is an essential nutrient that exists in low quantity in human milk. Whether or not iron in human milk will meet the developmental needs of the breastfed infant for the first 6 months of life is controversial [1,2]. Some countries recommend supplementation of iron as drops at 4 months, others do not [1,3,4]. This has bearing on the best time of introduction of solids as iron fortification of foods assists in meeting iron needs for the second half of infancy. Recent evidence has indicated that iron is not secreted into mother's milk, and what iron that is present is present in low quantities. In terms of supplying solid foods that are rich in iron, there are new recommendations but no consensus. We review the evidence to support the early introduction of iron-enriched solid foods or iron drops by 4 months of age. We discuss these issues in light of recent molecular biological information derived from our studies of iron transporters in human mammary epithelial cells.

2. Iron

2.1. *Biological Functions of Fe*

In the human body, iron is the most abundant trace element, and acts as a center for a broad spectrum of functions [4]. Its importance is derived from its redox activity, because iron exists mainly in ferrous (Fe^{2+}) and ferric (Fe^{3+}) oxidation states, which are interchangeable. The conversion of one state to the other forms part of the electron transport chain, essential in the generation of energy (ATP) during metabolism and in the reductions needed for synthesis [5]. There is little free iron in vivo. Iron is chelated to proteins or other molecules; this maintains solubility, limits participation in oxygen redox chemistry, and limits availability to microbes [6].

Proteins that bind iron act functionally as antioxidants [5,7]. An antioxidant is a substance that, when present at a low concentration compared with that of an oxidizable substrate, inhibits oxidation of the substrate, the process known as oxidative stress [5,7]. Iron is more known as an oxidant, a species that causes or promotes oxidation, whereas molecules that bind iron function as antioxidants. In contrast, vitamin C acts as a dietary iron reductant [5,7].

Hemoglobin (Hb) iron (60%), myoglobin iron (5%), both heme and non-heme enzymes (5%), and transferrin (less than 1%), are designated as functional iron. The remaining iron is found in the storage proteins ferritin (about 20%) and in hemosiderin (about 10%) [8]. The primary role of iron is for oxygen transport to assist in cell respiration. Myoglobin uses iron to store oxygen in muscle tissue. Enzyme iron functions in immune function and other metabolic actions [8]. An underappreciated role of iron is its importance in neurotransmitter function and myelination [9].

2.2. Fe Absorption and Transport

Fe uptake by enterocytes depends on the forms of the Fe. The sources of Fe include non-heme Fe, heme Fe, and ferritin. It has been proposed that heme Fe is transported by an intestinal heme transporter, heme carrier protein 1 (HCP1) [10], or another transporter [11]. This process has not yet been fully elucidated. Ferritin enters the enterocytes via an unknown mechanism, and it is likely then degraded in the lysosomes [12]. Non-heme ferric Fe must first be reduced to ferrous Fe by duodenal cytochrome b (DCYTB) [13] or other cell surface ferrireductases [14], and then be transported into the enterocytes by divalent metal transporter 1 (DMT1) [15]. Once it enters the cell, cellular Fe is stored as ferritin, used by the intracellular compartments, or exported into the blood for use by other tissues in the body [12]. Intracellular ferrous Fe is transferred across the basolateral membrane by ferroportin FPN [12], and is then oxidized to ferric Fe by hephaestin (HEPH), a membrane-anchored, multi-copper ferroxidase [16]. Then, ferric Fe binds to transferrin (TF) in the interstitial fluids and circulates throughout the body.

2.3. Fe Requirements of Infants

At birth, full-term healthy infants have an iron content of about 75 mg/kg, with high blood volume, and Hb concentration in proportion to their body weight [17]. During the first few months of life, they experience a physiological decline in their blood volume and Hb concentration, and an active shift from fetal Hb to adult type Hb [18]. There are conflicting thoughts on the Fe requirement of infants. For newborn infants, most of the Fe in the body is found in Hb and some smaller stores. When a newborn is transferred from the uterine environment into an oxygen-rich atmosphere, the Hb level falls from 170 g/L to 120 g/L during the first 6 weeks of life [18]. For exclusively breastfed infants, the major source of Fe comes from body stores because the Fe content in human milk is extremely low [18,19]. Some researchers conclude that a normal healthy full-term infant has a sufficient amount of Fe until about 4 to 6 months of age [20]. Based on the average Fe concentration in human milk, the Institute of Medicine Dietary Reference Intakes (DRIs) for Fe for infants before the age of 6 months is 0.27 mg/d [21]. By contrast, the American Academy of Pediatrics recommends that exclusively breastfed, full-term infants receive 1 mg/kg per day of Fe supplement beginning at the age of 4 months [1].

2.4. Iron Content of Human Milk

As the current recommendations for infants are based on the iron content of human milk, we need to examine milk more closely. Human breast milk has very little iron (0.4 mg/L) [19]. Since breast milk is designed for humans by humans, it can be concluded that what is in breast milk is optimal for developing infants. While there is no controversy that iron in human milk is low, the current thought is that the small amount present must in some way be sufficient. Indeed, breast milk is thought to have "a special form" of iron often stated to be "highly bioavailable" [22,23]. To support this concept, Lonnerdal has shown the presence of a receptor in the infant gut specifically for lactoferrin-iron [24]. The concept that "breast milk is the perfect food" is challenged by the shortfall in several nutrients, including iron [25]. This is not a popular concept as a door might be opened for supplementation of any and all nutrients as is done for the premature infant [26]. Nonetheless, vitamin D is given to breastfed infants, although there is controversy around this as well [27].

The Fe content in human breast milk is considered low in comparison to maternal serum Fe. The Fe concentration in human colostrum is approximately 0.8 μg/mL; in mature breast milk, it is 0.2–0.4 μg/mL [28]. In contrast, the Fe concentrations in the milk of other species are much higher [28,29]. The Fe concentration in mature milk in rat is 5–10 μg/mL, which is about 25 times higher than the Fe concentration of human milk [29]. Although the Fe concentration is low in human milk, it is thought to be independent of the mother's Fe status and it cannot be increased through maternal diet or Fe supplementation [30–32]. A recent study suggests the possibility that maternal iron status during pregnancy may affect the quantity of iron during lactation [33].

Human mammary epithelial cells do not secrete iron into breast milk. This surprising finding is based on the fact that the primary membrane iron exporter is not found in human lactating epithelial cells [34]. This accords with the prevailing view that body iron content is not controlled by excretion, but is controlled by absorption [35]. The iron content of human milk can be accounted in large amount by what is present in milk epithelial cells [19,36], which are the predominant cells in a healthy mother [37]. It may be that the infant gets all its needed iron from external sources as iron is ubiquitous, as it is the most common element on earth, and was readily available as contamination until recent times [38,39].

2.5. Supplementation with Iron Drops

The Fe status of exclusively breastfed infants and how it is maintained, remains a controversial topic in neonatal nutrition [40]. Some voices support Fe supplementation while others regard it as harmful due to potential Fe overload. Concerns have been expressed about Fe supplementation, as Fe is a potent pro-oxidant, and it cannot be actively excreted by humans [41]. Some studies have suggested that Fe supplementation may have adverse effects on iron-replete infants, including increased risk of infections and impaired growth [42]. Increased risk of severe infections seems to be restricted to malaria regions [43]. However, current evidence is not definitive, nor are the negative consequences of short-term impaired growth on long-term outcome.

We have found that iron supplementation in early infancy improves cognitive development [44]. Healthy breastfed infants who received iron drops between 1 and 6 months of age had improvements in both psychomotor development skills and visual acuity, in comparison to control infants. From these findings, the American Academy of pediatrics recommended all exclusively breastfed infants should receive iron drops of 1 mg/kg/day at 4 months of age [22] to augment the low levels of iron in mother's milk.

Results from a meta-analysis, which included four randomized control trials (RCT) involving 511 infants, supported early iron supplementation [45]. Current data suggests that though iron supplementation of healthy exclusively breastfed infants may improve their iron status and cognitive development, there may be a delay in their physical growth. There was no evidence to suggest iron supplementation could cause other adverse effects [45].

2.6. Iron Deficiency Anemia and Effects on Neurodevelopment

As iron supplements may be of benefit, maintaining an adequate level of Fe is critical to an infant's physical and neurological development. Iron deficiency (ID) is commonly considered to develop in three stages: iron depletion, iron-deficient erythropoiesis, and iron deficiency anemia (IDA) [46].

Fe is critical for the rapid development of the central nervous system during infancy. Animal studies have shown that Fe is critical for many aspects of brain development, including myelination, monoamine neurotransmitter function, and neuronal and glial energy metabolism [41]. Some human studies have suggested that early ID is associated with later neurodevelopmental impairments. A longitudinal study in Costa Rica assessed changes in cognitive functioning after ID in infancy by evaluating four subsequent follow-ups at 5, 11–14, 15–18, and 19 years of age [47–49]. The results indicated that participants who had ID in infancy had lower cognitive scores over time compared to participants in the group with good Fe status. The results of these studies have increased concerns that early ID may irreversibly affect long-term neurodevelopment. A meta-analysis of 17 randomized clinical trials in children indicated that Fe supplements have positive cognitive effects in iron-deficient children [50]. Consequently, early prevention of ID seems to be extremely important. However, whether or not Fe has positive neurodevelopment effects on exclusively breastfed infants still needs to be clarified.

2.7. Solids and Their Introduction

An important issue for the breastfed infant is the timing of the introduction of complementary feeding or solid foods. Once solids are started, the role of breast milk changes. Whereas breast milk was the only food the infant was receiving, the simplicity of the diet is now altered. Interactions between nutrients in different food items is now possible. When and what solids to introduce is controversial. Some [3] advocate delaying solids until 6 months of age, however, others suggest around 4 months is best [51,52]. In North America, the average age of introduction is around 4–5 months [53]. We think that there is some risk in being prescriptive about the timing of introduction of solids as some infants may or not need the energy and nutrients from solids at different times [52,54]. For health professionals to insist that 6 months is best for each and every infant is not biologically reasonable [55]. It is more reasonable for individual caregivers to base their decision of timing of introduction of solids on cues signifying physiological readiness provided by the infant [52]. It appears the main reason for recommending 6 months is an attempt to prolong the use of breastfeeding [4,54]. While a laudable goal, there are some infants who will need more nutrients than available from breast milk before 6 months of age [55].

2.8. Possible Adverse Effects of Fe in the Gastrointestinal Tract

There is evidence that unabsorbed iron in the gastrointestinal tract will lead to the generation of reactive oxygen species [56,57]. This may be particularly true for infants consuming iron-fortified cereals of low bioavailability [58]. It is known that antioxidant foods, including fruit, may ameliorate the consequences of reactive oxygen species (ROS) generation [59]. We conducted a study in adults who received a large dose of iron concurrently with an antioxidant supplement [60]. Those subjects receiving the antioxidant supplement had significantly less ROS generation. Infants receiving iron-fortified cereals are consuming similar levels of iron that may subject them to inflammation [61].

2.9. Iron and Microbiota

The gastrointestinal tract is home to thousands of species of bacteria collectively known as the microbiome [62], which plays a role in metabolism. Dysbiosis of the infant microbiome may have unwanted consequences long-term [63]. The gut microbiome has been shown to be altered in animals receiving iron supplementation, however, little work has been done in infants [64–66]. We completed a study assessing the effect of meat and cereal based diets in infants on the infant gut microbiome [67]. Choice of first complimentary foods may influence gut inflammation and microbiota, potentially due to variations in iron absorption from different foods. Our findings supported the use of meats as a first food as suggested by Krebs group [66].

3. Complementary Feeding (CF)

There are few large studies examining complementary feeding of infants in developed countries. A large study in Canadian infants indicated that infants started solids as early as 4 months, little meat was consumed, and primary sources of iron were from iron-fortified infant cereals [53]. These findings do not indicate mother's support of current recommendations to start solids at 6 months with meat as the first choice [3]. Mean iron intake from solids never met the 7- to 12-month recommendations for amounts of CF [53].

As there is little iron in mother's milk [19], the low intake of iron from complementary foods becomes an issue. Iron in solids foods is found primarily in meat and fortified cereal, with very little found in fruits and vegetables [68]. Significant sources of iron, including meat, poultry, fish, and eggs, are not routinely consumed until 8–9 months of age [53]. In a large American study, infant cereal was the major source of most minerals for infants [69]. However, the form of iron used by manufacturers is of low bioavailability [70]. It is not surprising that 24% of Canadian infants have low iron stores [53]. Novel ways of meeting iron needs will have to be considered.

Further reviews on iron content of mother's milk [18,19,23,28–30,32,33], iron metabolism [8,20,35,41], and timing of introduction of solid foods [52,54,55], address these issues as well.

4. Conclusions

(1) Is there enough iron in breast milk to meet infant needs for the first 6 months of life?
Not enough to meet estimated needs.
(2) Will iron given as either drops or fortified foods before 6 months of age be harmful?
Disturbed growth is not consistent, nor evidence of harm.
(3) When is the best time to introduce iron fortified solid foods?
No earlier than 4 months, no later than 7 months, depending on the infant.
(4) What is the best solid food to give the infant first?
Meat, no residual iron, to potentially induce ROS generation in gut.
(5) What is the best public health approach?
Screen all infants at 4 months: otherwise, flag for any abnormality of infant or mother. There may be benefit in creating a composite system including ferritin, haemoglobin, mean corpuscular volume, dietary intake, and maternal risk factors. This would have to be examined carefully in a prospective cohort study.

Acknowledgments: This work was carried out with support from the Canadian Institutes of Health Research.

Author Contributions: James Friel, Wafaa Qasem and Chenxi Cai participated in the preparation of this article.

Conflicts of Interest: The authors declare no conflict of interest.

References

1. Baker, R.D.; Greer, F.R.; Committee on Nutrition American Academy of Pediatrics. Diagnosis and prevention of iron deficiency and iron-deficiency anemia in infants and young children (0–3 years of age). *Pediatrics* **2010**, *126*, 1040–1050. [CrossRef] [PubMed]
2. Trumbo, P.; Yates, A.A.; Schlicker, S.; Poos, M. Dietary reference intakes: Vitamin A, vitamin K, arsenic, boron, chromium, copper, iodine, iron, manganese, molybdenum, nickel, silicon, vanadium, and zinc. *J. Am. Diet. Assoc.* **2001**, *101*, 294–301. [CrossRef]
3. Bank, J. Nutrition for Healthy Term Infants: Recommendations from Birth to Six Months. *Can. J. Diet. Pract. Res. Publ. Dietit. Can.* **2012**, *73*, 204. [CrossRef]
4. Qasem, W.; Friel, J. An Overview of Iron in Term Breast-Fed Infants. *Clin. Med. Insights Pediatr.* **2015**, *9*, 79–84. [CrossRef] [PubMed]
5. Halliwell, B. Commentary oxidative stress, nutrition and health. Experimental strategies for optimization of nutritional antioxidant intake in humans. *Free Radic. Res.* **1996**, *25*, 57–74. [CrossRef] [PubMed]
6. Caza, M.; Kronstad, J.M. Shared and Distinct Mechanisms of Iron Acquisition by Bacterial and Fungal Pathogens of Humans. *Front. Cell. Infect. Microbiol.* **2013**, *80*. [CrossRef] [PubMed]
7. Zhuang, T.; Han, H.; Yang, Z. Iron, oxidative stress and gestational diabetes. *Nutrients* **2014**, *6*, 3968–3980. [CrossRef] [PubMed]
8. McDermid, J.M.; Lonnerdal, B. Iron. *Adv. Nutr.* **2012**, *3*, 532–533. [CrossRef] [PubMed]
9. Tran, P.; Fretham, S.; Carlson, E.; Georgieff, M. Long-term reduction of hippocampal brain-derived neurotrophic factor activity after fetal-neonatal iron deficiency in adult rats. *Pediatr. Res.* **2009**, *65*, 493–498. [CrossRef] [PubMed]

10. Shayeghi, M.; Latunde-Dada, G.O.; Oakhill, J.S.; Laftah, A.H.; Takeuchi, K.; Halliday, N.; Khan, Y.; Warley, A.; McCann, F.E.; Hider, R.C.; et al. Identification of an intestinal heme transporter. *Cell* **2005**, *122*, 789–801. [CrossRef] [PubMed]
11. Qiu, A.; Jansen, M.; Sakaris, A.; Min, S.H.; Chattopadhyay, S.; Tsai, E.; Sandoval, C.; Zhao, R.; Akabas, M.H.; Goldman, I.D. Identification of an intestinal folate transporter and the molecular basis for hereditary folate malabsorption. *Cell* **2006**, *127*, 917–928. [CrossRef] [PubMed]
12. Gulec, S.; Anderson, G.; Collins, J. Mechanistic and regulatory aspects of intestinal iron absorption. *Am. J. Physiol. Gastrointest. Liver Physiol.* **2014**, *307*, G397–G409. [CrossRef] [PubMed]
13. McKie, A.T.; Barrow, D.; Latunde-Dada, G.O.; Rolfs, A.; Sager, G.; Mudaly, E.; Mudaly, M.; Richardson, C.; Barlow, D.; Bomford, A.; et al. An iron-regulated ferric reductase associated with the absorption of dietary iron. *Science* **2001**, *291*, 1755–1759. [CrossRef] [PubMed]
14. Ohgami, R.S.; Campagna, D.R.; McDonald, A.; Fleming, M.D. The Steap proteins are metalloreductases. *Blood* **2006**, *108*, 1388–1394. [CrossRef] [PubMed]
15. Mackenzie, B.; Garrick, M.D. Iron Imports. II. Iron uptake at the apical membrane in the intestine. *Am. J. Physiol. Gastrointest. Liver Physiol.* **2005**, *289*, G981–G986. [CrossRef] [PubMed]
16. Chen, H.; Attieh, Z.K.; Su, T.; Syed, B.A.; Gao, H.; Alaeddine, R.M.; Fox, T.C.; Usta, J.; Naylor, C.E.; Evans, R.W.; et al. Hephaestin is a ferroxidase that maintains partial activity in sex-linked anemia mice. *Blood* **2004**, *103*, 3933–3939. [CrossRef] [PubMed]
17. Siddappa, A.M.; Rao, R.; Long, J.D.; Widness, J.A.; Georgieff, M.K. The assessment of newborn iron stores at birth: A review of the literature and standards for ferritin concentrations. *Neonatology* **2007**, *92*, 73–82. [CrossRef] [PubMed]
18. Domellof, M. Iron Requirements, Absorption and Metabolism in Infancy and Childhood. *Curr. Opin. Clin. Nutr. Metab. Care* **2007**, *10*, 329–335. [CrossRef] [PubMed]
19. Cai, C.; Harding, S.V.; Friel, J.K. Breast milk iron concentrations may be lower than previously reported: implications for exclusively breastfed infants. *Matern Pediatr. Nutr.* **2015**, *2*, 2. [CrossRef]
20. Domellof, M.; Braegger, C.; Campoy, V.; Colomb, T.; Decsi, M.; Fewtrell, I.; Hojsak, A.; Mihatsch, W.; Molgaard, C.; Shamir, R.; et al. Iron Requirements of Infants and Toddlers. *J. Pediatr. Gastroenterol. Nutr.* **2014**, *58*, 119–129. [CrossRef] [PubMed]
21. Institute of Medicine. *Dietary Reference Intakes: The Essential Guide to Nutrient Requirements*; National Academy Press: Washington, DC, USA, 2006.
22. Saarinen, U.M.; Siimes, M.A.; Dallman, P.R. Iron absorption in infants: high bioavailability of breast milk iron as indicated by the extrinsic tag method of iron absorption and by the concentration of serum ferritin. *J. Pediatr.* **1977**, *91*, 36–39. [CrossRef]
23. Dewey, K.G.; Chaparro, C.M. Session 4: Mineral metabolism and body composition iron status of breast-fed infants. *Proc. Nutr. Soc.* **2007**, *66*, 412–422. [CrossRef] [PubMed]
24. Suzuki, Y.A.; Shin, K.; Lönnerdal, B. Molecular cloning and functional expression of a human intestinal lactoferrin receptor. *Biochemistry* **2001**, *40*, 15771–15779. [CrossRef] [PubMed]
25. Erick, M. Breast milk is conditionally perfect. *Med. Hypotheses* **2018**, *111*, 82–89. [CrossRef] [PubMed]
26. Agostoni, C.; Buonocore, G.; Carnielli, V.P.; De Curtis, M.; Darmaun, D.; Decsi, T.; Domellöf, M.; Embleton, N.D.; Fusch, C.; Genzel-Boroviczeny, O.; et al. Enteral nutrient supply for preterm infants: Commentary from the European Society of Paediatric Gastroenterology, Hepatology and Nutrition Committee on Nutrition. *J. Pediatr. Gastroenterol. Nutr.* **2010**, *50*, 85–91. [CrossRef] [PubMed]
27. Heinig, M.J. Vitamin D and the breastfed infant: Controversies and concerns. *J. Hum. Lact.* **2003**, *19*, 247–249. [CrossRef] [PubMed]
28. Lonnerdal, B.; Keen, C.L.; Hurley, L.S. Iron, copper, zinc, and manganese in milk. *Annu. Rev. Nutr.* **1981**, *1*, 149–174. [CrossRef] [PubMed]
29. Lonnerdal, B.; Keen, C.L.; Hurley, L.S. *Trace Element Metabolism in Man and Animals (TEMA)-4*, 1st ed.; Nestly Griffen Press: Hindmarsh, Australia, 1981.
30. Domellof, M.; Lonnerdal, B.; Dewey, K.G.; Cohen, R.J.; Hernell, O. Iron, zinc, and copper concentrations in breast milk are independent of maternal mineral status. *Am. J. Clin. Nutr.* **2004**, *79*, 111–115. [CrossRef] [PubMed]
31. Celada, A.; Busset, R.; Gutierrez, J.; Herreros, V. No correlation between iron concentration in breast milk and maternal iron stores. *Helv. Paediatr. Acta* **1982**, *37*, 11–16. [PubMed]

32. Dorea, J.G. Iron and copper in human milk. *Nutrition* **2000**, *16*, 209–220. [CrossRef]
33. Hampel, D.; Shahab-Ferdows, S.; Gertz, E.; Flax, V.L.; Adair, L.S.; Bentley, M.E.; Jamieson, D.J.; Tegha, G.; Chasela, C.S.; Kamwendo, D.; et al. The effects of a lipid-based nutrient supplement and antiretroviral therapy in a randomized controlled trial on iron, copper, and zinc in milk from HIV-infected Malawian mothers and associations with maternal and infant biomarkers. *Matern. Child Nutr.* **2017**, e12503. [CrossRef] [PubMed]
34. Cai, C.; Eck, P.; Friel, J.K. Gene Expression Profiles Suggest Iron Transport Pathway in the Lactating Human Epithelial Cell. *J. Pediatr. Gastroenterol. Nutr.* **2017**, *64*, 460–464. [CrossRef] [PubMed]
35. Lönnerdal, B.; Georgieff, M.K.; Hernell, O. Developmental Physiology of Iron Absorption, Homeostasis, and Metabolism in the Healthy Term Infant. *J. Pediatr.* **2015**, *167* (Suppl. 4), S8–S14. [CrossRef] [PubMed]
36. Calero, M.; Chiappi, M.; Lazaro-Carrillo, A.; Rodríguez, M.J.; Chichón, F.J.; Crosbie-Staunton, K.; Prina-Mello, A.; Volkov, Y.; Villanueva, A.; Carrascosa, J.L. Characterization of interaction of magnetic nanoparticles with breast cancer cells. *J. Nanobiotechnol.* **2015**, *13*, 16. [CrossRef] [PubMed]
37. Hassiotou, F.; Hepworth, A.R.; Metzger, P.; Lai, C.T.; Trengove, N.; Hartmann, P.E.; Filgueira, L. Maternal and infant infections stimulate a rapid leukocyte response in breastmilk. *Clin. Transl. Immunol.* **2013**, *2*, e3. [CrossRef] [PubMed]
38. Harvey, P.W.; Dexter, P.B.; Darnton-Hill, I. The impact of consuming iron from non-food sources on iron status in developing countries. *Public Health Nutr.* **2000**, *3*, 375–383. [CrossRef] [PubMed]
39. Strachan, D. Re: The "hygiene hypothesis" for allergic disease is a misnomer. *BMJ* **2014**, *349*, g5267. [CrossRef]
40. Friel, J.K. There Is No Iron in Human Milk. *J. Pediatr. Gastroenterol. Nutr.* **2017**, *64*, 339–340. [CrossRef] [PubMed]
41. Lonnerdal, B. Development of iron homeostasis in infants and young children. *Am. J. Clin. Nutr.* **2017**, *106* (Suppl. 6), 1575S–1580S. [CrossRef] [PubMed]
42. Lönnerdal, B. Excess iron intake as a factor in growth, infections, and development of infants and young children. *Am. J. Clin. Nutr.* **2017**, *106* (Suppl. 6), 1681S–1687S. [CrossRef] [PubMed]
43. Spottiswoode, N.; Duffy, P.E.; Drakesmith, H. Iron, anemia and hepcidin in malaria. *Front. Pharmacol.* **2014**, *5*, 125. [CrossRef] [PubMed]
44. Friel, J.K.; Aziz, K.; Andrews, W.L.; Harding, S.V.; Courage, M.L.; Adams, R.J. A double-masked, randomized control trial of iron supplementation in early infancy in healthy term breast-fed infants. *J. Pediatr.* **2003**, *143*, 582–586. [CrossRef]
45. Cai, C.; Granger, M.; Eck, P.; Friel, J. Effect of Daily Iron Supplementation in Healthy Exclusively Breastfed Infants: A Systematic Review with Meta-Analysis. *Breastfeed. Med.* **2017**, *12*, 597–603. [CrossRef] [PubMed]
46. WHO. *Iron Deficiency Anemia: Assessment, Prevention and Control. A Guide for Programme Managers*; World Health Organization: Geneva, Switzerland, 2001; Available online: http://www.who.int/nutrition/publications/micronutrients/anaemia_iron_deficiency/WHO_NHD_01.3/en/ (accessed on 4 October 2001).
47. Lozoff, B.; Smith, J.B.; Kaciroti, N.; Clark, K.M.; Guevara, S.; Jimenez, E. Functional significance of early-life iron deficiency: Outcomes at 25 years. *J. Pediatr.* **2013**, *163*, 1260–1266. [CrossRef] [PubMed]
48. Lozoff, B.; Beard, J.; Connor, J.; Barbara, F.; Georgieff, M.; Schaller, T. Long-lasting neural and behavioral effects of iron deficiency in infancy. *Nutr. Rev.* **2006**, *64 5 Pt 2*, S34–S43; discussion S72–S91. [CrossRef]
49. Lozoff, B.; Jimenez, E.; Hagen, J.; Mollen, E.; Wolf, A. Poorer behavioral and developmental outcome more than 10 years after treatment for iron deficiency in infancy. *Pediatrics* **2000**, *105*, E51. [CrossRef] [PubMed]
50. Sachdev, H.; Gera, T.; Nestel, P. Effect of iron supplementation on mental and motor development in children: Systematic review of randomised controlled trials. *Public Health Nutr.* **2005**, *8*, 117–132. [CrossRef] [PubMed]
51. Fewtrell, M.; Bronsky, J.; Campoy, C.; Domellöf, M.; Embleton, N.; Fidler Mis, N.; Hojsak, I.; Hulst, J.M.; Indrio, F.; Lapillonne, A.; et al. Complementary Feeding: A Position Paper by the European Society for Paediatric Gastroenterology, Hepatology, and Nutrition (ESPGHAN) Committee on Nutrition. *J. Pediatr. Gastroenterol Nutr.* **2017**, *64*, 119–132. [CrossRef] [PubMed]
52. Qasem, W.; Fenton, T.; Friel, J. Age of introduction of first complementary feeding for infants: A systematic review. *BMC Pediatr.* **2015**, *15*, 107. [CrossRef] [PubMed]
53. Friel, J.K.; Hanning, R.M.; Isaak, C.A.; Prowse, D.; Miller, A.C. Canadian infants' nutrient intakes from complementary foods during the first year of life. *BMC Pediatr.* **2010**, *10*, 43. [CrossRef] [PubMed]

54. Fewtrell, M.; Wilson, D.C.; Booth, I.; Lucas, A. Six months of exclusive breast feeding: How good is the evidence? *BMJ* **2010**, *13*, 342. [CrossRef] [PubMed]
55. Reilly, J.J.; Wells, J.C. Duration of exclusive breast-feeding: Introduction of complementary feeding may be necessary before 6 months of age. *Br. J. Nutr.* **2005**, *94*, 869–872. [CrossRef] [PubMed]
56. Lund, E.K.; Wharf, S.G.; Fairweather-Tait, S.J.; Johnson, I.T. Oral ferrous sulfate supplements increase the free radical-generating capacity of feces from healthy volunteers. *Am. J. Clin. Nutr.* **1999**, *69*, 250–255. [CrossRef] [PubMed]
57. Schümann, K.; Kroll, S.; Weiss, G.; Frank, J.; Biesalski, H.K.; Daniel, H.; Friel, J.; Solomons, N.W. Monitoring of hematological, inflammatory and oxidative reactions to acute oral iron exposure in human volunteers: Preliminary screening for selection of potentially-responsive biomarkers. *Toxicology* **2005**, *212*, 10–23. [CrossRef] [PubMed]
58. Kortman, G.A.; Raffatellu, M.; Swinkels, D.W.; Tjalsma, H. Nutritional iron turned inside out: Intestinal stress from a gut microbial perspective. *FEMS Microbiol. Rev.* **2014**, *38*, 1202–1234. [CrossRef] [PubMed]
59. Lotito, S.B.; Frei, B. Consumption of flavonoid-rich foods and increased plasma antioxidant capacity in humans: Cause, consequence, or epiphenomenon? *Free Radic. Biol. Med.* **2006**, *41*, 1727–1746. [CrossRef] [PubMed]
60. Orozco, M.N.; Solomons, N.W.; Schumann, K.; Friel, J.K.; de Montenegro, A.L. Antioxidant-rich oral supplements attenuate the effects of oral iron on in situ oxidation susceptibility of human feces. *J. Nutr.* **2010**, *140*, 1105–1110. [CrossRef] [PubMed]
61. Halliwell, B. Free radicals and antioxidants: A personal view. *Nutr. Rev.* **1994**, *52*, 253–265. [CrossRef] [PubMed]
62. Berg, R. The indigenous gastrointestinal microflora. *Trends Microbiol.* **1996**, *4*, 430–435. [CrossRef]
63. Xavier, R.; Podolsky, D. Unravelling the pathogenesis of inflammatory bowel disease. *Nature* **2007**, *448*, 427–434. [CrossRef] [PubMed]
64. Buhnik-Rosenblau, K.; Moshe-Belizowski, S.; Danin-Poleg, Y.; Meyron-Holtz, E.G. Genetic modification of iron metabolism in mice affects the gut microbiota. *Biometals* **2012**, *25*, 883–892. [CrossRef] [PubMed]
65. Jaeggi, T.; Kortman, G.A.; Moretti, D.; Chassard, C.; Holding, P.; Dostal, A.; Boekhorst, J.; Timmerman, H.M.; Swinkels, D.W.; Tjalsma, H.; et al. Iron fortification adversely affects the gut microbiome, increases pathogen abundance and induces intestinal inflammation in Kenyan infants. *Gut* **2015**, *64*, 731–742. [CrossRef] [PubMed]
66. Krebs, N.F.; Sherlock, L.G.; Westcott, J.; Culbertson, D.; Hambidge, K.M.; Feazel, L.M.; Robertson, C.E.; Frank, D.N. Effects of different complementary feeding regimens on iron status and enteric microbiota in breastfed infants. *J. Pediatr.* **2013**, *163*, 416–423. [CrossRef] [PubMed]
67. Qasem, W.; Azad, M.B.; Hossain, Z.; Azad, E.; Jorgensen, S.; Castillo San Juan, S.; Cai, C.; Khafipour, E.; Beta, T.; Roberts, L.J., 2nd; et al. Assessment of complementary feeding of Canadian infants: Effects on microbiome & oxidative stress, a randomized controlled trial. *BMC Pediatr.* **2017**, *17*, 54. [CrossRef]
68. Heinz Baby Canada. Step 1: Beginner Foods. Version Current 2003. Available online: http://www.heinzbaby.com/english/solid/beginner_foods.html (accessed on 23 December 2008).
69. Fox, M.K.; Reidy, K.; Novak, T.; Zeigler, P. Sources of energy and nutrients in the diets of infants and toddlers. *J. Am. Diet. Assoc.* **2006**, *106*, S28–S42. [CrossRef] [PubMed]
70. Davidsson, L.; Kastenmayer, P.; Szajewska, H.; Hurrell, R.F.; Barclay, D. Iron bioavailability in infants from an infant cereal fortified with ferric pyrophosphate or ferrous fumarate. *Am. J. Clin. Nutr.* **2000**, *71*, 1597–1602. [CrossRef] [PubMed]

11

A Review of the Catalytic Mechanism of Human Manganese Superoxide Dismutase

Jahaun Azadmanesh [1] and Gloria E. O. Borgstahl [1,2,*]

[1] Department of Biochemistry and Molecular Biology, 985870 Nebraska Medical Center, Omaha, NE 68198-5870, USA; jahaun.azadmanesh@unmc.edu
[2] Eppley Institute for Cancer and Allied Diseases, 986805 Nebraska Medical Center, Omaha, NE 68198-6805, USA
[*] Correspondence: gborgstahl@unmc.edu

Abstract: Superoxide dismutases (SODs) are necessary antioxidant enzymes that protect cells from reactive oxygen species (ROS). Decreased levels of SODs or mutations that affect their catalytic activity have serious phenotypic consequences. SODs perform their bio-protective role by converting superoxide into oxygen and hydrogen peroxide by cyclic oxidation and reduction reactions with the active site metal. Mutations of SODs can cause cancer of the lung, colon, and lymphatic system, as well as neurodegenerative diseases such as Parkinson's disease and amyotrophic lateral sclerosis. While SODs have proven to be of significant biological importance since their discovery in 1968, the mechanistic nature of their catalytic function remains elusive. Extensive investigations with a multitude of approaches have tried to unveil the catalytic workings of SODs, but experimental limitations have impeded direct observations of the mechanism. Here, we focus on human MnSOD, the most significant enzyme in protecting against ROS in the human body. Human MnSOD resides in the mitochondrial matrix, the location of up to 90% of cellular ROS generation. We review the current knowledge of the MnSOD enzymatic mechanism and ongoing studies into solving the remaining mysteries.

Keywords: superoxide dismutase; human; mechanism; anti-oxidant; reactive oxygen species; mitochondria; manganese; catalysis

---

1. Introduction

Superoxide ($O_2{\bullet}^-$) is a potent oxidizing agent. Excessive amounts lead to a cascade of reactions causing damage to important biological macromolecules such as DNA, lipids, and proteins. Excess superoxide plays a role in the pathogenesis of many disease states including cancers, cardiovascular disorders, and neurodegenerative diseases [1–3]. To protect cells from harmful amounts of superoxide, SODs convert two superoxide anions to oxygen and hydrogen peroxide using a cyclic reduction and oxidation reaction of the active site metal. This redox shuffling of the active site metal to perform catalysis, called dismutation, is dependent on two protons per cycle.

$$Mn^{3+} + O_2^{\bullet -} \leftrightarrow Mn^{2+} + O_2$$
$$Mn^{2+} + O_2^{\bullet -} + 2H^+ \leftrightarrow Mn^{3+} + H_2O_2$$

The coordinated metals at the active site classify SODs. FeSOD and NiSOD are prokaryotic whereas FeSOD is also present in chloroplasts. CuZnSODs are located in the extracellular matrix and cytosol of eukaryotes. MnSOD dwells within bacteria and all eukaryotes. Of note, FeSODs and MnSODs have near identical active site configurations [4]. In eukaryotes, MnSOD is in the mitochondrial matrix, an organelle compartment with a high rate of endogenous superoxide generation.

Electrons leak from the electron-transport chain and perform a one-electron reduction of diatomic oxygen to form superoxide [5]. The ability of MnSOD to decrease superoxide levels in the mitochondria is associated with longevity of eukaryotic organisms [6]. MnSOD knockout mice die within the first day of life due to dilated cardiomyopathy and neurodegeneration whereas overexpression of MnSOD in fruit flies increases lifespan [7,8]. Sequence comparison and conservation of the active site residues among all published MnSOD structures shows all MnSODs have identical active sites [9]. In humans, polymorphisms of MnSOD have been associated with type 2 diabetes, hypertension, and the onset of prostate cancer [10,11]. Due to its necessary antioxidant role in biological systems, characterization of the catalytic mechanism of MnSOD has been the goal of many research groups. However, the atomic mechanism has been elusive because of (1) the fast reaction rate of MnSOD; (2) the high reactivity and short half-life of superoxide; and (3) the difficulties in detecting protons and protonation states of amino acids in an enzyme [12,13]. This review describes the current knowledge of the MnSOD mechanism and ongoing studies, with a focus on the human variant for its medical relevance. Several articles review other SOD mechanisms [4,14,15].

2. Medical Relevance and Therapeutics

The presence of excessive superoxide and its derivatives, such as hydroxyl radical (OH•), peroxynitrite ($ONOO^-$), and nitrogen dioxide (NO_2), leads to oxidative stress and is prevalent during inflammation, mitochondrial degeneration, and tumorigenesis [16]. Chronic inflammation can lead to disease states such as atherosclerosis and type two diabetes whereas mitochondrial degeneration leads to neurological disorders such as cerebral palsy and Parkinson's disease. Cells undergoing oxidative stress are susceptible to transformation and metastasis in a wide variety of cell types [17]. This is partly due to superoxide acting as a signaling molecule to induce cell division and proliferation [18]. Articles of this special issue discuss the roles of oxidative stress, superoxide, and SODs in cancer [19–21], and further reviews describe how oxidative stress influences disease states [22–25]. Therapeutic approaches in pre-clinical and clinical studies have arisen from the ability of MnSOD to decrease levels of superoxide and mitigate oxidative stress. There are three types of therapeutics: (1) MnSOD as an administered drug; (2) MnSOD expression as a transgene; or (3) as a small molecule mimetic [16,26,27].

Using MnSOD as a drug has been appealing due to its bio-protective role and used over other SODs because Mn is not susceptible to Fenton chemistry like Fe and Cu. MnSOD administration has been tested for irradiation protection, immunosuppression for transplantations, reduction of inflammation, and fibrosis in vivo in rats and humans [28–30]. Of note, MnSOD use in pre-clinical studies using rats and mice are applicable to humans due to high sequence identity, with 93% and 94% conservation, respectively. While using MnSOD for treatments has shown promising results, practical issues arise from the short half-life of the enzyme (6 min) due to rapid renal clearance [31]. Protein engineering to increase longevity of MnSOD may overcome this issue [32,33]. An alternative method for increasing life-span is delivery via liposomes, which augments the half-life to 4 h [31]. While MnSOD is a powerful protectant against diseases, its use as a drug requires chronic administration.

Development of gene therapy-based delivery approaches for MnSOD hopes to circumvent the issues of its short half-life. These investigations aim to increase MnSOD levels by production within cells. MnSOD overexpression by vector delivery showed significant toxicity for tumor cells and radio-protective properties for healthy cells in vitro and in vivo in mice [34–36]. Tumors cells have deficient systems for tolerating hydrogen peroxide production from dismutation whereas healthy cells are tolerant. Human clinical trials are ongoing for utilizing MnSOD expression from a plasmid containing liposome to confer radioprotection to healthy cells during concurrent radiotherapy and chemotherapy treatment for non-small-cell lung cancer [26]. Further details of using MnSOD for therapeutic approaches can be found in a detailed review by Borrelli and colleagues [27].

An alternative to utilizing the MnSOD enzyme is to use a small molecule mimic. The most promising mimics are Mn porphyrins, resembling the Fe containing heme group. Other classes of mimics are discussed in a review by Miriyala and colleagues [16]. Mn porphyrins are attractive because they (1) lack antigenicity; (2) are extremely stable; (3) can penetrate subcellular membranes; (4) scavenge other ROS such as peroxynitrite; and (5) are modifiable to optimize efficacy for their desired approach, all while approaching the catalytic rate and efficiency of MnSOD [37]. Mn porphyrin mimetics MnTE–2–PyP^{5+} and MnTnBuOE–2–PyP^{5+} have shown promising results in irradiation protection of healthy cells during radiotherapy and for treating diabetes, as noted within articles of this special issue [38,39] and in phase I/II clinical trials [40,41].

As expected, the design principles of MnSOD mimetics used to achieve a high catalytic rate are derived from mechanistic studies of MnSOD, which include a configured electrostatic guidance, coordinated water ligands, and fine-tuned redox potential [42,43]. However, the means by which superoxide interacts with the mimetics and substrate protonations are not clear. Further understanding the details of MnSOD catalysis has the potential to optimize efficacy of mimetics and protein engineered constructs for treatment approaches.

3. Function of Active Site Residues

Human MnSOD functions as a homotetramer, with each subunit containing an active site surrounding a manganese ion (Figure 1a). The metal is coordinated by His26, His74, His163, Asp159, and a single oxygen-containing molecule (denoted WAT1), thought to be either H_2O or OH^- (Figure 1b) [44]. These amino acids and ligands, termed the "inner sphere" residues, form a direct interaction with the manganese. The next layer of contacting amino acids, called the "outer sphere" residues, are essential for efficient dismutation. These are His30, Tyr34, Phe77, Trp78, Trp123, Gln143, Trp161, and from across the dimer interface, Glu162 [45–50]. Each of these residues plays a role in catalysis.

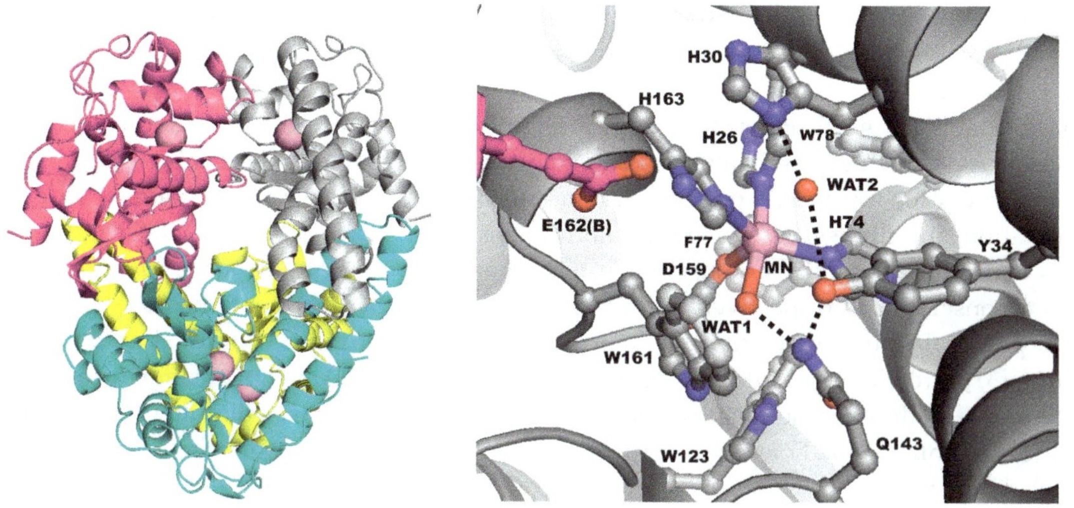

(a) (b)

Figure 1. Human MnSOD. (**a**) Each subunit contains a manganese ion at the catalytic center, indicated by pink spheres. (**b**) The active site. Red spheres denote oxygen atoms, blue denotes nitrogen atoms, grey denotes carbon atoms from one subunit of the tetramer, and magenta denotes carbon atoms from the adjacent subunit. The dashed lines represent the hydrogen bond network hypothesized to be the proton relay to the manganese ion used for catalysis. Glu162 hydrogen bonds with His163 across the dimer interface. Adapted from Azadmanesh et al., 2017, PDB entry 5VF9 [44]. WAT1: single oxygen-containing molecule; WAT2: single oxygen-containing molecule. Single letter amino acid code is used.

The outer sphere residues work together to promote the extremely fast catalysis of MnSOD. Substrate is thought to diffuse into the active site through residues His30 and Tyr34 where it most likely binds to the manganese ion in the position opposite Asp159 [44]. The ~5 Å gap between His30 and Tyr34 is the only solvent-accessible area that allows entry into the active site (occupied by a single oxygen-containing molecule, denoted WAT2 in Figure 1b). Residues of the outer sphere, Phe77, Trp78, Trp123, and Trp161, form a hydrophobic cage opposite the solvent-accessible portion of the active site to promote substrate interaction with the manganese ion [45]. Glu162 from the adjacent subunit hydrogen bonds with His163 to stabilize oligomerization [50]. Tyr34, His30, Gln143, and two single-oxygen containing molecules (denoted WAT1 and WAT2) form a hydrogen-bond network that is thought to serve as a proton relay to the manganese ion for proton-assisted electron transfer (dashed lines, Figure 1b) [46–49,51]. Investigations into the catalytic mechanism have been unable to determine the path of proton transfers owing to limitations in hydrogen detection.

4. Substrate Diffusion to the Active Site

MnSOD has one of the fastest and most efficient reaction rates of all enzymes, with a k_{cat} of 40,000 s^{-1} and a k_{cat}/K_M close to 10^9 M^{-1} s^{-1} [52]. Given that superoxide is a negatively charged substrate, MnSOD probably achieves rapid catalysis with the aid of electrostatic guidance. In 1983, Getzoff and colleagues were the first to calculate electrostatic field vectors for a SOD. For bovine Cu/ZnSOD, they found that superoxide guidance to the active site is a long-range process [53], which means that neutralization of a charged amino acid far from the active site, such as acetylation of a lysine, would perturb the net field vectors and hamper guidance of the substrate to the active site [44].

The active site of human MnSOD is within a cavity formed by two adjacent subunits (Figure 2a, arrow). Calculated electrostatic surfaces show that the cavity is positively charged, due to the presence of the manganese cation. Basic residues Lys29, and from the adjacent subunit, Lys170, Lys178, and Arg173 contribute to the positive surfaces near the active site cavity (Figure 2b). Interestingly, acetylated Lys29, Lys65, and Lys98 reduce measured enzyme activity [54–56]. At the outer ridge of the protein is a cluster of acidic residues contributing to negative electrostatic surfaces, such as Asp6, Asp10, and Glu15. The enrichment of positive electrostatic surfaces near and at the active site in conjunction with the negative surfaces at the edges of the protein explains the productive diffusion of superoxide to the active site. The negatively charged substrate is repelled from the outer areas of the tetramer and attracted to the positively charged cavity of the active site.

At the active site cavity there is an interesting pair of oppositely charged amino acids. Residues Glu162 and Arg173, are 7 and 12 Å from the active site manganese, respectively (Figure 2c). Efficient enzymatic activity requires this negative and positive pair. MnSODs, FeSODs, and CuZnSODs all conserve these residues. Mutation of Glu162 to alanine or aspartate in human MnSOD decreases enzymatic activity 5–25%, and increases product inhibition (discussed later) two-fold. While the Glu162Asp mutation maintains the charge, the side chain is one carbon shorter and breaks a hydrogen bond at the dimer interface, resulting in a packing defect. This decreased stability at the dimer interface may account for the activity loss [50]. Chemical modification of Arg173 with phenylglyoxal abolishes activity, suggesting a crucial role for a positive charge at this site [57,58]. Getzoff and colleagues studied the influence of the negative and positive amino acid configuration in the active site cavity of bovine CuZnSOD (consisting of Glu131 and Lys134) [53]. These amino acids direct the net positive electrostatic vectors into the active site, with mutations of either amino acid changing the net vector direction by at least 20 degrees. Glu131 also reduces non-productive association of a passing superoxide molecule with Lys134. These studies show that Glu162 and Arg173 that line the active site cavity play a significant role in productive entry of the substrate to the active site.

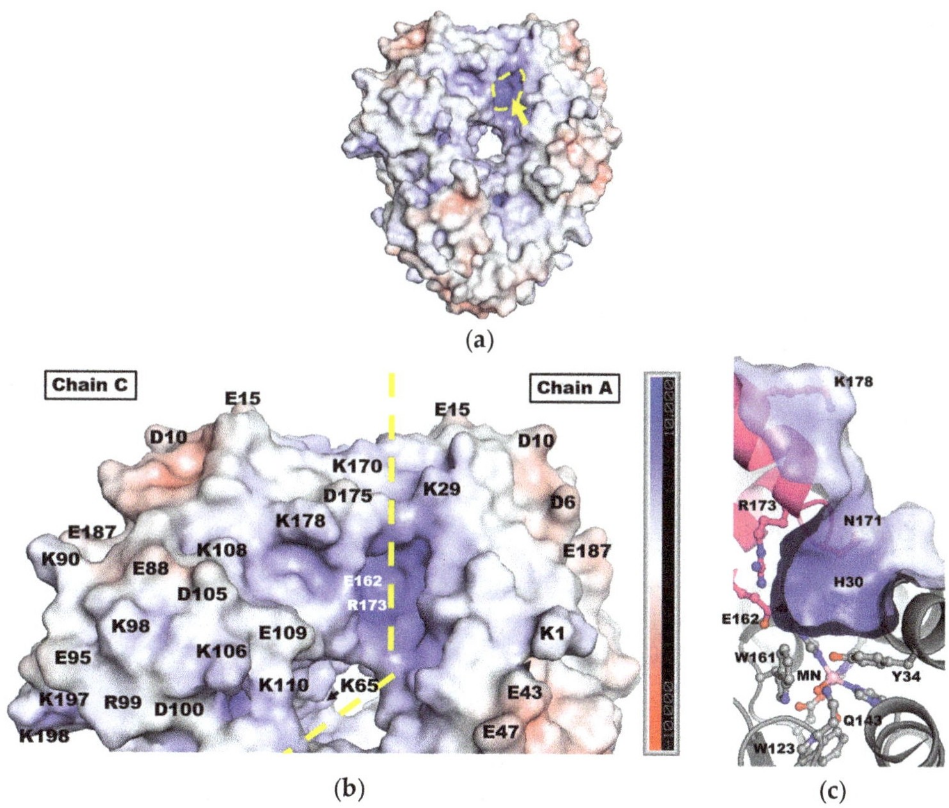

Figure 2. Electrostatic surfaces of human MnSOD. (**a**) The electrostatic surface of the tetramer with only one active site viewed in this orientation (yellow arrow and dashed lines). (**b**) A zoomed-in view of the dimer interface indicated by a yellow, dashed line. The labels for Glu162 and Arg173 are white to indicate their location on the concave surface within the active site pit. (**c**) A cross section-view of the active site across the dimer interface, rotated 90° along the horizontal axis in relation to (**a**,**b**). Glu162 is behind Arg173 in this view. Electrostatic surface is colored in kiloteslas. Adapted from Azadmanesh et al., 2017 [44]. Single letter amino acid code is used.

5. Superoxide Binding and Active Site Geometry

How superoxide interacts with the catalytic site has been difficult to investigate owing to the short half-life and high reactivity of superoxide in solution. Crystallographic and spectroscopic studies have instead used azide (N_3^-) as a substrate analog to study superoxide binding [59–61]. The azide anion is a potent competitive inhibitor of SODs and binds directly to the active site metal [62,63]. Of note, azide and superoxide are different enough in size that their binding to the active site could differ. Regardless, studies with azide suggest several mechanisms.

Lah and colleagues outlined a binding mechanism based on an azide-bound *Thermus thermophilus* MnSOD crystal structure (Protein Data Bank (PDB) entry code 1MNG) where the azide molecule binds to a sixth coordinate position opposite to the metal-bound aspartate. They propose that the resting state of the MnSOD active site is five-coordinate distorted trigonal bipyramidal which shifts to six-coordinate octahedral upon superoxide binding (Figure 3) [59]. Widening of the angle of two adjacent histidine-ligands (His74 and His163) accommodates binding opposite of the aspartate-ligand. *Caenorhabditis elegans* and human MnSOD crystal structures with azide bound also support this mode of binding (PDB entry 5AG2 and 5T30) [44,64]. A 100 K *Escherichia coli* MnSOD crystal structure at alkaline pH (8.5), in which the enzyme is inactive, shows a hydroxide anion at the sixth-coordinate position (PDB entry 1D5N) [65]. This further suggests that this position is the location of superoxide binding at the active site. However, so far no one has structurally captured the location of the highly reactive superoxide anion in the active site. The 5-6-5 mechanism describes the active site manganese dynamically changing its coordination during dismutation.

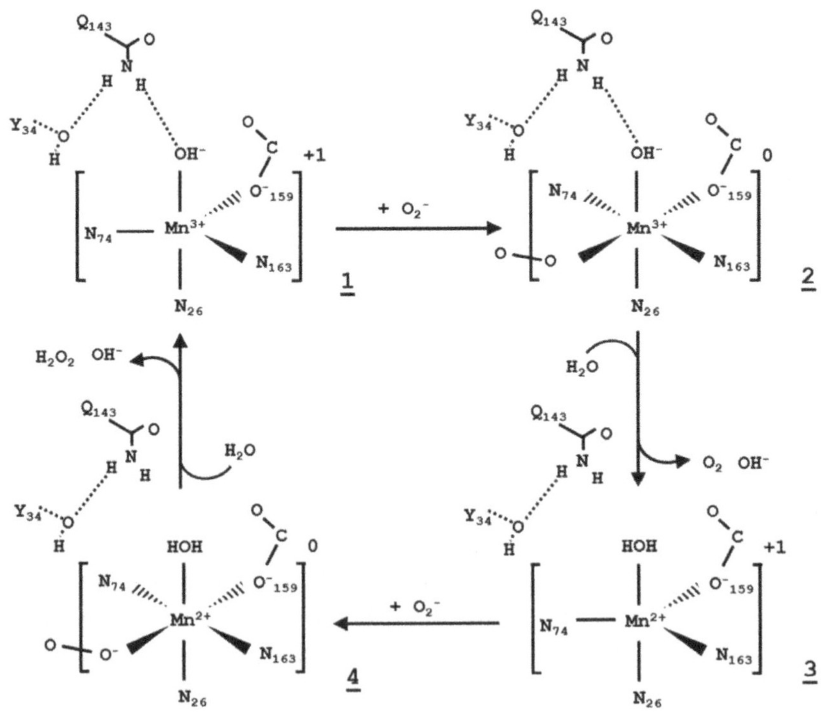

Figure 3. Human MnSOD 5-6-5 mechanism adapted from Lah et al., 1995 [59]. Dotted lines indicated hydrogen bonds.

Whittaker and Whittaker proposed the "associative displacement" mechanism from their thermochromism (temperature-dependent optical spectra) studies of *E. coli* MnSOD with azide [66,67]. The associative displacement mechanism is an alternative mode of superoxide binding, defined by a five-coordinate manganese ion in both the resting and substrate-bound forms. Their findings suggest that the active site of *E. coli* MnSOD remains five-coordinate trigonal bipyramidal at physiological temperature (295 K). Upon substrate binding, an unidentified manganese ligand displaces, with protonated aspartate or the solvent molecule being the most likely candidates. At low-temperatures (275–280 K), the coordination becomes six. These spectroscopic observations are in conflict with the six-coordinate azide-MnSOD structure from *T. thermophilus* (PDB 1MNG), where the crystallization and data collection was at room temperature [59]. Since *T. thermophilus* thrives in relatively high temperatures (320–350 K), room temperature may be a "cold" temperature for the thermophilic species. Whittaker and Whittaker do note that the six-coordinate complex is only marginally unstable at 295 K and suggest it could act as a kinetic intermediate [66,67]. Thus, the mechanism of superoxide dismutases studied with optical spectra suggests a differing mode of superoxide-substrate binding.

Density function theory (DFT) calculations performed by Jackson and co-workers with *E. coli* MnSOD indicate that the active site with azide adducts exists in a dynamic equilibrium between five and six coordinate states at 296 K. At 273 K, the coordination shifts to predominately six [68]. However, the active site states of either coordination were not supportive of displacement of metal bound ligands, indicating that these calculations are not favorable for the associative displacement mechanism. Instead, the authors propose that the superoxide substrate may convert to products without coordination to the metal. This could occur through hydrogen-bond interactions with Tyr34. In nuclear magnetic resonance (NMR) studies of *E. coli* FeSOD by the Miller group, azide did not bind to the reduced form of the active site metal, but instead was near Tyr34. These studies indicate that direct binding of superoxide to the active site metal for catalysis does not occur for at least some portions of the enzymatic mechanism [69].

6. Proton Transfers and the Hydrogen Bond Network

For MnSOD to perform its enzymatic function efficiently it must shuttle protons to the active site for proton-assisted electron transfer in a systematic manner. Extensive investigations through both experimental and theoretical approaches studied the proton-based mechanism and yielded several conflicting catalytic models [14,51,59,65,67,68,70–77]. The lack of consensus from the multitude of interdisciplinary approaches is a consequence of the experimental difficulty of directly detecting protons.

To date, insight into the proton-based mechanism has come from indirect observations. X-ray diffraction does not detect the hydrogen atom well, but analysis of X-ray crystal structures reveal a hydrogen bond network at the active site, consisting of His30–WAT2–Tyr34–Gln143–WAT1 (hereafter referred to as the superoxide-independent network, Figure 1b). This configuration is conserved in all Mn and FeSODs [78] and is thought to be involved in a proton relay for proton-assisted electron transfer at the active site metal [14,45–48,50,72,79]. Mutation of His30, Tyr34, or Gln143 disturbs catalysis drastically, indicating the importance of these residues in enzymatic function [14].

Theoretical studies of the proton-shuttling mechanism have been performed through quantum mechanical molecular modeling (QM/MM) and DFT [51,68,70,75,80,81]. Such approaches attempt to address the underlying complexity of how pK_as of amino acids and solvent are influenced at the active site to allow systematic proton transfers [82]. The positively charged manganese at the active site lowers the pK_as of amino acids and solvent allowing easier deprotonation. Conversely, positively charged ionization would be unfavorable and increase the pK_as of molecules with such capacity (protonation). The extent of influence that manganese has on the pK_as of molecules at the active site is dynamically changing through shuffling of its redox state (i.e., Mn^{3+} vs. Mn^{2+}). pK_as are further determined by whether ionization would make a non-covalent interaction more favorable. Together, the net changes in ionization (i.e., proton transfers) at the active site must be energetically downhill and be able to regenerate through cycling of the redox state of the manganese cation.

The metal-bound solvent molecule, WAT1, is probably a redox-linked proton accepter and perhaps the most studied component of the network [70,71,83]. QM/MM and DFT calculations indicate that in the Mn^{3+} state, the solvent ligand is hydroxide (OH^-), with its ionization stabilized by the electrostatic interaction with Mn^{3+}. Upon conversion to the Mn^{2+} state, the solvent ligand is protonated to H_2O, counterbalancing the changes in the metal charge (Figure 3). The second half reaction regenerates the Mn^{3+}–OH^- state, with the proton from the solvent ligand likely reducing superoxide to hydroperoxyl ion (HO_2^-), which accounts for one of the two protons needed for conversion to H_2O_2. The source of the second proton to convert HO_2^- to H_2O_2 is poorly understood and is hypothesized to come from His30, WAT2, Tyr34, or bulk solvent [59,70]. Protonation and deprotonation of the solvent ligand likely happens when a superoxide is bound at the active site (not necessarily directly to the manganese) as this makes product disassociation exergonic and enhances product formation [70]. These theoretical studies attempt to clarify the source of the two protons during the enzymatic reaction of MnSOD.

Second sphere residues appear to play critical roles in catalysis. Working backwards from WAT1 in the hydrogen bond network, Gln143 and Tyr34 are evolutionarily conserved and mutation abolishes SOD activity. Yet, their exact functional role is unresolved [14]. Proton shuttling through these amino acids to WAT1 would require their protonation or deprotonation. For Gln143, both possibilities are highly unfavorable in QM/MM calculations [70]. For Tyr34, its protonation (–OH_2^+) is chemically unlikely in both QM/MM and DFT but its deprotonation (–O^-) is plausible [51,70]. However, this deprotonation would interfere with superoxide binding due to electrostatic repulsion. Direct NMR observations by the Miller group have shown that Tyr34 likely remains in the neutral state (–OH) in both oxidized and reduced states of the enzyme but these studies do not take into account substrate binding effects [71]. These investigations suggest the roles for Gln143 and Tyr34 may be limited to orienting and positioning superoxide substrate and the solvent ligand.

DFT calculations indicate His30 and WAT2 could relay protons [51]. While protonation to a positive charge is unfavorable at the manganese-containing active site, the net sum of proton transfers is energetically favorable. Borgstahl and collaborators have recently employed the use of neutron diffraction to directly detect hydrogen positions and observed protonation of His30 (Figure 4) [84]. This also suggests that WAT2 can be protonated as it is the nearest hydrogen-bond acceptor/donor to His30 in the crystal structure. The proton shuttling through His30, WAT2 and WAT1 is feasible. It is noteworthy that protonation of His30 would change the electrostatic surface potentials at the active site opening to be more positive (Figure 2c).

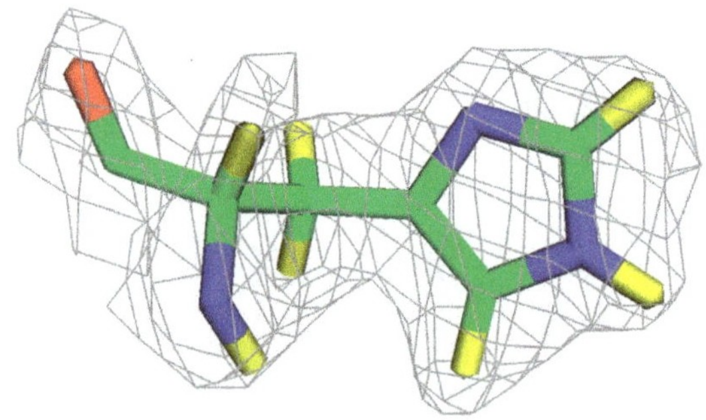

(a)

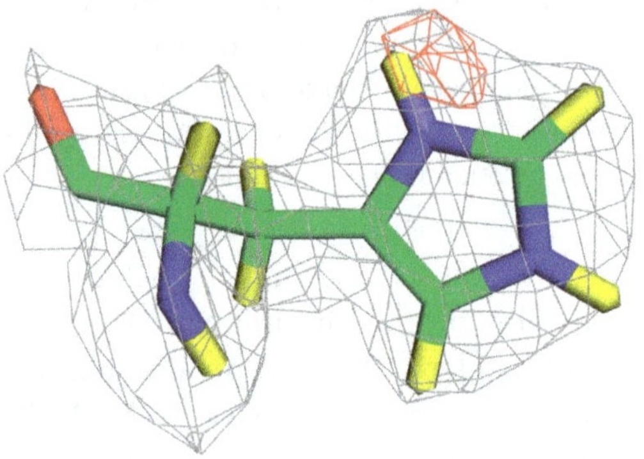

(b)

Figure 4. Protonation state of His30 in human MnSOD revealed by neutron diffraction. Carbons are green, nitrogens are blue, and oxygens are red. Deuterium (yellow) replaced hydrogen in the sample to increase diffraction signal. The $2F_o$-F_c grey nuclear density is 1.0 σ. The red omit positive F_o-F_C nuclear density is at 2.5 σ. (**a**) Chain A of the neutron crystal structure displays an unprotonated His30. (**b**) Chain B shows a protonated His30. Methods and statistics for crystal growth, deuterium exchange, data collection, and data reduction are found in Azadmanesh et al., 2017 [84]. Data was refined to 2.30 Å using PHENIX.REFINE with R_{work} and R_{free} values of 0.28, and 0.31, respectively (unpublished) [85,86].

A superoxide-dependent proton shuttling network is thought to exist because superoxide binding to the active site allows different hydrogen-bonding and more energetically favorable conditions for proton transfers [51,70] (Figure 5). Such a pathway, His30–WAT2–$O_2\bullet^-$–WAT1 or His30–$O_2\bullet^-$–WAT1, could involve superoxide binding at the active site either directly to the manganese or by non-covalent interactions with Tyr34, Gln143, WAT2, and/or WAT1. QM/MM calculations by Srnec and colleagues suggest that superoxide binding differs between half-reactions, with superoxide directly binding to the manganese in the oxidized state but not in the reduced state [70]. These results are supported by NMR experiments which observe substrate-analog binding to the metal of FeSOD only in the oxidized state [69]. These investigations indicate that superoxide binding to the active site forms an alternative hydrogen-bond network that allows for exergonic proton shuttling.

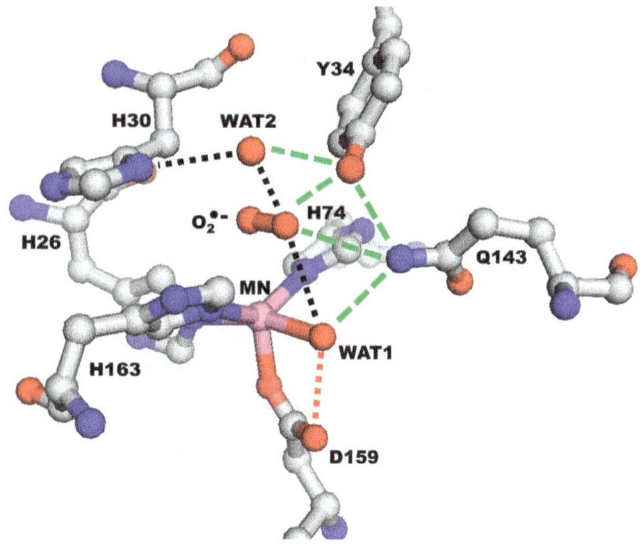

Figure 5. Putative superoxide-dependent proton shuttling mechanism. Black dashed lines indicate the proton transfer relay during catalysis. Red dashed line indicates the proton transfer from WAT1 to Asp159 that results in the inactive complex whereas the backwards transfer restores activity of the enzyme (model based on PDB entry 5T30). Green dashed lines indicate stabilizing hydrogen-bond interactions for molecules of the proton relay. Of note, superoxide is thought to bind Mn^{3+} directly but not Mn^{2+}, where it is instead bound to the active site solely through hydrogen bonding to members of the hydrogen-bond network. Single letter amino acid code is used.

Studies of combined pulse radiolysis and metal visible absorption spectra experiments have shown that all MnSODs exhibit product-inhibition. An inactive complex can form when manganese is in the reduced state. Here, the superoxide-bound complex, $O_2\bullet^-$–Mn^{2+}–(H_2O), is converted to oxidized peroxide-bound manganese, $O_2{}^{2-}$–Mn^{3+}–(OH^-), and peroxide does not disassociate [73,87,88]. In contrast, the active enzyme converts into oxidized hydroperoxyl-bound manganese, $HO_2{}^-$–Mn^{3+}–(OH^-), and hydroperoxyl radical disassociation is favorable. In both cases, an electron transfer occurs between the manganese and superoxide substrate, with the differences between these two outcomes being the fate of the WAT1 proton. During the active state, superoxide gains a proton from the solvent ligand to form hydroperoxyl radical, whereas the inactive complex forms due to proton donation from the solvent ligand to an alternative proton acceptor. The most probable acceptor is the carboxylate group (–COO^-) of metal-bound Asp159 as it is within hydrogen-bond distance of the solvent ligand. Protonation of Asp159 would likely lead to disassociation from the metal. Mutagenesis and QM calculations support this inactivation mechanism [89,90]. To regenerate the active enzyme, the proton from the carboxylic acid group (–COOH) of Asp159 is donated back to the WAT1 ligand to reform superoxide-bound reduced manganese, $O_2\bullet^-$–Mn^{2+}(H_2O), in conjunction with an electron transfer between the substrate and the metal. The reaction can then move forward to dismute superoxide.

A cryotrapped hydrogen peroxide-soaked X-ray crystal structure of *E. coli* MnSOD provides three-dimensional visualization of the putative product-inhibited complex (PDB entry 3K9S) [77]. A molecule containing two oxygen atoms is bound side-on to the manganese cation at the active site. This molecule had two differing orientations. However, the resolution of the diffraction data limited the identification of the protonation states of the amino acids and ligated molecules. Oxidized MnSOD in the presence of excess hydrogen peroxide is known to instigate a backwards enzymatic reaction of MnSOD, in which hydrogen peroxide is converted to superoxide [73]. This puts the identity of the double-oxygen containing molecules into question. Hydrogen positions of this structure would be informative in deciphering a product-inhibited mechanism.

Of note, FeSODs, which have identical active site amino acid configurations that are nearly superimposable on those of MnSODs, do not exhibit a reversible inactive, product-inhibited complex [4]. Instead, FeSOD inactivation occurs through the Fenton reaction. Regardless, the catalysis of superoxide into oxygen and hydrogen peroxide products likely follows extremely similar proton-shuttling mechanisms for both Fe and MnSODs.

7. Discussion

MnSOD is of great interest to the medical field because of its protection against the deleterious effects of excessive superoxide in disease states [22–25]. A defense against the pro-oxidant insults of superoxide has brought the potential of treating a plethora of human dysfunctions, including neurodegenerative diseases, diabetes, and cancer within reach [91]. Identifying the multi-step means of catalysis would provide atomic details useful for the design of mimetics and engineered protein constructs for therapeutics.

The MnSOD mechanism includes three categories: (1) the means of highly efficient substrate and product diffusion; (2) the mode of superoxide binding to the active site; and (3) the proton-shuttling mechanism for proton-assisted electron transfer. An intricately fine-tuned electrostatic surface and long-range electrostatic vectors guide superoxide substrate to the active site and products away. Substrate-analog binding provides clues as to how superoxide binds to the active site of MnSOD, yet there is no consensus, with direct or indirect binding to the manganese with or without Mn-ligand displacement being possible modes. The difference in molecular length of superoxide and substrate analogs makes it possible that they do not bind exactly the same way. Two protonations occur during each redox cycle of catalysis that involve rapid catalytic turnover and a high catalytic efficiency [52]. This points to protonations as a particularly orderly process, most likely through a hydrogen-bond relay at the active site. Theoretical calculations point to a proton-relay forming upon superoxide binding to the active site as the most energetically favorable means of proton shuttling [51,70]. From the culmination of experimental and theoretical data, four proton shuttling mechanisms are possible for MnSOD, depending on the stage of catalysis (Figure 5).

$$\begin{gathered} \mathrm{Mn}^{3+} + \mathrm{O}_2^{\bullet-} \rightarrow \mathrm{Mn}^{2+} + \mathrm{O}_2 \\ \mathrm{H}^+ \text{ from bulk solvent} \rightarrow \text{His30} \rightarrow \text{WAT2} \rightarrow \mathrm{O}_2^{\bullet-} \rightarrow \text{WAT1 } (\mathrm{OH}^-) \\ \text{Final proton acceptor}: \text{ WAT1 } (\mathrm{OH}^-) \rightarrow \text{ WAT1 } (\mathrm{H_2O}) \end{gathered} \tag{1}$$

$$\begin{gathered} \mathrm{Mn}^{2+} + \mathrm{O}_2^{\bullet-} + 2\mathrm{H}^+ \rightarrow \mathrm{Mn}^{3+} + \mathrm{H_2O_2} \\ \mathrm{H}^+ \text{from WAT1 } (\mathrm{H_2O}) \rightarrow \mathrm{O}_2^{\bullet-} \\ \text{Final proton acceptor}: \mathrm{O}_2^{\bullet-} \rightarrow \mathrm{HO}_2^- \end{gathered} \tag{2}$$

$$\begin{gathered} \mathrm{Mn}^{2+} + \mathrm{O}_2^{\bullet-} \rightarrow \mathrm{Mn}^{3+} + \mathrm{O}_2^{2-} \text{ [Inactive Complex]} \\ \mathrm{H}^+ \text{from WAT1 } (\mathrm{H_2O}) \rightarrow \text{Asp159}(\mathrm{COO}^-) \\ \text{Final proton acceptor}: \text{ Asp159}(\mathrm{COO}^-) \rightarrow \text{Asp159}(\mathrm{COOH}), \text{ Asp159 disassociates from Mn} \end{gathered} \tag{3}$$

$$\begin{gathered} \mathrm{Mn}^{3+} + \mathrm{O}_2^{2-} \text{ [Inactive Complex]} \rightarrow \mathrm{Mn}^{2+} + \mathrm{O}_2^{\bullet-} \\ \mathrm{H}^+ \text{from Asp159}(\mathrm{COOH}) \rightarrow \text{ WAT1 } (\mathrm{OH}^-) \\ \text{Final proton acceptor}: \text{WAT1 } (\mathrm{OH}^-) \rightarrow \text{ WAT1 } (\mathrm{H_2O}), \text{ Asp159 reassociates to Mn} \end{gathered} \tag{4}$$

The source of the second proton to convert hydroperoxyl radical to hydrogen peroxide is hypothesized to come from other players of the proton relay, His30 and WAT2, and/or bulk solvent [59,70]. Even 50 years after their discovery by Irwin Fridovich in 1968, the question of how SODs work is still unanswered [92].

8. Conclusions

The mechanistic SOD field would benefit from direct observation of the binding mode of superoxide and the proton relay. Observing the manner of superoxide binding has not been possible due to the exceedingly short half-life of superoxide and the fast catalytic rate of SODs. Visualization of protonation states through conventional structural biology techniques is difficult. NMR and X-ray crystallography are not very sensitive to revealing the positions of hydrogen, especially on solvent molecules. Recently, neutron diffraction experiments, which can reveal hydrogen positions, have been employed to investigate human MnSOD [84]. The experiments use a neutron diffractometer tailored to biological samples called the Macromolecular Neutron Diffractometer (MaNDi), which opened for academic use at Oak Ridge National Laboratory in 2014 [93]. It would be intriguing to couple the backwards reaction of the enzyme in the presence of excess hydrogen peroxide with cryo-neutron crystallography. These technological developments are making this experimentally elegant question addressable.

Acknowledgments: We would like to thank Carol Kolar, William Lutz, Kevin Weiss, and Leighton Coates for useful discussion, technical assistance, and expertise. This work was supported by NASA EPSCoR funding (44-0307-1021-201) and the Fred & Pamela Buffett Cancer Center Support Grant (P30CA036727). Jahaun Azadmanesh also acknowledges University of Nebraska Medical Center and Nebraska EPSCoR and Space Grant for fellowships.

Author Contributions: Jahaun Azadmanesh wrote the paper and created the figures. Gloria E. O. Borgstahl provided guidance and assisted in the critical revision of the manuscript for the intellectual content.

Conflicts of Interest: The authors declare no conflicts of interests.

References

1. Warner, H.R. Superoxide Dismutase, Aging, and Degenerative Disease. *Free Radic. Biol. Med.* **1994**, *17*, 249–258. [CrossRef]
2. Fukai, T.; Ushio-Fukai, M. Superoxide Dismutases: Role in Redox Signaling, Vascular Function, and Diseases. *Antioxid. Redox Signal.* **2011**, *15*, 1583–1606. [CrossRef] [PubMed]
3. Miao, L.; St Clair, D.K. Regulation of Superoxide Dismutase Genes: Implications in Disease. *Free Radic. Biol. Med.* **2009**, *47*, 344–356. [CrossRef] [PubMed]
4. Perry, J.J.; Shin, D.S.; Getzoff, E.D.; Tainer, J.A. The Structural Biochemistry of the Superoxide Dismutases. *Biochim. Biophys. Acta* **2010**, *1804*, 245–262. [CrossRef] [PubMed]
5. Jastroch, M.; Divakaruni, A.S.; Mookerjee, S.; Treberg, J.R.; Brand, M.D. Mitochondrial Proton and Electron Leaks. *Essays Biochem.* **2010**, *47*, 53–67. [CrossRef] [PubMed]
6. Landis, G.N.; Tower, J. Superoxide Dismutase Evolution and Life Span Regulation. *Mech. Ageing Dev.* **2005**, *126*, 365–379. [CrossRef] [PubMed]
7. Li, Y.; Huang, T.T.; Carlson, E.J.; Melov, S.; Ursell, P.C.; Olson, J.L.; Noble, L.J.; Yoshimura, M.P.; Berger, C.; Chan, P.H.; et al. Dilated Cardiomyopathy and Neonatal Lethality in Mutant Mice Lacking Manganese Superoxide Dismutase. *Nat. Genet.* **1995**, *11*, 376–381. [CrossRef] [PubMed]
8. Sun, J.; Folk, D.; Bradley, T.J.; Tower, J. Induced Overexpression of Mitochondrial Mn-Superoxide Dismutase Extends the Life Span of Adult Drosophila Melanogaster. *Genetics* **2002**, *161*, 661–672. [PubMed]
9. Perera, N.C.N.; Godahewa, G.I.; Lee, S.; Kim, M.J.; Hwang, J.Y.; Kwon, M.G.; Hwang, S.D.; Lee, J. Manganese-Superoxide Dismutase (MnSOD), a Role Player in Seahorse (Hippocampus Abdominalis) Antioxidant Defense System and Adaptive Immune System. *Fish Shellfish Immunol.* **2017**, *68*, 435–442. [CrossRef] [PubMed]
10. Nakanishi, S.; Yamane, K.; Ohishi, W.; Nakashima, R.; Yoneda, M.; Nojima, H.; Watanabe, H.; Kohno, N. Manganese Superoxide Dismutase Ala16Val Polymorphism Is Associated with the Development of Type 2 Diabetes in Japanese-Americans. *Diabetes Res. Clin. Pract.* **2008**, *81*, 381–385. [CrossRef] [PubMed]
11. Arsova-Sarafinovska, Z.; Matevska, N.; Petrovski, D.; Banev, S.; Dzikova, S.; Georgiev, V.; Sikole, A.; Sayal, A.; Aydin, A.; Suturkova, L.; et al. Manganese Superoxide Dismutase (MnSOD) Genetic Polymorphism is Associated with Risk of Early-Onset Prostate Cancer. *Cell Biochem. Funct.* **2008**, *26*, 771–777. [CrossRef] [PubMed]

12. Bannister, W.H.; Bannister, J.V. Factor Analysis of the Activities of Superoxide Dismutase, Catalase and Glutathione Peroxidase in Normal Tissues and Neoplastic Cell Lines. *Free Radic. Res. Commun.* **1987**, *4*, 1–13. [CrossRef] [PubMed]
13. Hayyan, M.; Hashim, M.A.; AlNashef, I.M. Superoxide Ion: Generation and Chemical Implications. *Chem. Rev.* **2016**, *116*, 3029–3085. [CrossRef] [PubMed]
14. Abreu, I.A.; Cabelli, D.E. Superoxide Dismutases—A Review of the Metal-Associated Mechanistic Variations. *Biochim. Biophys. Acta* **2010**, *1804*, 263–274. [CrossRef] [PubMed]
15. Hart, P.J.; Balbirnie, M.M.; Ogihara, N.L.; Nersissian, A.M.; Weiss, M.S.; Valentine, J.S.; Eisenberg, D. A Structure-Based Mechanism for Copper-Zinc Superoxide Dismutase. *Biochemistry* **1999**, *38*, 2167–2178. [CrossRef] [PubMed]
16. Miriyala, S.; Spasojevic, I.; Tovmasyan, A.; Salvemini, D.; Vujaskovic, Z.; St Clair, D.; Batinic-Haberle, I. Manganese Superoxide Dismutase, MnSOD and Its Mimics. *Biochim. Biophys. Acta* **2012**, *1822*, 794–814. [CrossRef] [PubMed]
17. Hempel, N.; Carrico, P.M.; Melendez, J.A. Manganese Superoxide Dismutase (SOD2) and Redox-Control of Signaling Events that Drive Metastasis. *Anticancer Agents Med. Chem.* **2011**, *11*, 191–201. [CrossRef] [PubMed]
18. Buetler, T.M.; Krauskopf, A.; Ruegg, U.T. Role of superoxide as a signaling molecule. *News Physiol. Sci.* **2004**, *19*, 120–123. [CrossRef] [PubMed]
19. Kim, Y.S.; Gupta Vallur, P.; Phaeton, R.; Mythreye, K.; Hempel, N. Insights into the Dichotomous Regulation of SOD2 in Cancer. *Antioxidants* **2017**, *6*, 86. [CrossRef] [PubMed]
20. Case, A.J. On the Origin of Superoxide Dismutase: An Evolutionary Perspective of Superoxide-Mediated Redox Signaling. *Antioxidants* **2017**, *6*, 82. [CrossRef] [PubMed]
21. Wilkes, J.G.; Alexander, M.S.; Cullen, J.J. Superoxide Dismutases in Pancreatic Cancer. *Antioxidants* **2017**, *6*, 66. [CrossRef] [PubMed]
22. Adly, A.A. Oxidative Stress and Disease: An Updated Review. *Res. J. Immunol.* **2010**, *3*, 129–145.
23. Seifried, H.; Anderson, D.; Milner, J.; Greenwald, P. Reactive Oxygen Species and Dietary Antioxidants: Double-Edged Swords? In *New Developments in Antioxidants Research*; Panglossi, H.V., Ed.; Nova Science Publishers: New York, NY, USA, 2007; pp. 1–24.
24. Uttara, B.; Singh, A.V.; Zamboni, P.; Mahajan, R.T. Oxidative Stress and Neurodegenerative Diseases: A Review of Upstream and Downstream Antioxidant Therapeutic Options. *Curr. Neuropharmacol.* **2009**, *7*, 65–74. [CrossRef] [PubMed]
25. Liou, G.Y.; Storz, P. Reactive Oxygen Species in Cancer. *Free Radic. Res.* **2010**, *44*, 479–496. [CrossRef] [PubMed]
26. Tarhini, A.A.; Belani, C.P.; Luketich, J.D.; Argiris, A.; Ramalingam, S.S.; Gooding, W.; Pennathur, A.; Petro, D.; Kane, K.; Liggitt, D.; et al. A Phase I Study of Concurrent Chemotherapy (Paclitaxel and Carboplatin) and Thoracic Radiotherapy with Swallowed Manganese Superoxide Dismutase Plasmid Liposome Protection in Patients with Locally Advanced Stage Iii Non-Small-Cell Lung Cancer. *Hum. Gene Ther.* **2011**, *22*, 336–342. [CrossRef] [PubMed]
27. Borrelli, A.; Schiattarella, A.; Bonelli, P.; Tuccillo, F.M.; Buonaguro, F.M.; Mancini, A. The Functional Role of MnSOD as a Biomarker of Human Diseases and Therapeutic Potential of a New Isoform of a Human Recombinant MnSOD. *Biomed. Res. Int.* **2014**, *2014*, 476789. [CrossRef] [PubMed]
28. Emerit, J.; Michelson, A.M.; Robert, H.G.; Chomette, G.; Guerin, R.A.; Blondon, J.; Bertrand, M. Superoxide Dismutase Treatment of 2 Cases of Radiation-Induced Sclerosis. *Sem. Hop.* **1983**, *59*, 277–281. [PubMed]
29. Land, W.; Schneeberger, H.; Schleibner, S.; Illner, W.D.; Abendroth, D.; Rutili, G.; Arfors, K.E.; Messmer, K. The Beneficial Effect of Human Recombinant Superoxide Dismutase on Acute and Chronic Rejection Events in Recipients of Cadaveric Renal Transplants. *Transplantation* **1994**, *57*, 211–217. [CrossRef] [PubMed]
30. Guillaume, M.; Rodriguez-Vilarrupla, A.; Gracia-Sancho, J.; Rosado, E.; Mancini, A.; Bosch, J.; Garcia-Pagan, J.C. Recombinant Human Manganese Superoxide Dismutase Reduces Liver Fibrosis and Portal Pressure in CCl_4-Cirrhotic Rats. *J. Hepatol.* **2013**, *58*, 240–246. [CrossRef] [PubMed]
31. Turrens, J.F.; Crapo, J.D.; Freeman, B.A. Protection against Oxygen Toxicity by Intravenous Injection of Liposome-Entrapped Catalase and Superoxide Dismutase. *J. Clin. Investig.* **1984**, *73*, 87–95. [CrossRef] [PubMed]

32. Gao, B.; Flores, S.C.; Leff, J.A.; Bose, S.K.; McCord, J.M. Synthesis and Anti-Inflammatory Activity of a Chimeric Recombinant Superoxide Dismutase: SOD2/3. *Am. J. Physiol. Lung Cell. Mol. Physiol.* **2003**, *284*, L917–L925. [CrossRef] [PubMed]
33. Borrelli, A.; Schiattarella, A.; Mancini, R.; Morrica, B.; Cerciello, V.; Mormile, M.; d'Alesio, V.; Bottalico, L.; Morelli, F.; D'Armiento, M.; et al. A Recombinant Mnsod is Radioprotective for Normal Cells and Radiosensitizing for Tumor Cells. *Free Radic. Biol. Med.* **2009**, *46*, 110–116. [CrossRef] [PubMed]
34. Ough, M.; Lewis, A.; Zhang, Y.; Hinkhouse, M.M.; Ritchie, J.M.; Oberley, L.W.; Cullen, J.J. Inhibition of Cell Growth by Overexpression of Manganese Superoxide Dismutase (MnSOD) in Human Pancreatic Carcinoma. *Free Radic. Res.* **2004**, *38*, 1223–1233. [CrossRef] [PubMed]
35. Yang, J.Q.; Buettner, G.R.; Domann, F.E.; Li, Q.; Engelhardt, J.F.; Weydert, C.D.; Oberley, L.W. V-Ha-Ras Mitogenic Signaling through Superoxide and Derived Reactive Oxygen Species. *Mol. Carcinog.* **2002**, *33*, 206–218. [CrossRef] [PubMed]
36. Epperly, M.W.; Gretton, J.A.; DeFilippi, S.J.; Greenberger, J.S.; Sikora, C.A.; Liggitt, D.; Koe, G. Modulation of Radiation-Induced Cytokine Elevation Associated with Esophagitis and Esophageal Stricture by Manganese Superoxide Dismutase-Plasmid/Liposome (SOD2-Pl) Gene Therapy. *Radiat. Res.* **2001**, *155*, 2–14. [CrossRef]
37. Batinic-Haberle, I.; Reboucas, J.S.; Spasojevic, I. Superoxide Dismutase Mimics: Chemistry, Pharmacology, and Therapeutic Potential. *Antioxid. Redox Signal.* **2010**, *13*, 877–918. [CrossRef] [PubMed]
38. Coudriet, G.M.; Delmastro-Greenwood, M.M.; Previte, D.M.; Marre, M.L.; O'Connor, E.C.; Novak, E.A.; Vincent, G.; Mollen, K.P.; Lee, S.; Dong, H.H.; et al. Treatment with a Catalytic Superoxide Dismutase (SOD) Mimetic Improves Liver Steatosis, Insulin Sensitivity, and Inflammation in Obesity-Induced Type 2 Diabetes. *Antioxidants* **2017**, *6*, 85. [CrossRef] [PubMed]
39. Shrishrimal, S.; Kosmacek, E.A.; Chatterjee, A.; Tyson, M.J.; Oberley-Deegan, R.E. The SOD Mimic, Mnte-2-PyP, Protects from Chronic Fibrosis and Inflammation in Irradiated Normal Pelvic Tissues. *Antioxidants* **2017**, *6*, 87. [CrossRef] [PubMed]
40. Gala-Lopez, B.L.; Kin, T.; O'Gorman, D.; Malcolm, A.J.; Pepper, A.R.; Pawlick, R.L.; Bruni, A.; Abualhassan, N.; Bral, M.; Jones, C.; et al. The Metalloporphyrin BMX-010 in Human Islet Isolationand Clinical Transplantation. *CellR4* **2016**, *4*, e2066.
41. Batinic-Haberle, I.; Tovmasyan, A.; Roberts, E.R.; Vujaskovic, Z.; Leong, K.W.; Spasojevic, I. SOD Therapeutics: Latest Insights into Their Structure-Activity Relationships and Impact on the Cellular Redox-Based Signaling Pathways. *Antioxid. Redox Signal.* **2014**, *20*, 2372–2415. [CrossRef] [PubMed]
42. Ferrer-Sueta, G.; Batinic-Haberle, I.; Spasojevic, I.; Fridovich, I.; Radi, R. Catalytic Scavenging of Peroxynitrite by Isomeric Mn(III) *N*-Methylpyridylporphyrins in the Presence of Reductants. *Chem. Res. Toxicol.* **1999**, *12*, 442–449. [CrossRef] [PubMed]
43. Batinic-Haberle, I.; Tovmasyan, A.; Spasojevic, I. An Educational Overview of the Chemistry, Biochemistry and Therapeutic Aspects of Mn Porphyrins—From Superoxide Dismutation to H_2O_2-Driven Pathways. *Redox Biol.* **2015**, *5*, 43–65. [CrossRef] [PubMed]
44. Azadmanesh, J.; Trickel, S.R.; Borgstahl, G.E.O. Substrate-Analog Binding and Electrostatic Surfaces of Human Manganese Superoxide Dismutase. *J. Struct. Biol.* **2017**, *199*, 68–75. [CrossRef] [PubMed]
45. Hearn, A.S.; Stroupe, M.E.; Cabelli, D.E.; Lepock, J.R.; Tainer, J.A.; Nick, H.S.; Silverman, D.N. Kinetic Analysis of Product Inhibition in Human Manganese Superoxide Dismutase. *Biochemistry* **2001**, *40*, 12051–12058. [CrossRef] [PubMed]
46. Edwards, R.A.; Whittaker, M.M.; Whittaker, J.W.; Baker, E.N.; Jameson, G.B. Outer Sphere Mutations Perturb Metal Reactivity in Manganese Superoxide Dismutase. *Biochemistry* **2001**, *40*, 15–27. [CrossRef] [PubMed]
47. Leveque, V.J.; Stroupe, M.E.; Lepock, J.R.; Cabelli, D.E.; Tainer, J.A.; Nick, H.S.; Silverman, D.N. Multiple Replacements of Glutamine 143 in Human Manganese Superoxide Dismutase: Effects on Structure, Stability, and Catalysis. *Biochemistry* **2000**, *39*, 7131–7137. [CrossRef] [PubMed]
48. Perry, J.J.; Hearn, A.S.; Cabelli, D.E.; Nick, H.S.; Tainer, J.A.; Silverman, D.N. Contribution of Human Manganese Superoxide Dismutase Tyrosine 34 to Structure and Catalysis. *Biochemistry* **2009**, *48*, 3417–3424. [CrossRef] [PubMed]
49. Ramilo, C.A.; Leveque, V.; Guan, Y.; Lepock, J.R.; Tainer, J.A.; Nick, H.S.; Silverman, D.N. Interrupting the Hydrogen Bond Network at the Active Site of Human Manganese Superoxide Dismutase. *J. Biol. Chem.* **1999**, *274*, 27711–27716. [CrossRef] [PubMed]

50. Quint, P.S.; Domsic, J.F.; Cabelli, D.E.; McKenna, R.; Silverman, D.N. Role of a Glutamate Bridge Spanning the Dimeric Interface of Human Manganese Superoxide Dismutase. *Biochemistry* **2008**, *47*, 4621–4628. [CrossRef] [PubMed]
51. Abreu, I.A.; Rodriguez, J.A.; Cabelli, D.E. Theoretical Studies of Manganese and Iron Superoxide Dismutases: Superoxide Binding and Superoxide Oxidation. *J. Phys. Chem. B* **2005**, *109*, 24502–24509. [CrossRef] [PubMed]
52. Guan, Y.; Hickey, M.J.; Borgstahl, G.E.; Hallewell, R.A.; Lepock, J.R.; O'Connor, D.; Hsieh, Y.; Nick, H.S.; Silverman, D.N.; Tainer, J.A. Crystal Structure of Y34F Mutant Human Mitochondrial Manganese Superoxide Dismutase and the Functional Role of Tyrosine 34. *Biochemistry* **1998**, *37*, 4722–4730. [CrossRef] [PubMed]
53. Getzoff, E.D.; Tainer, J.A.; Weiner, P.K.; Kollman, P.A.; Richardson, J.S.; Richardson, D.C. Electrostatic Recognition between Superoxide and Copper, Zinc Superoxide Dismutase. *Nature* **1983**, *306*, 287–290. [CrossRef] [PubMed]
54. Ozden, O.; Park, S.H.; Kim, H.S.; Jiang, H.; Coleman, M.C.; Spitz, D.R.; Gius, D. Acetylation of MnSOD Directs Enzymatic Activity Responding to Cellular Nutrient Status or Oxidative Stress. *Aging* **2011**, *3*, 102–107. [CrossRef] [PubMed]
55. Tao, R.; Coleman, M.C.; Pennington, J.D.; Ozden, O.; Park, S.H.; Jiang, H.; Kim, H.S.; Flynn, C.R.; Hill, S.; Hayes McDonald, W.; et al. Sirt3-Mediated Deacetylation of Evolutionarily Conserved Lysine 122 Regulates MnSOD Activity in Response to Stress. *Mol. Cell* **2010**, *40*, 893–904. [CrossRef] [PubMed]
56. Qiu, X.; Brown, K.; Hirschey, M.D.; Verdin, E.; Chen, D. Calorie Restriction Reduces Oxidative Stress by Sirt3-Mediated SOD2 Activation. *Cell Metab.* **2010**, *12*, 662–667. [CrossRef] [PubMed]
57. Borders, C.L., Jr.; Chain, V.W.; Bjerrum, M.J. The Positive Charge at Position 189 is Essential for the Catalytic Activity of Iron- and Manganese-Containing Superoxide Dismutases. *Free Radic. Res. Commun.* **1991**, *12–13 Pt 1*, 279–285. [CrossRef] [PubMed]
58. Chan, V.W.; Bjerrum, M.J.; Borders, C.L., Jr. Evidence That Chemical Modification of a Positively Charged Residue at Position 189 Causes the Loss of Catalytic Activity of Iron-Containing and Manganese-Containing Superoxide Dismutases. *Arch. Biochem. Biophys.* **1990**, *279*, 195–201. [CrossRef]
59. Lah, M.S.; Dixon, M.M.; Pattridge, K.A.; Stallings, W.C.; Fee, J.A.; Ludwig, M.L. Structure-Function in *Escherichia Coli* Iron Superoxide Dismutase: Comparisons with the Manganese Enzyme from Thermus Thermophilus. *Biochemistry* **1995**, *34*, 1646–1660. [CrossRef] [PubMed]
60. Ludwig, M.L.; Metzger, A.L.; Pattridge, K.A.; Stallings, W.C. Manganese Superoxide Dismutase from Thermus Thermophilus. A Structural Model Refined at 1.8 a Resolution. *J. Mol. Biol.* **1991**, *219*, 335–358. [CrossRef]
61. Tierney, D.L.; Fee, J.A.; Ludwig, M.L.; Penner-Hahn, J.E. X-ray Absorption Spectroscopy of the Iron Site in *Escherichia Coli* Fe(III) Superoxide Dismutase. *Biochemistry* **1995**, *34*, 1661–1668. [CrossRef] [PubMed]
62. Bull, C.; Fee, J.A. Steady-State Kinetic Studies of Superoxide Dismutases: Properties of the Iron Containing Protein from Escherichia Coli. *J. Am. Chem. Soc.* **1985**, *107*, 3295–3304. [CrossRef]
63. Misra, H.P.; Fridovich, I. Inhibition of Superoxide Dismutases by Azide. *Arch. Biochem. Biophys.* **1978**, *189*, 317–322. [CrossRef]
64. Hunter, G.J.; Trinh, C.H.; Bonetta, R.; Stewart, E.E.; Cabelli, D.E.; Hunter, T. The Structure of the Caenorhabditis Elegans Manganese Superoxide Dismutase MnSOD-3-Azide Complex. *Protein Sci.* **2015**, *24*, 1777–1788. [CrossRef] [PubMed]
65. Borgstahl, G.E.; Pokross, M.; Chehab, R.; Sekher, A.; Snell, E.H. Cryo-Trapping the Six-Coordinate, Distorted-Octahedral Active Site of Manganese Superoxide Dismutase. *J. Mol. Biol.* **2000**, *296*, 951–959. [CrossRef] [PubMed]
66. Whittaker, M.M.; Whittaker, J.W. A "Thermophilic Shift" in Ligand Interactions for Thermus Thermophilus Manganese Superoxide Dismutase. *J. Biol. Inorg. Chem.* **1997**, *2*, 667–671. [CrossRef]
67. Whittaker, M.M.; Whittaker, J.W. Low-Temperature Thermochromism Marks a Change in Coordination for the Metal Ion in Manganese Superoxide Dismutase. *Biochemistry* **1996**, *35*, 6762–6770. [CrossRef] [PubMed]
68. Jackson, T.A.; Karapetian, A.; Miller, A.F.; Brunold, T.C. Spectroscopic and Computational Studies of the Azide-Adduct of Manganese Superoxide Dismutase: Definitive Assignment of the Ligand Responsible for the Low-Temperature Thermochromism. *J. Am. Chem. Soc.* **2004**, *126*, 12477–12491. [CrossRef] [PubMed]
69. Surekha, V.; Byrd, R.A.; Miller, A. Mapping the Effects of Metal Ion Reduction and Substrate Analog Binding to Fe-Superoxide Dismutase by NMR Spectroscopy. *Magn. Reson. Chem.* **2000**, 5329–5339.

70. Srnec, M.; Aquilante, F.; Ryde, U.; Rulísek, L. Reaction Mechanism of Manganese Superoxide Dismutase Studied by Combined Quantum and Molecular Mechanical Calculations and Multiconfigurational Methods. *J. Phys. Chem. B* **2009**, *113*, 6074–6086. [CrossRef] [PubMed]
71. Miller, A.F.; Padmakumar, K.; Sorkin, D.L.; Karapetian, A.; Vance, C.K. Proton-Coupled Electron Transfer in Fe-Superoxide Dismutase and Mn-Superoxide Dismutase. *J. Inorg. Biochem.* **2003**, *93*, 71–83. [CrossRef]
72. Hearn, A.S.; Stroupe, M.E.; Cabelli, D.E.; Ramilo, C.A.; Luba, J.P.; Tainer, J.A.; Nick, H.S.; Silverman, D.N. Catalytic and Structural Effects of Amino Acid Substitution at Histidine 30 in Human Manganese Superoxide Dismutase: Insertion of Valine C Gamma into the Substrate Access Channel. *Biochemistry* **2003**, *42*, 2781–2789. [CrossRef] [PubMed]
73. Hearn, A.S.; Tu, C.; Nick, H.S.; Silverman, D.N. Characterization of the Product-Inhibited Complex in Catalysis by Human Manganese Superoxide Dismutase. *J. Biol. Chem.* **1999**, *274*, 24457–24460. [CrossRef] [PubMed]
74. Leveque, V.J.; Vance, C.K.; Nick, H.S.; Silverman, D.N. Redox Properties of Human Manganese Superoxide Dismutase and Active-Site Mutants. *Biochemistry* **2001**, *40*, 10586–10591. [CrossRef] [PubMed]
75. Noodleman, L.; Lovell, T.; Han, W.G.; Li, J.; Himo, F. Quantum Chemical Studies of Intermediates and Reaction Pathways in Selected Enzymes and Catalytic Synthetic Systems. *Chem. Rev.* **2004**, *104*, 459–508. [CrossRef] [PubMed]
76. Li, J.; Fisher, C.L.; Konecny, R.; Bashford, D.; Noodleman, L. Density Functional and Electrostatic Calculations of Manganese Superoxide Dismutase Active Site Complexes in Protein Environments. *Inorg. Chem.* **1999**, *38*, 929–939. [CrossRef] [PubMed]
77. Porta, J.; Vahedi-Faridi, A.; Borgstahl, G.E. Structural Analysis of Peroxide-Soaked MnSOD Crystals Reveals Side-on Binding of Peroxide to Active-Site Manganese. *J. Mol. Biol.* **2010**, *399*, 377–384. [CrossRef] [PubMed]
78. Wintjens, R.; Noel, C.; May, A.C.; Gerbod, D.; Dufernez, F.; Capron, M.; Viscogliosi, E.; Rooman, M. Specificity and Phenetic Relationships of Iron- and Manganese-Containing Superoxide Dismutases on the Basis of Structure and Sequence Comparisons. *J. Biol. Chem.* **2004**, *279*, 9248–9254. [CrossRef] [PubMed]
79. Edwards, R.A.; Whittaker, M.M.; Whittaker, J.W.; Baker, E.N.; Jameson, G.B. Removing a Hydrogen Bond in the Dimer Interface of *Escherichia Coli* Manganese Superoxide Dismutase Alters Structure and Reactivity. *Biochemistry* **2001**, *40*, 4622–4632. [CrossRef] [PubMed]
80. Konecny, R.; Li, J.; Fisher, C.L.; Dillet, V.; Bashford, D.; Noodleman, L. Cuzn Superoxide Dismutase Geometry Optimization, Energetics, and Redox Potential Calculations by Density Functional and Electrostatic Methods. *Inorg. Chem.* **1999**, *38*, 940–950. [CrossRef] [PubMed]
81. Heimdal, J.; Kaukonen, M.; Srnec, M.; Rulisek, L.; Ryde, U. Reduction Potentials and Acidity Constants of Mn Superoxide Dismutase Calculated by Qm/Mm Free-Energy Method. *Chem. Phys. Chem.* **2011**, 3337–3347. [CrossRef] [PubMed]
82. Nielsen, J.E.; McCammon, J.A. Calculating Pka Values in Enzyme Active Sites. *Protein Sci.* **2003**, *12*, 1894–1901. [CrossRef] [PubMed]
83. Stallings, W.C.; Metzger, A.L.; Pattridge, K.A.; Fee, J.A.; Ludwig, M.L. Structure-Function Relationships in Iron and Manganese Superoxide Dismutases. *Free Radic. Res. Commun.* **1991**, *12–13 Pt 1*, 259–268. [CrossRef] [PubMed]
84. Azadmanesh, J.; Trickel, S.R.; Weiss, K.L.; Coates, L.; Borgstahl, G.E. Preliminary Neutron Diffraction Analysis of Challenging Human Manganese Superoxide Dismutase Crystals. *Acta Crystallogr. Sect. F* **2017**, *73*, 235–240. [CrossRef] [PubMed]
85. Adams, P.D.; Afonine, P.V.; Bunkoczi, G.; Chen, V.B.; Davis, I.W.; Echols, N.; Headd, J.J.; Hung, L.W.; Kapral, G.J.; Grosse-Kunstleve, R.W.; et al. Phenix: A Comprehensive Python-Based System for Macromolecular Structure Solution. *Acta Crystallogr. Sect. D* **2010**, *66*, 213–221. [CrossRef] [PubMed]
86. Afonine, P.V.; Mustyakimov, M.; Grosse-Kunstleve, R.W.; Moriarty, N.W.; Langan, P.; Adams, P.D. Joint X-ray and Neutron Refinement with Phenix.Refine. *Acta Crystallogr. Sect. D* **2010**, *66*, 1153–1163. [CrossRef] [PubMed]
87. Bull, C.; Niederhoffer, E.C.; Yoshida, T.; Fee, J.A. Kinetic Studies of Superoxide Dismutases: Properties of the Manganese-Containing Protein from Thermus Thermophilus. *J. Am. Chem. Soc.* **1991**, *113*, 4069–4076. [CrossRef]
88. McAdam, M.E.; Levelle, F.; Fox, R.A.; Fielden, E.M. A Pulse-Radiolysis Study of the Manganese-Containing Superoxide Dismutase from Bacillus Stearothermophilus. *Biochem. J.* **1977**, *165*, 81–87. [CrossRef] [PubMed]

89. Whittaker, M.M.; Whittaker, J.W. Mutagenesis of a Proton Linkage Pathway in *Escherichia Coli* Manganese Superoxide Dismutase. *Biochemistry* **1997**, *36*, 8923–8931. [CrossRef] [PubMed]
90. Rulisek, L.; Jensen, K.P.; Lundgren, K.; Ryde, U. The Reaction Mechanism of Iron and Manganese Superoxide Dismutases Studied by Theoretical Calculations. *J. Comput. Chem.* **2006**, *27*, 1398–1414. [CrossRef] [PubMed]
91. Macmillan-Crow, L.A.; Cruthirds, D.L. Invited Review: Manganese Superoxide Dismutase in Disease. *Free Radic. Res.* **2001**, *34*, 325–336. [CrossRef] [PubMed]
92. McCord, J.M.; Fridovich, I. Superoxide Dismutase: The First Twenty Years (1968–1988). *Free Radic. Biol. Med.* **1988**, *5*, 363–369. [CrossRef]
93. Coates, L.; Cuneo, M.J.; Frost, M.J.; He, J.; Weiss, K.L.; Tomanicek, S.J.; McFeeters, H.; Vandavasi, V.G.; Langan, P.; Iverson, E.B. The Macromolecular Neutron Diffractometer Mandi at the Spallation Neutron Source. *J. Appl. Crystallogr.* **2015**, *48*, 1302–1306. [CrossRef]

12

Mitochondria-Targeted Antioxidants and Skeletal Muscle Function

Sophie C. Broome [1], Jonathan S. T. Woodhead [1] and Troy L. Merry [1,2,*]

[1] Discipline of Nutrition, Faculty of Medical and Health Sciences, The University of Auckland, Auckland 1023, New Zealand; s.broome@auckland.ac.nz (S.C.B.); j.woodhead@auckland.ac.nz (J.S.T.W.)
[2] Maurice Wilkins Centre for Molecular Biodiscovery, The University of Auckland, Auckland 1023, New Zealand
* Correspondence: t.merry@auckland.ac.nz

Abstract: One of the main sources of reactive oxygen species (ROS) in skeletal muscle is the mitochondria. Prolonged or very high ROS exposure causes oxidative damage, which can be deleterious to muscle function, and as such, there is growing interest in targeting antioxidants to the mitochondria in an effort to prevent or treat muscle dysfunction and damage associated with disease and injury. Paradoxically, however, ROS also act as important signalling molecules in controlling cellular homeostasis, and therefore caution must be taken when supplementing with antioxidants. It is possible that mitochondria-targeted antioxidants may limit oxidative stress without suppressing ROS from non-mitochondrial sources that might be important for cell signalling. Therefore, in this review, we summarise literature relating to the effect of mitochondria-targeted antioxidants on skeletal muscle function. Overall, mitochondria-targeted antioxidants appear to exert beneficial effects on mitochondrial capacity and function, insulin sensitivity and age-related declines in muscle function. However, it seems that this is dependent on the type of mitochondrial-trageted antioxidant employed, and its specific mechanism of action, rather than simply targeting to the mitochondria.

Keywords: mitochondria; reactive oxygen species; oxidative stress; skeletal muscle; antioxidant

---

1. Introduction

Reactive oxygen species (ROS) are continuously produced by skeletal muscle from a number of mitochondrial and non-mitochondrial sources, with production being increased during contractile activity [1]. Skeletal muscle fibers contain a well-developed endogenous antioxidant defence network consisting of the primary antioxidant enzymes superoxide dismutase (SOD), glutathione peroxidase (GPX) and catalase, in addition to other antioxidant enzymes such as thioredoxins, glutaredoxins and peroxiredoxins, and nonenzymatic antioxidants, such as glutathione [1]. Under most conditions, these cellular antioxidants work as a complex unit to regulate ROS, maintain oxidative balance and protect cells against oxidative damage. However, prolonged exposure to high levels of ROS can overwhelm the antioxidant defense system leading to oxidative damage of proteins, nucleic acids and lipids, resulting in cellular dysfunction, and has been associated with the pathogenesis of muscle related diseases such as type 2 diabetes, cachexia, and several dystrophies [2–5], as well as impaired exercise performance and recovery [1,6,7]. For this reason, the use of oral antioxidant supplements to support the endogenous antioxidant defence system has received much attention as a potential strategy to limit oxidative stress and promote muscle health and performance [1,7,8]. Somewhat paradoxically, ROS are increasingly being recognised as important signalling molecules that regulate skeletal muscle function and adaptation, and are required for optimal cell functioning [9–12]. As such, it is probably not surprising that supplementation with non-targeted antioxidants have had little impact on disease development and progression [9,13–15] and exercise performance [16,17] and in some instances have been reported to be deleterious [18–21]. This has driven the development of inhibitors [4,11,22,23] and cellular organelle-targeted antioxidants that are aimed at decreasing ROS levels from specific production sites in the cell.

It is clear that skeletal muscle produces ROS from numerous subcellular sites in a controlled and regulated manner in response to physiological stimuli, and may become unregulated under pathophysiological stimuli. The mitochondria have been cited as the major site of superoxide production in skeletal muscle, with approximately 0.15% of the oxygen consumed by the mitochondria undergoing one electron reduction to generate superoxide [24]. A number of potential alternative sites of ROS production have been identified including nicotinamide adenine dinucleotide phosphate (NADPH) oxidases, xanthine oxidases, and phospholipase A2 dependent processes. It is beyond the scope of this review to discuss the production of ROS from these non-mitochondrial sources, and readers are directed to the following comprehensive reviews [1,25]. The production of ROS from these non-mitochondrial sources appears to be linked to the signalling processes that modulate skeletal muscle adaptation, whereas excess mitochondrial ROS are more often associated with oxidative damage and disease states [26–28]. There has been extensive research focusing on transgenic mice with targeted overexpression of the human catalase gene to mitochondria, which has highlighted the role of mitochondrial ROS production in numerous disease states [29–31]. As a result, mitochondria-targeted antioxidants are increasingly being developed as a potential strategy to limit mitochondrial ROS production and oxidative damage, potentially without suppressing ROS that are important for signalling, and are becoming more widely available as an over the counter supplement. Compared with general antioxidants, mitochondria-targeted antioxidants are chemically modified to enable their transport across biological membranes where they accumulate several-hundred fold within the mitochondria and decrease ROS [32]. The purpose of this review is to discuss the literature that relates to exogenous mitochondria-targeted products that primarily act as antioxidants, specifically, MitoQ (10-(4,5-dimethoxy-2-methyl-3,6-dioxo-1,4-cyclohexadien-1-yl)decyl) triphenylphosphonium mesylate), and SkQ1 (10-(6′-plastoquinonyl) decyltriphenylphosphonium), which are antioxidants that are targeted to the mitochondria, as well as the mitochondria locating peptides SS-31 (d-Arg-2′, 6′-dimethyltyrosine-Lys-Phe-NH_2) and XJB-5-131, and their effects on muscle function.

2. Targeting Antioxidants to the Mitochondria

2.1. Conjugation of Antioxidants to Lipophilic Cations

Antioxidants such as ubiquinone and plastoquinone have been targeted to the mitochondria through conjugation to a lipophilic cation, such as the triphenylphosphonium (TPP^+) cation, which can pass easily through phospholipid bilayers. The ability of these positively charged cations to cross the plasma membrane allows them to accumulate substantially within the mitochondria owing to the large membrane potential [33,34]. As the plasma membrane potential is approximately 30–60 mV (negative inside), lipophilic cations accumulate 5–10 fold within the cytoplasm. The mitochondrial membrane potential is typically 140–180 mV, therefore the cations further accumulate several hundredfold within the mitochondria. It is important to consider that accumulation of the lipophilic cation within the mitochondria can result in the dissipation of the mitochondrial membrane potential when targeting antioxidants to the mitochondria using lipophilic cations, as this may have implications for their transport into the mitochondria and, thus, impact on their therapeutic capacity.

MitoQ, which consists of a ubiquinone moiety, is targeted to the mitochondria by conjugation to the TPP^+ cation. Within the mitochondria, MitoQ localises to the inner mitochondrial membrane and is reduced to the active antioxidant ubiquinol by complex II of the respiratory chain. In acting as an antioxidant, the ubiquinol form of MitoQ is oxidised to form ubiquinone, which is then reduced by complex II to ubiquinol. MitoQ is an effective antioxidant against lipid peroxidation and has also been shown to detoxify peroxynitrite [35] (Figure 1).

Similarly, SkQ1, which comprises a plastoquinone moiety, is also targeted to the mitochondria via the conjugation of the TPP^+ cation [36]. Within the mitochondria, SkQ1 is reduced to $SkQ1H_2$ by the respiratory chain. SkQ1 acts as an antioxidant by preventing peroxidation of the mitochondrial phospholipid cardiolipin [37] and inhibiting the formation of superoxide [38]. In acting as an antioxidant $SkQH_2$ is oxidised to SkQ1, which is reduced by the respiratory chain to $SkQH_2$ (Figure 1).

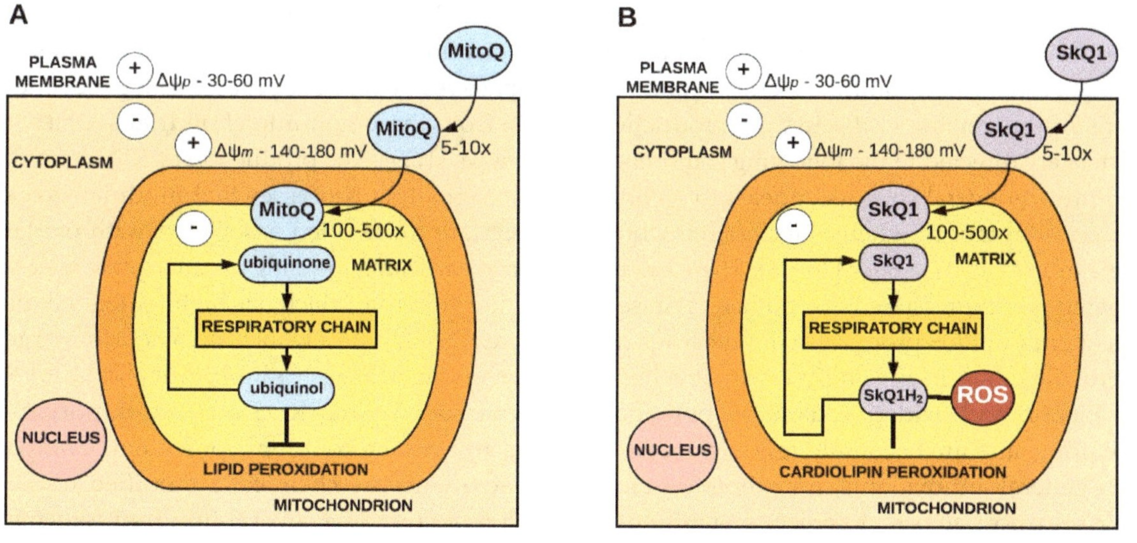

Figure 1. Accumulation and antioxidant mechanism of 10-(4,5-dimethoxy-2-methyl-3,6-dioxo-1,4-cyclohexadien-1-yl)decyl) triphenylphosphonium mesylate (MitoQ) (**A**) and 10-(6′-plastoquinonyl) decyltriphenylphosphonium (SkQ1) (**B**). Driven by the plasma membrane potential ($\Delta\psi_p$), MitoQ and SkQ1 pass through the plasma membrane and accumulate 5-10 fold within the cytosol. MitoQ and SkQ1 then accumulate several-hundredfold within the mitochondria driven by the mitochondrial membrane potential ($\Delta\psi_m$).Within the mitochondria, MitoQ is reduced to ubiquinol and SkQ1 is reduced to $SkQH_2$ by the respiratory chain. In acting as an antioxidant, ubiquinol is oxidised to ubiquinone and $SkQH_2$ is oxidised to SkQ1, both of which are rereduced by the respiratory chain. MitoQ is effective at preventing lipid peroxidation. SkQ1 is effective at preventing peroxidation of cardiolipin and inhibits the production of superoxide. (adapted from Murphy and Smith, 2007 [39]).

2.2. Mitochondria-Targeted Peptides that Incorporate Antioxidants

Szeto-Schiller (SS) peptides are a series of antioxidant peptides that contain an amino acid sequence, which allows them to pass through plasma membranes independent of the membrane potential and localise to the inner mitochondrial membrane [40]. Data suggests that SS-31 targets cardiolipin [41] and that its antioxidant mechanism likely involves decreased mitochondrial ROS production rather than direct savaging of ROS [42] (Figure 2). In addition to SS peptides, several peptides that consist of an electron and ROS scavenger (4-NH_2-TEMPO) conjugated to fragments of the gramicidin S cyclopeptide antibiotic, known as XJB peptides, have been used to limit oxidative stress [43,44] (Figure 2).

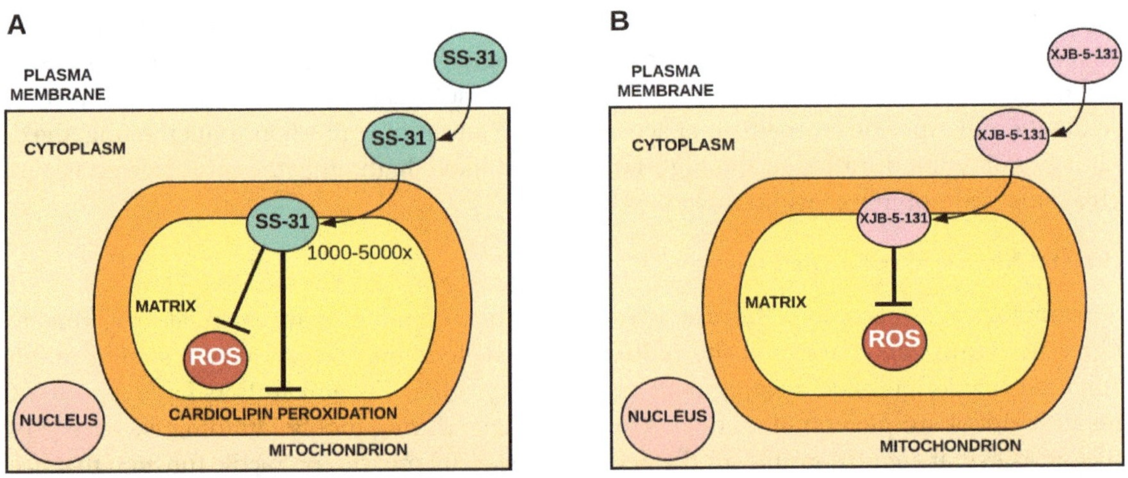

Figure 2. Accumulation and antioxidant mechanism of Szeto-Schiller-31 (SS-31) (**A**) and XJB-5-131 (**B**). SS-31 accumulates several-thousand fold within the mitochondria where it binds to cardiolipin. In acting as an antioxidant, it is likely that SS-31 prevents peroxidation of cardiolipin and decreases mitochondrial ROS production. XJB-5-131 accumulates within the mitochondria independent of the membrane potential, where it acts as an antioxidant by scavenging mitochondrial ROS.

3. Mitochondrial Biogenesis and Function

General antioxidants have been shown to attenuate mitochondrial biogenesis, particularly in response to exercise [19–21]. However, the ROS that signal the initiation of mitochondrial biogenesis during exercise may not be coming from the mitochondria. Indeed, exercise has been shown to increase skeletal muscle mitochondrial capacity during concurrent MitoQ supplementation [45], which supports previous studies that suggest that non-mitochondrial ROS production plays a central role in mediating exercise training-induced adaptations [1,24,46,47]. Similarly to exercise, high-fat diets have been reported to initiate mitochondrial biogenesis via a ROS dependent activation of CaMKII [48]. During high-fat feeding, mitochondrial biogenesis may promote a higher reliance on fatty acids as a fuel source and may actually decrease mitochondrial ROS production by dissipating proton-motive force over a greater mitochondrial volume. This potentially compensatory effect can be reversed by SkQ1 administration [48], which suggests that mitochondria-targeted antioxidants may not be beneficial under all conditions of metabolic stress. This is supported by the finding that high fat diet-induced mitochondrial dysfunction was not improved following SkQ1 administration [49]. In contrast, however, MitoQ has been shown to restore mitochondrial function during high-fat feeding [50], which suggests that the effect of mitochondrial-targeted antioxidants on mitochondrial function during high-fat feeding may be dependent on a number of factors including its mechanism of action, dose, and the duration and type of metabolic stress.

4. Insulin Sensitivity

Transient increases in ROS, such as those that occur during exercise, have been implicated in the promotion of insulin sensitivity, and general antioxidants have been shown to attenuate the improvements in insulin signalling and sensitivity that are associated with acute and chronic (training) exercise [20,51]. On the contrary, high levels of mitochondrial ROS production and oxidative stress have been implicated in the development of insulin resistance [26,52]. As such, the effect of mitochondria-targeted antioxidants on insulin sensitivity during times of increased oxidative stress, such as during high-fat feeding, is being increasingly investigated. SS-31 preserved insulin sensitivity in mice fed a high-fat diet [26], and MitoQ has been shown to partially reverse high-fat diet-induced glucose intolerance [50,53]. This suggests that clearance of mitochondrial ROS through the use of mitochondria-targeted antioxidants is associated with improved glucose homeostasis under conditions of metabolic stress. However, whilst SkQ1 treatment attenuated high fat diet-induced oxidative stress, there was no effect on glucose tolerance or insulin signalling [49]. This again suggests that the effect of the mitochondria-targeted antioxidant employed on insulin sensitivity during high-fat feeding is dependent on the specific mechanism of action rather than simply mitochondrial targeting, the dose used or possibly the duration of the high-fat diet, and likely highlights the multifaceted nature of mechanisms underpinning insulin resistance.

5. Skeletal Muscle Contractile Function

Physiological levels of ROS that are present under basal conditions are essential for normal force production. However, changes in the redox state of skeletal muscle can have a significant effect on force production, fatigue development and recovery [1,6,7]. Several authors have reported that acute antioxidant supplementation delays muscle fatigue during highly fatiguing exercise [54–57]. However, ROS that are responsible for the decrease in skeletal muscle contractile function that occurs during fatiguing stimulation potentially come from non-mitochondrial sources. Indeed, SS-31 had no effect on force production during fatiguing stimulation in isolated muscle fibres [58], nor did it affect fatigue-induced decreases in contractile force [59]. During recovery, SS-31 restored the fatigue-induced decrease in sarcoplasmic Ca^{2+} release but did not improve force recovery in isolated muscle fibres [59]. The specific action of the mitochondria-targeted antioxidant employed appears to be an important factor in a number of other parameters of muscle function. Therefore, more studies implementing other mitochondria-targeted antioxidants are needed to further substantiate these findings.

6. Ageing, Sarcopenia and Disuse Muscle Atrophy

Ageing is associated with a progressive decline in muscular function and the development of diseases such as sarcopenia (muscle loss) and mitochondrial dysfunction [60]. The free-radical theory of ageing states that these changes may be driven by an increased production of ROS [61,62]. Levels of mitochondrial ROS have been shown to increase with age and have been suggested to damage mitochondria resulting in lower adenosine triphosphate (ATP) production and mitochondrial respiration capacity [30]. These shifts are hypothesised to contribute to the metabolically dysfunctional phenotype (muscular atrophy and decreased cellular respiration) seen with ageing [30,63]. Therefore, targeting mitochondrial ROS production with mitochondria-targeted antioxidants may be an effective strategy to prevent muscular dysfunction associated with ageing.

Mitochondria-targeted antioxidants have been shown to exert largely beneficial effects on measures of muscular function with age. SS-31, XJB-5-131, and SkQ1 have shown promise in protecting/restoring muscle from the ageing phenotype [64–66]. However, disappointingly MitoQ has failed to attenuate age-related decline in muscle function of mice, but this may relate to no observable effects on muscle oxidative balance at the doses given [67]. Whereas, SS-31 and XJB-5-131 supplementation have been reported to increase respiratory complex activity (CI, III, and IV) and muscle fiber contractile properties (indicating maintained protein quality) in aged rodents in comparison to age-matched controls [65,66], however, whether this translated to improvements in vivo health and life span remains unclear. Additionally, SS-31 supplementation restores time to muscular fatigue, ATP production capacity, oxidative phosphorylation (phosphate/oxygen ratio), and energy state (PCr/ATP ratio) to levels comparable to that of younger mice, 1 hour following a single dose. Extended treatment with SS-31 further showed significantly lowered mitochondrial H_2O_2 emissions, indicating enhanced redox status, which is thought to be contributing to the restoration of mitochondrial function. Therefore, early research suggests great promise for these mitochondria-targeted antioxidants as potential supplements to attenuate aged related functional decline.

Oxidative damage is also associated with muscular atrophy in ageing, and interestingly, SkQ1 supplementation has been shown to decrease pathological changes in mitochondrial structure including myofibril structural retardation and autophagosome accumulation in 24-month old rats.

Supplemented rats suffered less degradation of mitochondrial reticulum and cristae structures, which are involved in maintaining electron transport chain activity and ATP synthesis capacity [68]. Similar findings are seen in muscular atrophy models utilising limb immobilisation, where increased mitochondrial oxidative damage associates with muscle atrophy [64,69,70]. Mice with immobilised hind-limbs and supplemented with SS-31 had reduced H_2O_2 production which was comparable to age-matched ambulatory controls. This effect also translated to a retention of muscle to body-weight ratio, muscle fiber cross-sectional area and mitochondrial energetic state activity similar to that of ambulatory controls.

Taken together, targeted inhibition of mitochondrial sources of ROS by SS-31, SkQ1, and XJB-5-131 have shown promising restorative and protective effects that could be implemented in ageing and immobilization-induced muscular atrophy/dysfunction therapies. However, these findings have largely been demonstrated in rodent models and, therefore, there is a clear need for human clinical trials investigating the effects of these antioxidants within an ageing and muscle wasting context.

7. Mitochondria-Targeted Antioxidants in the Clinic

In general, mitochondria-targeted antioxidants have been shown to exert beneficial effects on muscle function through the improvement or attenuation of declines in mitochondrial capacity and function, insulin sensitivity and age or immobilisation induced-atrophy (Table 1). These findings suggest that mitochondria-targeted antioxidants may be a useful therapy for skeletal muscle related diseases that involve mitochondrial ROS production and oxidative damage. However, to date, studies that have investigated the effects of mitochondria-targeted antioxidants on skeletal muscle function have mostly employed rodent models, and there are very few studies that have translated these findings to a human population or clinical setting. Given that ROS are beginning to be implicated in the pathogenesis of several muscular dystrophies [5], investigating the utility of mitochondria-targeted antioxidants in the treatment of muscle diseases in a clinical setting requires further investigation. Antipodean Pharmaceuticals Inc. developed MitoQ as a pharmaceutical and now MitoQ is available as an over the counter supplement, and has been shown to be well tolerated and safe in doses up to 80 mg twice daily [71]. Originally MitoQ was investigated for its ability to act as a disease-modifying agent in newly diagnosed patients with Parkinson's disease (PD) [71] but appeared to be ineffective in altering disease progression over 12 months. It seems likely that by the time PD is clinically evident, the fate of the remaining dopaminergic neurons is already determined and neuroprotection cannot prevent their death. In contrast, MitoQ has been shown to be effective in reducing serum alanine transaminase in patients with Hepatitis C virus (HCV) infection [72], indicating that it may be effective in reducing liver damage in HCV infection. Furthermore, MitoQ has also been shown to improve endothelial function and aortic stiffness in individuals with elevated baseline levels [73], suggesting that MitoQ and other therapeutic strategies that target mitochondrial ROS hold promise for treating age-related vascular dysfunction. To date, the results from human studies indicate that MitoQ can be safely administered to patients for up to a year [71] and that these doses are effective in decreasing liver damage and improving endothelial function.

SS-31 has been in clinical development with Stealth BioTherapeutics Inc. since 2010 using the acetate salt form (MTP-131), and has been shown to be safe and well tolerated [74–77]. SS-31 (also referred to as elamipretide or Bendavia) was originally investigated for its ability to prevent ischemia-reperfusion injury in patients with acute ST-segment elevation myocardial infarction undergoing percutaneous coronary intervention, however, disappointingly SS-31 failed to decrease myocardial infarct size [75]. Conversely, SS-31 has been shown to attenuate the development of transient hypoxia after renal stenting in patients with atherosclerotic renal artery stenosis [78], suggesting that targeted mitochondrial protection may minimise the ischemic injury associated with such procedures. Other researchers investigating the effectiveness of SS-31 in the treatment of acute heart failure have shown that a single infusion can induce favourable changes in cardiac structure and function [76]. Furthermore, 5 days of SS-31 treatment has been shown to increase exercise performance in patients with primary mitochondrial myopathy [77]. The results from this study suggest that SS-31 improves ATP synthesis regardless of the underlying genetic defect impairing mitochondrial respiration [77]. The results from human studies involving SS-31 have been overwhelmingly positive, indicating that it may be a promising treatment in a wide range of human diseases and disorders that involve mitochondrial oxidative damage.

These results clearly highlight a role for mitochondria-targeted antioxidants in a clinical setting for the treatment of diseases involving mitochondrial oxidative damage. Future studies are needed to translate the results of animal studies indicating that mitochondria-targeted antioxidants may be an effective treatment for skeletal muscle-related diseases, such as type 2 diabetes, and age-related declines in muscle function to humans in a clinical setting.

Table 1. The effect of mitochondria-targeted antioxidants on different parameters of muscle function.

Measure Parameter	Antioxidant	Model	Supplementation Protocol	Result
Mitochondrial biogenesis and function	MitoQ	Exercise training, humans	10 mg/day	No effect [45].
		High fat diet, rats	375 μmol/kg for 8 weeks	↑ Mitochondrial function [50].
	SkQ1	High fat diet, mice	250 nmol/kg for 16 weeks	↓ Mitochondrial biogenesis [51].
		High-fat diet, rats	250 nmol/kg for 16 weeks	No effect [48].
Insulin sensitivity	MitoQ	High-fat diet, rats	375 μmol /kg for 8 weeks	↑ Glucose tolerance [50,53]
	SkQ1	High-fat diet, rats	250 nmol/kg for 16 weeks	No effect [49].
	SS-31	High-fat diet, rats	1.5 mg/kg for 6 weeks	↑ Insulin sensitivity [26].
Contractile function	SS-31	Fatiguing stimulation of isolated skeletal muscle fibers	3 μmol	No effect [58].
			200 nM	No effect [59]
				No effect [59].
Ageing, sarcopenia and disuse muscle atrophy	MitoQ	Ageing, mice	100 μmol for 15 weeks	No effect [67].
	SkQ	Ageing, rats	250 nmol/kg	↓ Age-associated pathological changes in mitochondrial structure [68].
	SS-31	Ageing, mice	3mg/kg	↑ Time to muscular fatigue, ATP production capacity, oxidative phosphorylation, and energy state [65].
		Hind limb immobilisation, rats [64] and mice [70]	3 mg/kg for 7 days [64], 1.5 mg/kg for 14 days [70]	↓ Oxidative damage, mitochondrial dysfunction and atrophy [64,70].
	XJB-5-131	Aged rats	3 mg/kg for 4 weeks	↑ Respiratory complex activity and muscle fiber contractile properties [66].

8. Conclusions

To date, the results from human clinical trials suggest that mitochondria-targeted antioxidants, specifically MitoQ and SS-31, may be effective treatments in the pathology of a variety of human diseases that involve mitochondrial oxidative damage. In general, studies that have investigated the effect of mitochondria-targeted antioxidants on different parameters of muscle function indicate that they exert a beneficial effect on muscle function by improving or attenuating declines in mitochondrial capacity and function, atrophy, and insulin sensitivity (Figure 3). However, their effects appear to be dependent on the specific mechanism through which they limit mitochondrial ROS, the doses used, and possibly the context in which ROS production is increased. Future studies should focus on translating the findings from animal studies, which indicate that mitochondria-targeted antioxidants may be a beneficial strategy for the treatment of skeletal muscle related diseases involving mitochondrial ROS production and oxidative damage, to a human population in a clinical setting.

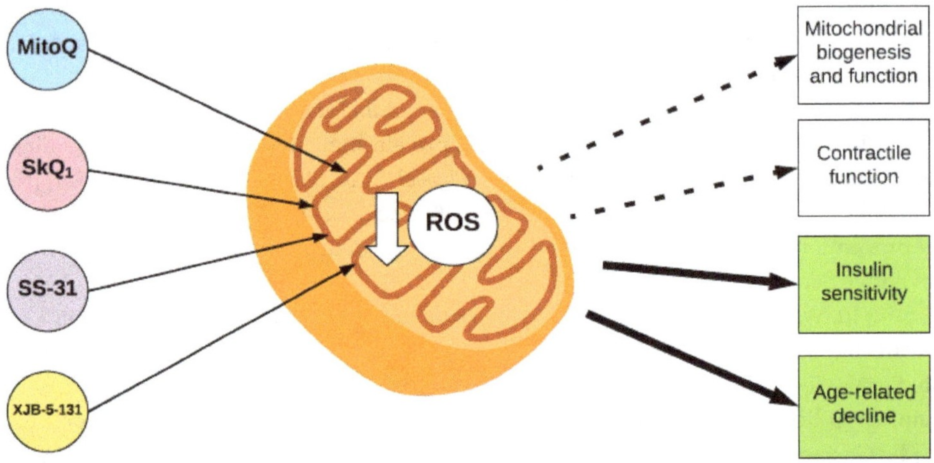

Figure 3. The effect of mitochondria-targeted antioxidants on parameters of skeletal muscle function. The mitochondria-targeted antioxidants MitoQ and SkQ1, and the mitochondria-locating peptides SS-31 and XJB-5-131 accumulate within the inner membrane of the mitochondrion, where they decrease ROS. Mitochondria-targeted antioxidants have a beneficial effect on insulin sensitivity and age-related declines in muscle function (indicated by green squares). However, their effects on mitochondrial biogenesis and function and skeletal muscle contractile function are still unclear (indicated by white squares).

Author Contributions: S.C.B., J.S.T.W., and T.L.M. co-wrote the manuscript.

Funding: The writing of this review was supported by the Marsden Fund Fast Start Grant (16-UOA-313 to T.L.M.), and T.L.M. is supported by a Rutherford Discovery Fellowship (15-UOA-020). S.C.B. is supported by a Callaghan Innovation R and D Fellowship.

Conflicts of Interest: The authors declare no conflict of interest.

References

1. Powers, S.K.; Jackson, M.J. Exercise-induced oxidative stress: Cellular mechanisms and impact on muscle force production. *Physiol. Rev.* **2008**, *88*, 1243–1276. [CrossRef] [PubMed]
2. Houstis, N.; Rosen, E.D.; Lander, E.S. Reactive oxygen species have a causal role in multiple forms of insulin resistance. *Nature* **2006**, *440*, 944–948. [CrossRef] [PubMed]
3. Kojda, G.; Harrison, D. Interactions between NO and reactive oxygen species: Pathophysiological importance in atherosclerosis, hypertension, diabetes and heart failure. *Cardiovasc. Res.* **1999**, *43*, 562–571. [CrossRef]
4. Buck, M.; Chojkier, M. Muscle wasting and dedifferentiation induced by oxidative stress in a murine model of cachexia is prevented by inhibitors of nitric oxide synthesis and antioxidants. *EMBO J.* **1996**, *15*, 1753–1765. [PubMed]
5. Tidball, J.G.; Wehling-Henricks, M. The role of free radicals in the pathophysiology of muscular dystrophy. *J. Appl. Physiol.* **2007**, *102*, 1677–1686. [CrossRef] [PubMed]
6. Lamb, G.D.; Westerblad, H. Acute effects of reactive oxygen and nitrogen species on the contractile function of skeletal muscle. *J. Physiol.* **2011**, *589*, 2119–2127. [CrossRef] [PubMed]
7. Reid, M.B. Invited review: Redox modulation of skeletal muscle contraction: What we know and what we don't. *J. Appl. Physiol.* **2001**, *90*, 724–731. [CrossRef] [PubMed]
8. Gomez-Cabrera, M.C.; Domenech, E.; Vina, J. Moderate exercise is an antioxidant: Upregulation of antioxidant genes by training. *Free Radic. Biol. Med.* **2008**, *44*, 126–131. [CrossRef] [PubMed]
9. Ristow, M. Unraveling the truth about antioxidants: Mitohormesis explains ros-induced health benefits. *Nat. Med.* **2014**, *20*, 709–711. [CrossRef] [PubMed]
10. Yun, J.; Finkel, T. Mitohormesis. *Cell Metab.* **2014**, *19*, 757–766. [CrossRef] [PubMed]

11. Gomez-Cabrera, M.C.; Borras, C.; Pallardo, F.V.; Sastre, J.; Ji, L.L.; Vina, J. Decreasing xanthine oxidase-mediated oxidative stress prevents useful cellular adaptations to exercise in rats. *J. Physiol.* **2005**, *567*, 113–120. [CrossRef] [PubMed]
12. Paulsen, G.; Hamarsland, H.; Cumming, K.T.; Johansen, R.E.; Hulmi, J.J.; Borsheim, E.; Wiig, H.; Garthe, I.; Raastad, T. Vitamin C and E supplementation alters protein signalling after a strength training session, but not muscle growth during 10 weeks of training. *J. Physiol.* **2014**, *592*, 5391–5408. [CrossRef] [PubMed]
13. Fortmann, S.P.; Burda, B.U.; Senger, C.A.; Lin, J.S.; Whitlock, E.P. Vitamin and mineral supplements in the primary prevention of cardiovascular disease and cancer: An updated systematic evidence review for the U.S. Preventive Services Task Force. *Ann. Intern. Med.* **2013**, *159*, 824–834. [CrossRef] [PubMed]
14. Myung, S.K.; Ju, W.; Cho, B.; Oh, S.W.; Park, S.M.; Koo, B.K.; Park, B.J. Efficacy of vitamin and antioxidant supplements in prevention of cardiovascular disease: Systematic review and meta-analysis of randomised controlled trials. *BMJ* **2013**, *346*. [CrossRef] [PubMed]
15. Grodstein, F.; O'Brien, J.; Kang, J.H.; Dushkes, R.; Cook, N.R.; Okereke, O.; Manson, J.E.; Glynn, R.J.; Buring, J.E.; Gaziano, M.; et al. Long-term multivitamin supplementation and cognitive function in men: A randomized trial. *Ann. Intern. Med.* **2013**, *159*, 806–814. [CrossRef] [PubMed]
16. Roberts, L.A.; Beattie, K.; Close, G.L.; Morton, J.P. Vitamin C consumption does not impair training-induced improvements in exercise performance. *Int. J. Sports Physiol. Perform.* **2011**, *6*, 58–69. [CrossRef] [PubMed]
17. Yfanti, C.; Akerstrom, T.; Nielsen, S.; Nielsen, A.R.; Mounier, R.; Mortensen, O.H.; Lykkesfeldt, J.; Rose, A.J.; Fischer, C.P.; Pedersen, B.K. Antioxidant supplementation does not alter endurance training adaptation. *Med. Sci. Sports Exerc.* **2010**, *42*, 1388–1395. [CrossRef] [PubMed]
18. Bjelakovic, G.; Nikolova, D.; Gluud, L.L.; Simonetti, R.G.; Gluud, C. Mortality in randomized trials of antioxidant supplements for primary and secondary prevention: Systematic review and meta-analysis. *JAMA* **2007**, *297*, 842–857. [CrossRef] [PubMed]
19. Paulsen, G.; Cumming, K.T.; Holden, G.; Hallen, J.; Ronnestad, B.R.; Sveen, O.; Skaug, A.; Paur, I.; Bastani, N.E.; Ostgaard, H.N.; et al. Vitamin C and E supplementation hampers cellular adaptation to endurance training in humans: A double-blind, randomised, controlled trial. *J. Physiol.* **2014**, *592*, 1887–1901. [CrossRef] [PubMed]
20. Ristow, M.; Zarse, K.; Oberbach, A.; Kloting, N.; Birringer, M.; Kiehntopf, M.; Stumvoll, M.; Kahn, C.R.; Bluher, M. Antioxidants prevent health-promoting effects of physical exercise in humans. *Proc. Natl. Acad. Sci. USA* **2009**, *106*, 8665–8670. [CrossRef] [PubMed]
21. Gomez-Cabrera, M.C.; Domenech, E.; Romagnoli, M.; Arduini, A.; Borras, C.; Pallardo, F.V.; Sastre, J.; Vina, J. Oral administration of vitamin c decreases muscle mitochondrial biogenesis and hampers training-induced adaptations in endurance performance. *Am. J. Clin. Nutr.* **2008**, *87*, 142–149. [CrossRef] [PubMed]
22. Ryan, M.J.; Jackson, J.R.; Hao, Y.; Leonard, S.S.; Alway, S.E. Inhibition of xanthine oxidase reduces oxidative stress and improves skeletal muscle function in response to electrically stimulated isometric contractions in aged mice. *Free Radic. Biol. Med.* **2011**, *51*, 38–52. [CrossRef] [PubMed]
23. Rochette, L.; Lorin, J.; Zeller, M.; Guilland, J.C.; Lorgis, L.; Cottin, Y.; Vergely, C. Nitric oxide synthase inhibition and oxidative stress in cardiovascular diseases: Possible therapeutic targets? *Pharmacol. Ther.* **2013**, *140*, 239–257. [CrossRef] [PubMed]
24. St-Pierre, J.; Buckingham, J.A.; Roebuck, S.J.; Brand, M.D. Topology of superoxide production from different sites in the mitochondrial electron transport chain. *J. Biol. Chem.* **2002**, *277*, 44784–44790. [CrossRef] [PubMed]
25. Sakellariou, G.K.; Jackson, M.J.; Vasilaki, A. Redefining the major contributors to superoxide production in contracting skeletal muscle. The role of NAD(P)H oxidases. *Free Radic. Res.* **2014**, *48*, 12–29. [CrossRef] [PubMed]
26. Anderson, E.J.; Lustig, M.E.; Boyle, K.E.; Woodlief, T.L.; Kane, D.A.; Lin, C.T.; Price, J.W., III; Kang, L.; Rabinovitch, P.S.; Szeto, H.H.; et al. Mitochondrial H_2O_2 emission and cellular redox state link excess fat intake to insulin resistance in both rodents and humans. *J. Clin. Investig.* **2009**, *119*, 573–581. [CrossRef] [PubMed]
27. Lin, M.T.; Beal, M.F. Mitochondrial dysfunction and oxidative stress in neurodegenerative diseases. *Nature* **2006**, *443*, 787–795. [CrossRef] [PubMed]
28. Nishikawa, T.; Araki, E. Impact of mitochondrial ROS production in the pathogenesis of diabetes mellitus and its complications. *Antioxid. Redox Signal.* **2007**, *9*, 343–353. [CrossRef] [PubMed]

29. Schriner, S.E.; Linford, N.J.; Martin, G.M.; Treuting, P.; Ogburn, C.E.; Emond, M.; Coskun, P.E.; Ladiges, W.; Wolf, N.; Van Remmen, H.; et al. Extension of murine life span by overexpression of catalase targeted to mitochondria. *Science* **2005**, *308*, 1909–1911. [CrossRef] [PubMed]
30. Lee, H.Y.; Choi, C.S.; Birkenfeld, A.L.; Alves, T.C.; Jornayvaz, F.R.; Jurczak, M.J.; Zhang, D.; Woo, D.K.; Shadel, G.S.; Ladiges, W.; et al. Targeted expression of catalase to mitochondria prevents age-associated reductions in mitochondrial function and insulin resistance. *Cell Metab.* **2010**, *12*, 668–674. [CrossRef] [PubMed]
31. Chen, T.; Wanagat, J.; Laflamme, M.; Marcinek, D.J.; Emond, M.J.; Ngo, C.P.; Prolla, T.A.; Rabinovitch, P.S. Age-dependent cardiomyopathy in mitochondrial mutator mice is attenuated by overexpression of catalase targeted to mitochondria. *Aging Cell* **2010**, *9*, 536–544.
32. Ostojic, S.M. Mitochondria-targeted nutraceuticals in sports medicine: A new perspective. *Res. Sports Med.* **2017**, *25*, 91–100. [CrossRef] [PubMed]
33. Ross, M.F.; Kelso, G.F.; Blaikie, F.H.; James, A.M.; Cocheme, H.M.; Filipovska, A.; Da Ros, T.; Hurd, T.R.; Smith, R.A.; Murphy, M.P. Lipophilic triphenylphosphonium cations as tools in mitochondrial bioenergetics and free radical biology. *Biochemistry* **2005**, *70*, 222–230. [CrossRef] [PubMed]
34. Liberman, E.A.; Topaly, V.P.; Tsofina, L.M.; Jasaitis, A.A.; Skulachev, V.P. Mechanism of coupling of oxidative phosphorylation and the membrane potential of mitochondria. *Nature* **1969**, *222*, 1076–1078. [CrossRef] [PubMed]
35. Murphy, M.P. Targeting lipophilic cations to mitochondria. *Biochim. Biophys. Acta* **2008**, *1777*, 1028–1031. [CrossRef] [PubMed]
36. Skulachev, V.P. A biochemical approach to the problem of aging: "Megaproject" on membrane-penetrating ions. The first results and prospects. *Biochemistry* **2007**, *72*, 1385–1396. [CrossRef] [PubMed]
37. Antonenko, Y.N.; Roginsky, V.A.; Pashkovskaya, A.A.; Rokitskaya, T.I.; Kotova, E.A.; Zaspa, A.A.; Chernyak, B.V.; Skulachev, V.P. Protective effects of mitochondria-targeted antioxidant SKQ in aqueous and lipid membrane environments. *J. Membr. Biol.* **2008**, *222*, 141–149. [CrossRef] [PubMed]
38. Severin, F.F.; Severina, I.I.; Antonenko, Y.N.; Rokitskaya, T.I.; Cherepanov, D.A.; Mokhova, E.N.; Vyssokikh, M.Y.; Pustovidko, A.V.; Markova, O.V.; Yaguzhinsky, L.S.; et al. Penetrating cation/fatty acid anion pair as a mitochondria-targeted protonophore. *Proc. Natl. Acad. Sci. USA* **2010**, *107*, 663–668. [CrossRef] [PubMed]
39. Murphy, M.P.; Smith, R.A. Targeting antioxidants to mitochondria by conjugation to lipophilic cations. *Annu. Rev. Pharmacol. Toxicol.* **2007**, *47*, 629–656. [CrossRef] [PubMed]
40. Zhao, K.; Zhao, G.M.; Wu, D.; Soong, Y.; Birk, A.V.; Schiller, P.W.; Szeto, H.H. Cell-permeable peptide antioxidants targeted to inner mitochondrial membrane inhibit mitochondrial swelling, oxidative cell death, and reperfusion injury. *J. Biol. Chem.* **2004**, *279*, 34682–34690. [CrossRef] [PubMed]
41. Birk, A.V.; Liu, S.; Soong, Y.; Mills, W.; Singh, P.; Warren, J.D.; Seshan, S.V.; Pardee, J.D.; Szeto, H.H. The mitochondrial-targeted compound SS-31 re-energizes ischemic mitochondria by interacting with cardiolipin. *J. Am. Soc. Nephrol.* **2013**, *24*, 1250–1261. [CrossRef] [PubMed]
42. Brown, D.A.; Hale, S.L.; Baines, C.P.; del Rio, C.L.; Hamlin, R.L.; Yueyama, Y.; Kijtawornrat, A.; Yeh, S.T.; Frasier, C.R.; Stewart, L.M.; et al. Reduction of early reperfusion injury with the mitochondria-targeting peptide bendavia. *J. Cardiovasc. Pharmacol. Ther.* **2014**, *19*, 121–132. [CrossRef] [PubMed]
43. Xun, Z.; Rivera-Sanchez, S.; Ayala-Pena, S.; Lim, J.; Budworth, H.; Skoda, E.M.; Robbins, P.D.; Niedernhofer, L.J.; Wipf, P.; McMurray, C.T. Targeting of XJB-5-131 to mitochondria suppresses oxidative DNA damage and motor decline in a mouse model of huntington's disease. *Cell Rep.* **2012**, *2*, 1137–1142. [CrossRef] [PubMed]
44. Fink, M.P.; Macias, C.A.; Xiao, J.; Tyurina, Y.Y.; Delude, R.L.; Greenberger, J.S.; Kagan, V.E.; Wipf, P. Hemigramicidin-TEMPO conjugates: Novel mitochondria-targeted antioxidants. *Crit. Care Med.* **2007**, *35*, S461–S467. [CrossRef] [PubMed]
45. Shill, D.D.; Southern, W.M.; Willingham, T.B.; Lansford, K.A.; McCully, K.K.; Jenkins, N.T. Mitochondria-specific antioxidant supplementation does not influence endurance exercise training-induced adaptations in circulating angiogenic cells, skeletal muscle oxidative capacity or maximal oxygen uptake. *J. Physiol.* **2016**, *594*, 7005–7014. [CrossRef] [PubMed]

46. Herrero, A.; Barja, G. Adp-regulation of mitochondrial free radical production is different with complex i- or complex ii-linked substrates: Implications for the exercise paradox and brain hypermetabolism. *J. Bioenerg. Biomembr.* **1997**, *29*, 241–249. [CrossRef] [PubMed]
47. Di Meo, S.; Venditti, P. Mitochondria in exercise-induced oxidative stress. *Biol. Signals Recept.* **2001**, *10*, 125–140. [CrossRef] [PubMed]
48. Jain, S.S.; Paglialunga, S.; Vigna, C.; Ludzki, A.; Herbst, E.A.; Lally, J.S.; Schrauwen, P.; Hoeks, J.; Tupling, A.R.; Bonen, A.; et al. High-fat diet–induced mitochondrial biogenesis is regulated by mitochondrial-derived reactive oxygen species activation of camkii. *Diabetes* **2014**, *63*, 1907–1913. [CrossRef] [PubMed]
49. Paglialunga, S.; van Bree, B.; Bosma, M.; Valdecantos, M.P.; Amengual-Cladera, E.; Jorgensen, J.A.; van Beurden, D.; den Hartog, G.J.M.; Ouwens, D.M.; Briede, J.J.; et al. Targeting of mitochondrial reactive oxygen species production does not avert lipid-induced insulin resistance in muscle tissue from mice. *Diabetologia* **2012**, *55*, 2759–2768. [CrossRef] [PubMed]
50. Coudray, C.; Fouret, G.; Lambert, K.; Ferreri, C.; Rieusset, J.; Blachnio-Zabielska, A.; Lecomte, J.; Ebabe Elle, R.; Badia, E.; Murphy, M.P.; et al. A mitochondrial-targeted ubiquinone modulates muscle lipid profile and improves mitochondrial respiration in obesogenic diet-fed rats. *Br. J. Nutr.* **2016**, *115*, 1155–1166. [CrossRef] [PubMed]
51. Loh, K.; Deng, H.; Fukushima, A.; Cai, X.; Boivin, B.; Galic, S.; Bruce, C.; Shields, B.J.; Skiba, B.; Ooms, L.M.; et al. Reactive oxygen species enhance insulin sensitivity. *Cell Metab.* **2009**, *10*, 260–272. [CrossRef] [PubMed]
52. Haber, C.A.; Lam, T.K.T.; Yu, Z.; Gupta, N.; Goh, T.; Bogdanovic, E.; Giacca, A.; Fantus, I.G. *N*-acetylcysteine and taurine prevent hyperglycemia-induced insulin resistance in vivo: Possible role of oxidative stress. *Am. J. Physiol. Endocrinol. Metab.* **2003**, *285*, E744–E753. [CrossRef] [PubMed]
53. Feillet-Coudray, C.; Fouret, G.; Ebabe Elle, R.; Rieusset, J.; Bonafos, B.; Chabi, B.; Crouzier, D.; Zarkovic, K.; Zarkovic, N.; Ramos, J. The mitochondrial-targeted antioxidant mitoq ameliorates metabolic syndrome features in obesogenic diet-fed rats better than apocynin or allopurinol. *Free Radic. Res.* **2014**, *48*, 1232–1246. [CrossRef] [PubMed]
54. Medved, I.; Brown, M.J.; Bjorksten, A.R.; McKenna, M.J. Effects of intravenous *N*-acetylcysteine infusion on time to fatigue and potassium regulation during prolonged cycling exercise. *J. Appl. Physiol.* **2004**, *96*, 211–217. [CrossRef] [PubMed]
55. Matuszczak, Y.; Farid, M.; Jones, J.; Lansdowne, S.; Smith, M.A.; Taylor, A.A.; Reid, M.B. Effects of *N*-acetylcysteine on glutathione oxidation and fatigue during handgrip exercise. *Muscle Nerve* **2005**, *32*, 633–638. [CrossRef] [PubMed]
56. McKenna, M.J.; Medved, I.; Goodman, C.A.; Brown, M.J.; Bjorksten, A.R.; Murphy, K.T.; Petersen, A.C.; Sostaric, S.; Gong, X. *N*-acetylcysteine attenuates the decline in muscle Na^+,K^+-pump activity and delays fatigue during prolonged exercise in humans. *J. Physiol.* **2006**, *576*, 279–288. [CrossRef] [PubMed]
57. Cobley, J.N.; McGlory, C.; Morton, J.P.; Close, G.L. *N*-acetylcysteine's attenuation of fatigue after repeated bouts of intermittent exercise: Practical implications for tournament situations. *Int. J. Sport Nutr. Exerc. Metab.* **2011**, *21*, 451–461. [CrossRef] [PubMed]
58. Katz, A.; Hernandez, A.; Caballero, D.M.; Briceno, J.F.; Amezquita, L.V.; Kosterina, N.; Bruton, J.D.; Westerblad, H. Effects of *N*-acetylcysteine on isolated mouse skeletal muscle: Contractile properties, temperature dependence, and metabolism. *Pflugers Arch. Eur. J. Physiol.* **2014**, *466*, 577–585. [CrossRef] [PubMed]
59. Cheng, A.J.; Bruton, J.D.; Lanner, J.T.; Westerblad, H. Antioxidant treatments do not improve force recovery after fatiguing stimulation of mouse skeletal muscle fibres. *J. Physiol.* **2015**, *593*, 457–472. [CrossRef] [PubMed]
60. Bonomini, F.; Rodella, L.F.; Rezzani, R. Metabolic syndrome, aging and involvement of oxidative stress. *Aging Dis.* **2015**, *6*, 109–120. [CrossRef] [PubMed]
61. Harman, D. Free radical theory of aging. *Mutat. Res./DNAging* **1992**, *275*, 257–266. [CrossRef]
62. Wickens, A.P. Ageing and the free radical theory. *Respir. Physiol.* **2001**, *128*, 379–391. [CrossRef]
63. Doughan, A.K.; Dikalov, S.I. Mitochondrial redox cycling of mitoquinone leads to superoxide production and cellular apoptosis. *Antioxid. Redox Signal.* **2007**, *9*, 1825–1836. [CrossRef] [PubMed]
64. Talbert, E.E.; Smuder, A.J.; Min, K.; Kwon, O.S.; Szeto, H.H.; Powers, S.K. Immobilization-induced activation of key proteolytic systems in skeletal muscles is prevented by a mitochondria-targeted antioxidant. *J. Appl. Physiol.* **2013**, *115*, 529–538. [CrossRef] [PubMed]

65. Siegel, M.P.; Kruse, S.E.; Percival, J.M.; Goh, J.; White, C.C.; Hopkins, H.C.; Kavanagh, T.J.; Szeto, H.H.; Rabinovitch, P.S.; Marcinek, D.J. Mitochondrial-targeted peptide rapidly improves mitochondrial energetics and skeletal muscle performance in aged mice. *Aging Cell* **2013**, *12*, 763–771. [CrossRef] [PubMed]
66. Javadov, S.; Jang, S.; Rodriguez-Reyes, N.; Rodriguez-Zayas, A.E.; Hernandez, J.S.; Krainz, T.; Wipf, P.; Frontera, W. Mitochondria-targeted antioxidant preserves contractile properties and mitochondrial function of skeletal muscle in aged rats. *Oncotarget* **2015**, *6*, 39469–39481. [CrossRef] [PubMed]
67. Sakellariou, G.K.; Pearson, T.; Lightfoot, A.P.; Nye, G.A.; Wells, N.; Giakoumaki, I.I.; Griffiths, R.D.; McArdle, A.; Jackson, M.J. Long-term administration of the mitochondria-targeted antioxidant mitoquinone mesylate fails to attenuate age-related oxidative damage or rescue the loss of muscle mass and function associated with aging of skeletal muscle. *FASEB J.* **2016**, *30*, 3771–3785. [CrossRef] [PubMed]
68. Vays, V.B.; Eldarov, C.M.; Vangely, I.M.; Kolosova, N.G.; Bakeeva, L.E.; Skulachev, V.P. Antioxidant SKQ1 delays sarcopenia-associated damage of mitochondrial ultrastructure. *Aging* **2014**, *6*, 140–148. [CrossRef] [PubMed]
69. Powers, S.K. Can antioxidants protect against disuse muscle atrophy? *Sports Med.* **2014**, *44*, 155–165. [CrossRef] [PubMed]
70. Min, K.; Smuder, A.J.; Kwon, O.-S.; Kavazis, A.N.; Szeto, H.H.; Powers, S.K. Mitochondrial-targeted antioxidants protect skeletal muscle against immobilization-induced muscle atrophy. *J. Appl. Physiol.* **2011**, *111*, 1459–1466. [CrossRef] [PubMed]
71. Snow, B.J.; Rolfe, F.L.; Lockhart, M.M.; Frampton, C.M.; O'Sullivan, J.D.; Fung, V.; Smith, R.A.; Murphy, M.P.; Taylor, K.M. A double-blind, placebo-controlled study to assess the mitochondria-targeted antioxidant mitoq as a disease-modifying therapy in parkinson's disease. *Mov. Disord.* **2010**, *25*, 1670–1674. [CrossRef] [PubMed]
72. Gane, E.J.; Weilert, F.; Orr, D.W.; Keogh, G.F.; Gibson, M.; Lockhart, M.M.; Frampton, C.M.; Taylor, K.M.; Smith, R.A.; Murphy, M.P. The mitochondria-targeted anti-oxidant mitoquinone decreases liver damage in a phase ii study of hepatitis c patients. *Liver Int.* **2010**, *30*, 1019–1026. [CrossRef] [PubMed]
73. Rossman, M.J.; Santos-Parker, J.R.; Steward, C.A.C.; Bispham, N.Z.; Cuevas, L.M.; Rosenberg, H.L.; Woodward, K.A.; Chonchol, M.; Gioscia-Ryan, R.A.; Murphy, M.P.; et al. Chronic supplementation with a mitochondrial antioxidant (MitoQ) improves vascular function in healthy older adults. *Hypertension* **2018**, *71*, 1056–1063. [CrossRef] [PubMed]
74. Szeto, H.H.; Birk, A.V. Serendipity and the discovery of novel compounds that restore mitochondrial plasticity. *Clin. Pharmacol. Ther.* **2014**, *96*, 672–683. [CrossRef] [PubMed]
75. Gibson, C.M.; Giugliano, R.P.; Kloner, R.A.; Bode, C.; Tendera, M.; Janosi, A.; Merkely, B.; Godlewski, J.; Halaby, R.; Korjian, S.; et al. Embrace stemi study: A phase 2a trial to evaluate the safety, tolerability, and efficacy of intravenous MTP-131 on reperfusion injury in patients undergoing primary percutaneous coronary intervention. *Eur. Heart J.* **2016**, *37*, 1296–1303. [CrossRef] [PubMed]
76. Daubert, M.A.; Yow, E.; Dunn, G.; Marchev, S.; Barnhart, H.; Douglas, P.S.; O'Connor, C.; Goldstein, S.; Udelson, J.E.; Sabbah, H.N. Novel mitochondria-targeting peptide in heart failure treatment. A Randomized, Placebo-Controlled Trial Elamipretide. *Circ. Heart Fail.* **2017**, *10*, e004389. [CrossRef] [PubMed]
77. Karaa, A.; Haas, R.; Goldstein, A.; Vockley, J.; Weaver, W.D.; Cohen, B.H. Randomized dose-escalation trial of elamipretide in adults with primary mitochondrial myopathy. *Neurology* **2018**, *90*, e1212–e1221. [CrossRef] [PubMed]
78. Saad, A.; Herrmann, S.M.S.; Eirin, A.; Ferguson, C.M.; Glockner, J.F.; Bjarnason, H.; McKusick, M.A.; Misra, S.; Lerman, L.O.; Textor, S.C. Phase 2a clinical trial of mitochondrial protection (elamipretide) during stent revascularization in patients with atherosclerotic renal artery stenosis. *Circ. Cardiovasc. Interv.* **2017**, *10*, e005478. [CrossRef] [PubMed]

13

Fluid Intake and Beverage Consumption Description and their Association with Dietary Vitamins and Antioxidant Compounds in Italian Adults from the Mediterranean Healthy Eating, Aging and Lifestyles (MEAL) Study

Armando Platania [1], Dora Castiglione [1], Dario Sinatra [1], Maurizio D' Urso [2] and Marina Marranzano [1,*]

1 Department of Medical and Surgical Sciences and Advanced Technologies "G.F. Ingrassia", University of Catania, 95123 Catania, Italy; armplt@hotmail.it (A.P.); doracastiglione29@gmail.com (D.C.); sinatradario@gmail.com (D.S.)
2 Provincial Health Authority of Catania, 95127 Catania, Italy; ma.durso76@gmail.com
* Correspondence: marranz@unict.it

Abstract: The aim of the present study was to investigate the total water intake (TWI) from drinks and foods and to evaluate the correlation between the different types of drinks on energy and antioxidant intake. The cohort comprised 1602 individuals from the city of Catania in Southern Italy. A food frequency questionnaire was administered to assess dietary and water intake. The mean total water intake was 2.7 L; more than about two thirds of the sample met the European recommendations for water intake. Water and espresso coffee were the most consumed drinks. Alcohol beverages contributed about 3.0% of total energy intake, and sugar sweetened beverages contributed about 1.4%. All antioxidant vitamins were significantly correlated with TWI. However, a higher correlation was found for water from food rather than water from beverages, suggesting that major food contributors to antioxidant vitamin intake might be fruits and vegetables, rather than beverages other than water. A mild correlation was found between fruit juices and vitamin C; coffee, tea and alcohol, and niacin and polyphenols; and milk and vitamin B12. The findings from the present study show that our sample population has an adequate intake of TWI and that there is a healthy association between beverages and dietary antioxidants.

Keywords: beverages; antioxidants; water; coffee; alcohol

1. Introduction

Water comprises from 75% body weight in infants to 55% in the elderly and is an essential nutrient that is involved in all body functions—cellular homeostasis, thermoregulation and chemical reactions to name just a few. Hydration status is regulated by a complex sensitive network of physiological controls, which aims to balance water intake and loss [1]. Proper hydration status is essential in order to preserve physical and mental functions; as a matter of fact, even slight dehydration can alter these two functions [2,3]. The importance of an adequate water intake has long been recognized, and guidelines have been established by the European Food Safety Authority (EFSA). Total water intake from all sources for men and women should be about 2.5 L and 2.0 L, respectively [4]. However, it must be stated that water requirements can change according to climatic state, salt intake and physical activity as well as health status, metabolism and age. However, it has been reported that the percentage of the population with an inadequate water intake may vary from 5% to 35% among European countries [5].

Fluid intake in all age groups depends not only on water, but also on a variety of beverages, such as tea, coffee, milk, sugar-sweetened soft drinks, juice and alcoholic drinks, that may contribute, to a various extent, to the level of hydration of an individual. The percentage of water intake in a typical Western diet has been estimated to be nearly 20–30% from food and 70–80% from fluids (including water and the aforementioned beverages) [5]. Moreover, there is plenty of scientific literature regarding the investigation of the role of specific beverages on health conditions, for instance, the adverse impact of sugar-sweetened soft drinks on metabolic disorders [6–8], the potential beneficial effects of milk on cardiovascular diseases [9,10], the positive impact on cardio-metabolic outcomes and decreased risk of certain cancers associated with coffee [11,12] and tea consumption [13–15], and the increased risk of cancer related to excessive alcohol drinking [16,17]. In addition, understanding the pattern of water contribution from food and beverages as well as beverages is essential for estimating individual or population-level adherence to recommended water intakes and the appropriateness of beverage habits. In fact, it is desirable to develop specific recommendations that take into account the hydration capability and potential effects related to energy and antioxidant content of beverages [18]. A previous report [19] attempted to summarize current knowledge regarding the relationship between water intake and human health, but the authors emphasized the scarcity of scientific literature on this matter, especially with respect to how rarely fluid intake is collected in epidemiological studies. The aim of the present study was to quantify the total water and beverage intake in a cohort of Southern Italian adults in order to test their compliance with the international guidelines of the European Food Safety Authority (EFSA). Correlations between beverages, energy and dietary antioxidant intake were further explored.

2. Materials and Methods

2.1. Study Design and Population

This study was a cross-sectional investigation of fluid intake and beverage patterns in the Mediterranean healthy eating, ageing, and lifestyle (MEAL) cohort. The total sample consisted of 2044 men and women, aged 18 to >70 years old, living in the city of Catania in Southern Italy. The sample was stratified by gender and 10-year age groups. The survey was conducted between the years 2014 and 2015; subjects and their clinical information were extracted randomly from a pool made up of general practitioners' databases. More detailed information on the study protocol has been published elsewhere [20]. The aim of the study was explained to all participants, and a written informed consent was filled in by the subjects involved. The conduction of the study and all of its procedures were performed in accordance with the Declaration of Helsinki (1989) of the World Medical Association. The study protocol has been approved by the ethical committee of the University of Catania (protocol number: 802/23 December 2014).

2.2. Data Collection

The survey consisted of a face-to-face computer-assisted personal interview with tablet computers. Participants were also provided with a paper copy of the survey to read the response options, and the interviewer filled in the digital copy of the survey on the tablet computer with the final answers from the interviewee. A section of the survey collected demographic data such as gender, age at recruitment, educational status, occupation (the main source of employment during the year before the survey was collected in more detail) or last occupation before retirement, and marital status. Participants were categorized into 3 age groups: (i) 18–35 years; (ii) 35–50 years; and (iii) >50 years. Educational status was categorized in 3 groups: (i) low (primary/secondary); (ii) medium (high school); and (iii) high (university). Occupational status was categorized in 4 groups: (i) unemployed; (ii) low (unskilled workers); (iii) medium (partially skilled workers); and (iv) high (skilled workers). Physical activity status was assessed through the International Physical Activity Questionnaires (IPAQ) [21]. This is a set of questionnaires (5 domains) collecting information about the time spent practicing physical activity in the last 7 days; following the IPAQ guidelines, final scores were used to categorize physical activity level in 3 groups: (i) low; (ii) moderate; and (iii) high. Smoking status was categorized in 3 groups: (i) non-smoker; (ii) ex-smoker; and (iii) current smoker. Alcohol consumption was categorized in 3 groups: (i) none; (ii) moderate drinker (0.1–12 g/day) and (iii) regular drinker (>12 g/day). Anthropometric measurements were collected using standardized methods [22]. Height was measured to the nearest 0.5 cm without shoes, with the back square against the wall tape, eyes looking straight ahead, and a right-angle triangle resting on the scalp and against the wall. Body mass index (BMI) was calculated, and patients were categorized as under/normal weight (BMI < 25 kg/m^2), overweight (BMI 25 to 29.9 kg/m^2), and obese (BMI > 30 kg/m^2) [23].

2.3. Dietary Assessment

Two food frequency questionnaires (a long and a short version) were administered to assess dietary and water intakes. These questionnaires have been previously tested for validity and reliability in the Sicilian population [24,25]. Beverages were combined into eight categories for further analysis: (i) alcohol beverages; (ii) sugar-sweetened beverages (including sugar-sweetened fruit juices); (iii) tea; (iv) coffee; (v) fruit juices (only 100% fruit juices); (vi) milk (all types of milk without separation by fat percentage); (vii) soy milk; (viii) water (including tap water and bottled water). Seasonal food consumption was registered during the period when the food was available; then it was adjusted by its proportional intake in one year. Food composition tables from the Research Center for Foods and Nutrition (CREA; *Consiglio per la ricerca in agricoltura e l'analisi dell'economia agraria*) [26] were used to assess the water content of food and beverages as well as energy and nutrient intakes. Total polyphenol and phytoestrogen (isoflavones and lignans) intake was calculated through a comparison with the Phenol-Explorer database (www.phenol-explorer.eu) [27]. The process of identification and calculation of the polyphenol content in foods is described in detail elsewhere [28]. Finally, intakes were adjusted for total energy intake (kcal/day) using the residual method in line with the Global Nutrition and Policy Consortium guidelines [29]. FFQs (Food Frequency Questionnaires) with unreliable intakes (<1000 or >6000 kcal/day) (n = 107) as well as missing items for the purposes of this study (n = 335) were excluded from the analyses, leaving a total of 1602 individuals included in the analysis. Total water intake (TWI) was compared with the EFSA Dietary Reference Values (DRV) regarding the Adequate Intake (AI) of water for men and women (2.5 L and 2.0 L). However, Nordic countries consider inadequate to be an intake of less than 1 g of water per 1 kcal of energy. For this reason, a combined classification was used to provide a more comprehensive evaluation of water intake: a classification based on the EFSA AI value (criterion 1), a ratio between water intake in g and energy intake in kcal (criterion 2), and a combination of criterion 1 and criterion 2 (criterion 3).

2.4. Statistical Analysis

Absolute numbers and percentages were used to show all frequencies, while means and standard errors were used to show continuous variables. Chi-square tests were used to compare categorical variables between groups, Student's t-test and ANOVA were used to compare continuous variables distributed normally, and the Mann–Whitney U-test and Kruskall–Wallis test were used to compare variables that were not normally distributed. An analysis of partial correlations, adjusted for age, gender, body weight, and physical activity, was performed between water intake, energy intake, beverage consumption, vitamins and polyphenols. All analyses were based on two-sided tests and significance was set to a p-value of 0.05. SPSS 17 (SPSS Inc., Chicago, IL, USA) software was used for all the statistical computations.

3. Results

Our sample comprised 1602 participants, ranging from 18 to >70 years old, with more women than men (Table 1). One quarter were current smokers, with men being more physically active than women. On average, BMI levels suggested a certain degree of overweight individuals in the sample, though women had slightly lower BMI levels. When considering BMI in categories, there was a higher prevalence of overweight men than women, while the opposite was observed for obesity prevalence.

Table 1. Descriptive statistics of the Mediterranean healthy eating, ageing, and lifestyle (MEAL) sample.

	Male (n = 669) (41.8% column)	Female (n = 933) (58.2% column)	Total (n = 1602)
Age groups, n (%)			
18–35	210 (31.4)	260 (27.9)	470 (29.3)
35–50	199 (29.7)	273 (29.3)	472 (29.5)
>50	260 (38.9)	400 (42.9)	660 (41.2)
Education, n (%)			
Elementary or Middle school	157 (23.5)	314 (33.7)	471 (29.4)
Diploma	308 (46.0)	341 (36.5)	649 (40.5)
Graduate	204 (30.5)	278 (29.8)	482 (30.1)
Occupation, n (%)			
Unemployed	66 (11.7)	299 (37.8)	365 (26.9)
Low (unskilled workers)	96 (17.1)	122 (15.4)	218 (16.1)
Medium (partially skilled workers)	170 (30.2)	153 (19.3)	323 (23.8)
High (skilled workers)	231 (41.0)	218 (27.5)	449 (33.1)
Smoking, n (%)			
Yes	173 (25.9)	225 (24.1)	398 (24.8)
No	374 (55.9)	648 (69.5)	1022 (63.8)
Ex-smoker	122 (18.2)	60 (6.4)	182 (11.4)
Body Mass Index (BMI) (kg/m^2) mean (SE)	26.3 (3.7)	25.1 (4.9)	25.6 (4.5)
BMI category (kg/m^2) n (%)			
Underweight/Normal (<18.5–24.9)	237 (39.4)	486 (55.7)	723 (49.1)
Overweight (25–29.9)	280 (46.5)	231 (26.5)	511 (34.7)
Obese (>29.9)	85 (14.1)	155 (17.8)	240 (15.0)
Physical activity (scale) n (%)			
Low	76 (11.4)	201 (21.5)	277 (17.3)
Moderate	317 (47.4)	481 (51.6)	798 (49.8)
High	276 (41.3)	247 (26.5)	523 (32.6)
Total Water Intake (L) mean (SE)	2729 (25.4)	2682 (23.6)	2701 (17.4)

The frequency distribution of total water intake (TWI) showed an average of 2.7 L for both men and women (Figure 1).

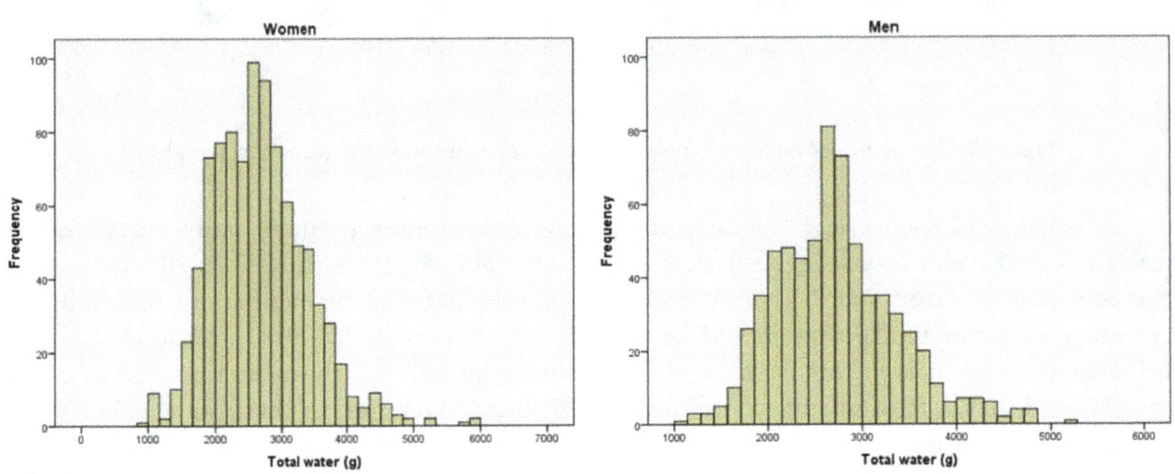

Figure 1. The frequency distribution of total water intake (TWI).

The combined classification including the EFSA AI recommendations was evaluated for both sexes (Table 2). Sixty-four percent of men and 83% of women met EFSA criterion 1 (total water intake >2.5 L in men, >2.0 L in women), while 88% of men and 86% of women met EFSA criterion 2 (water/energy intake >1).

Table 2. Combined classification for total water intake (TWI) following established criteria.

Criteria Classification	Men (n = 669)	Women (n = 933)
Criterion 1: (%)	63.7	82.7
Criterion 2: (%)	88.3	86.4
Criterion 3: (%)	59.8	75.1

EFSA: European Food Safety Authority. (1) Criterion 1: TWI >2.5 L men, >2 L women; (2) Criterion 2: ratio of total water intake and total energy >1; (3) Criterion 3: both criteria 1 and 2.

The major contribution to TWI was given by total beverages (73%), for which preference of consumption was assessed in both men and women (Figure 2). Water was consumed by all participants, followed by coffee (91% by both genders), alcohol beverages (85% by men, 79% by women) and sugar-sweetened beverages (83% by men, 75% by women). Tea and soy milk beverages were the less preferred, being consumed, respectively, by 35% of men and 30% of women (tea), and 12% of men and 15% of women (soy milk).

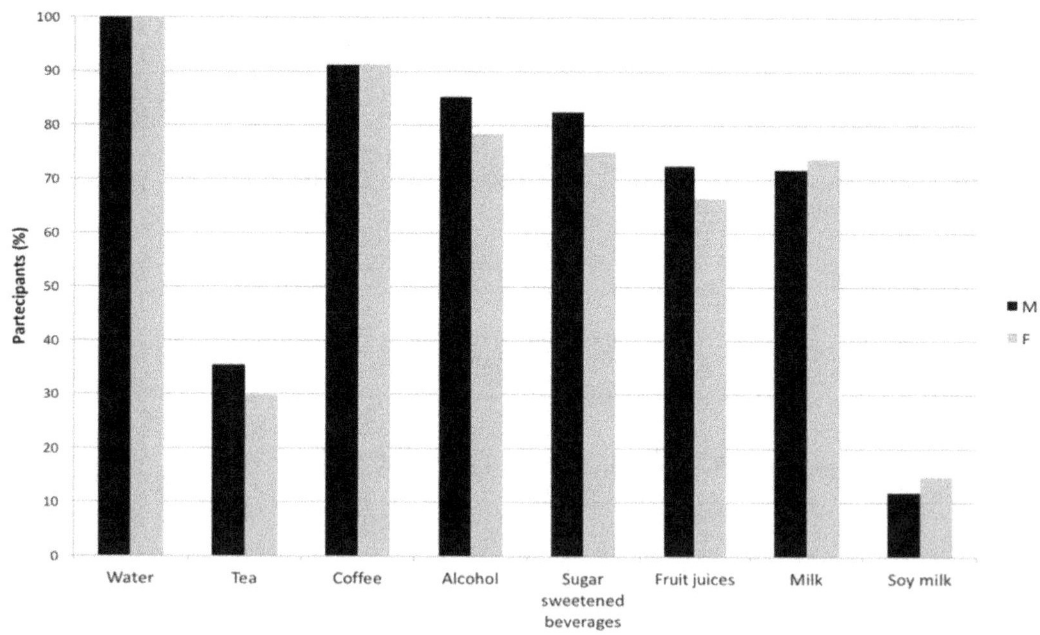

Figure 2. Prevalence of beverage consumption (% consumption by males and females).

Percentages of total weight (food and beverages) consumed (g/day), daily energy intake (kcal/day), and water intake (g/day) were calculated (Table 3). Regarding TWI, 73% came from beverages and 27% from food. These percentages met the EFSA recommendations regarding the percentage of water intake that should be provided by beverages (70–80%) and food (20–30%). Furthermore, water was the main source of TWI with a score of 55%. The mean total energy intake was 1951 kcal/day, with a relative contribution of 9% from beverages. Of these, alcohol beverages contributed 3.0% for men and 2.7% for women, while sugar-sweetened beverages contributed 1.4% for men and 1.3% for women. Little difference was found between the total weight percentage of alcohol beverages consumed by men and women (respectively, 3.5% and 3.0%).

Table 3. Contribution of food and beverages to total water and energy intake.

	Total Weight Consumed (g/day)			Contribution to Energy Intake (kcal/day)			Contribution to Water Intake (g/day)		
	Total	Men	Women	Total	Men	Women	Total	Men	Women
All food and drink, mean (SE)	3072.70 (19.76)	3102.36 (28.07)	3051.43 (27.31)	1950.53 (16.89)	1975.22 (24.81)	1932.83 (22.90)	2701.71 (17.35)	2729.08 (25.40)	2682.08 (23.57)
Food only, mean (SE)	36.0% (0.3%)	35.3% (0.4%)	36.5% (0.3%)	91.3% (0.1%)	91.4% (0.2%)	91.2% (0.2%)	27.4% (0.3%)	26.6% (0.4%)	28.0% (0.3%)
Beverages only, mean (SE)	64.0% (0.3%)	64.7% (0.4%)	63.5% (0.3%)	8.7% (0.1%)	8.6% (0.2%)	8.8% (0.2%)	72.6% (0.3%)	73.4% (0.4%)	72.0% (0.4%)
Alcohol beverages, mean (SE)	3.2% (0.1%)	3.5% (0.2%)	3.0% (0.2%)	2.8% (0.1%)	3.0% (0.1%)	2.7% (0.1%)	3.7% (0.1%)	4.0% (0.2%)	3.5% (0.2%)
Sugar-sweetened beverages, mean (SE)	2.1% (0.1%)	2.2% (0.1%)	2.0% (0.1%)	1.3% (0.1%)	1.4% (0.1%)	1.3% (0.1%)	2.5% (0.1%)	2.6% (0.2%)	2.4% (0.2%)
Tea, mean (SE)	2.4% (0.1%)	2.0% (0.2%)	2.7% (0.1%)	0.0% (0.0%)	0.0% (0.0%)	0.0% (0.0%)	2.7% (0.1%)	2.3% (0.2%)	3.0% (0.2%)
Coffee, mean (SE)	1.9% (0.0%)	1.9% (0.1%)	1.9% (0.0%)	0.3% (0.0%)	0.3% (0.0%)	0.3% (0.0%)	2.1% (0.0%)	2.2% (0.1%)	2.1% (0.1%)
Fruit juices, mean (SE)	1.1% (0.0%)	1.2% (0.1%)	1.1% (0.1%)	0.7% (0.0%)	0.8% (0.1%)	0.7% (0.0%)	1.3% (0.1%)	1.4% (0.1%)	1.2% (0.1%)
Milk, mean (SE)	4.3% (0.1%)	4.0% (0.2%)	4.5% (0.2%)	3.2% (0.1%)	2.9% (0.1%)	3.4% (0.1%)	4.9% (0.1%)	4.5% (0.2%)	5.2% (0.2%)
Soy milk, mean (SE)	0.5% (0.0%)	0.3% (0.0%)	0.6% (0.1%)	0.3% (0.0%)	0.2% (0.0%)	0.4% (0.0%)	0.5% (0.0%)	0.3% (0.0%)	0.7% (0.1%)
Water, mean (SE)	48.4% (0.3%)	49.5% (0.4%)	47.7% (0.4%)	/ /	/ /	/ /	54.9% (0.3%)	56.2% (0.5%)	54.0% (0.4%)

Water intake was also calculated separately by age group (Table 4).

Table 4. Total water intake and beverage consumption (g/day) by age group.

	Men				Women			
	Age Group			*p*	Age Group			*p*
	1	2	3		1	2	3	
Total water intake from food and beverages, mean (SE)	2804 53	2676 43	2709 37	0.12	2686 43	2739 44	2640 36	0.22
Water from food, mean (SE)	745 30	720 24	738 19	0.77	770 23	772 30	755 18	0.83
Water from beverages, mean (SE)	2059 40	1956 32	1971 29	0.07	1916 32	1967 32	1885 26	0.11
Alcoholic beverages, mean (SE)	112 9	91 7	127 12	0.05	93 8	78 7	98 8	0.20
Sugar-sweetened beverages, mean (SE)	84 9	65 8	66 7	0.18	76 9	71 8	55 6	0.13
Tea, mean (SE)	84 13	60 11	67 10	0.34	74 7	102 12	84 7	0.10
Coffee, mean (SE)	52 3	57 3	61 3	0.07	53 3	50 2	56 2	0.14
Fruit juices, mean (SE)	39 4	32 3	44 5	0.10	36 4	41 5	31 3	0.19
Milk, mean (SE)	126 10	117 11	114 9	0.68	129 10	144 11	132 8	0.52
Soy milk, mean (SE)	11 3	9 3	7 2	0.48	27 5	25 5	16 3	0.10
Water, mean (SE)	1552 31	1525 29	1485 26	0.22	1428 27	1456 27	1413 24	0.48

p-values were obtained through ANOVA tests.

The amount of water consumed in beverages did not change with age, while alcohol beverage consumption was higher in the elderly, followed by younger participants and then middle-aged ones. TWI correlated highly with the consumption of water from beverages ($r = 0.82$) and mildly with food weight ($r = 0.68$) (Table 5).

Table 5. Partial correlations between water intake, energy intake and beverage consumption.

	Total Water	Water from Beverages	Water from Food	Food Weight	Total Energy	Energy from Beverages	Energy from Food
Total water	1.00	0.82 **	0.66 **	0.68 **	0.53 **	0.37 **	0.49 **
Water from beverages	0.82 **	1.00	0.12 **	0.18 **	0.25 **	0.40 **	0.19 **
Water from food	0.66 **	0.12 **	1.00	0.96 **	0.60 **	0.11 **	0.61 **
Food weight	0.68 **	0.18 **	0.96 **	1.00	0.73 **	0.22 **	0.73 **
Total energy	0.53 **	0.25 **	0.60 **	0.73 **	1.00	0.39 **	0.98 **
Energy from beverages	0.37 **	0.40 **	0.11 **	0.22 **	0.39 **	1.00	0.22 **
Energy from food	0.49 **	0.19 **	0.61 **	0.73 **	0.98 **	0.22 **	1.00
Alcohol beverages	0.22 **	0.23 **	0.08 **	0.10 **	0.21 **	0.64 **	0.10 **
Sugar-sweetened beverages	0.20 **	0.24 **	0.05 *	0.20 **	0.35 **	0.47 **	0.28 **
Tea	0.34 **	0.23 **	0.16 **	0.15 **	0.03	0.06 *	0.02
Coffee	0.08 **	0.06 *	0.05 *	0.03	0.07 **	0.14 **	0.05 *
Fruit juices	0.29 **	0.21 **	0.22 **	0.27 **	0.18 **	0.28 **	0.14 **
Milk	0.12 **	0.20 **	−0.04	0.00	0.12 **	0.51 **	0.03
Soy milk	0.16 **	0.14 **	0.09 **	0.10 **	0.05 *	0.10 **	0.04
Water	0.61 **	0.81 **	0.02	0.02	0.03	−0.14 **	0.06 *

** Correlation is significant at the 0.01 level (bilateral); * Correlation is significant at the 0.05 level (bilateral).

Alcohol beverages, milk and sugar-sweetened beverages had the highest correlations with total energy from beverages ($r = 0.64$, $r = 0.51$, and $r = 0.47$, respectively), while the scores were low for the other beverages and near zero for water and tea. All antioxidant vitamins were significantly correlated with TWI (Table 6).

However, a higher correlation with TWI was found for water from food than for water from beverages, suggesting that the major food contributors to antioxidant vitamin intake might be fruits and vegetables, rather than beverages other than water. Another strong correlation was found between total phytoestrogen intake and soy milk intake ($r = 0.78$), suggesting that soy milk is a major contributor to phytoestrogen intake in this cohort. A mild correlation was found between fruit juices and vitamin C ($r = 0.42$), and tea and polyphenols ($r = 0.37$), and other correlations were found between coffee, and niacin ($r = 0.31$) and polyphenols ($r = 0.20$); milk and vitamin B12 ($r = 0.32$); and alcohol and polyphenols ($r = 0.31$).

Table 6. Partial correlations between water intake, energy intake, beverage consumption, vitamins and polyphenols.

Title	Total Water	Water from Beverages	Water from Food	Food Weight	Total Energy	Energy from Beverages	Energy from Food	Alcohol Beverages	Sugar-Sweetened Beverages	Tea	Coffee	Fruit Juices	Milk	Soy Milk	Water
Vitamin A	0.60 **	0.21 **	0.75 **	0.74 **	0.54 **	0.25 **	0.52 **	0.11 **	0.01	0.23 **	0.05	0.21 **	0.01	0.15 **	0.03
Vitamin B1	0.48 **	0.22 **	0.54 **	0.56 **	0.76 **	0.27 **	0.75 **	0.15 **	0.23 **	0.15 **	0.05	0.09 **	0.08 **	0.11 **	0.07 **
Vitamin B2	0.51 **	0.27 **	0.52 **	0.53 **	0.72 **	0.39 **	0.69 **	0.17 **	0.19 **	0.18 **	0.12 **	0.06 *	0.27 **	0.17 **	0.04
Niacin	0.54 **	0.27 **	0.60 **	0.69 **	0.77 **	0.25 **	0.76 **	0.12 **	0.16 **	0.11 **	0.31 **	0.10 **	0.00	0.14 **	0.10 **
Vitamin B6	0.66 **	0.29 **	0.73 **	0.82 **	0.83 **	0.30 **	0.82 **	0.08 **	0.12 **	0.25 **	0.02	0.17 **	0.05 *	0.18 **	0.08 **
Folate	0.59 **	0.23 **	0.73 **	0.79 **	0.69 **	0.25 **	0.68 **	0.12 **	0.06 *	0.20 **	0.06 *	0.23 **	0.01	0.21 **	0.06 *
Vitamin B12	0.35 **	0.21 **	0.35 **	0.41 **	0.44 **	0.14 **	0.44 **	0.06 *	0.27 **	0.11 **	−0.03	0.11 **	0.32 **	0.04	0.20 **
Vitamin C	0.62 **	0.18 **	0.84 **	0.85 **	0.50 **	0.29 **	0.47 **	0.12 **	0.06 *	0.18 **	0.02	0.42 **	0.00	0.13 **	−0.03
Vitamin D	0.31 **	0.17 **	0.32 **	0.36 **	0.35 **	0.04	0.37 **	−0.02	0.15 **	0.14 **	−0.05	0.14 **	0.06*	0.10 **	0.20 **
Vitamin E	0.57 **	0.21 **	0.71 **	0.74 **	0.76 **	0.28 **	0.76 **	0.15 **	0.14 **	0.19 **	0.01	0.15 **	−0.05 *	0.19 **	0.02
Total polyphenols	0.46 **	0.24 **	0.43 **	0.44 **	0.42 **	0.32 **	0.39 **	0.31 **	−0.07 **	0.37 **	0.20 **	0.13 **	−0.11 **	0.14 **	0.04
Total phytoestrogens	0.34 **	0.14 **	0.40 **	0.39 **	0.38 **	0.05 *	−0.05 *	0.15	0.01	0.12 *	−0.05 *	0.11 **	-0.08 **	0.78 **	0.04

** Correlation is significant at the 0.01 level (bilateral); * Correlation is significant at the 0.05 level (bilateral).

4. Discussion

This study analysed the total water intake from both food and beverages among the MEAL cohort, a representative sample of Southern Italian adults. Our study is one of the few attempts to describe the consumption of water and beverages in Italy, the relationship between energy intake and beverages, as well as being a reference for the role of some antioxidant vitamins and polyphenols contained in beverages. The EFSA Scientific Opinion on Dietary Reference Values for Water states that the dietary reference intake values for water should include water from drinking water (tap or bottled), all kinds of beverages, and food moisture. The adequate total water intake suggested by EFSA guidelines (2 L for women and 2.5 L for men) was met by the majority of our sample population.

Comparisons with similar studies are not easy to perform due to the use of different populations with different dietary habits, as well as different tools administered. Nonetheless, it can be stated that participants from two previous studies on hydration (Spanish and Italian) did not reach the EFSA guidelines recommended intake for water, while participants in another one (English) did reach the recommended intake [30–32]. In our study, the main contributor to TWI was plain water. Our results are only partially in line with previous studies in which the main source of TWI was either food (Italy and Spain) or hot beverages (UK); this can be explained by the hotter seasonal temperatures in Southern Italy, which stimulate thirst induction, and the preference for plain water over sugar-sweetened beverages due to the cultural heritage of adults living in Southern Italy who are still adherent, at least in part, to traditional dietary patterns [33,34]. The main benefit from a hydration pattern which mainly focuses on plain water intake is the fulfillment of its purpose without adding caloric intake, while providing mineral micronutrients. In line with other studies [30–32], water intake from beverages decreased with age, underlining a common trend which sees the elderly drinking less. Evidence from studies conducted in Mediterranean populations shows that adherence to traditional dietary patterns (including beverage consumption) might be beneficial for body composition in young, adult and elderly individuals [35–37]. However, more studies are needed to evaluate whether this trend could be linked with a risk of dehydration in the elderly or if it is a harmless manifestation of the lower physiological water needs of the metabolism in late years.

The second most popular beverage was coffee, namely as espresso coffee, which was drunk by 91% of our sample, but still had a low contribution to TWI (2%) due to the small quantity contained in a serving. In our analysis, we found a statistically significant correlation between coffee and niacin and total polyphenols. Coffee contains around 5 mg of niacin and thus can be an important source of this vitamin [38]. Moreover, previous studies have demonstrated that coffee is among the highest source of polyphenols in individuals living in Northern and Eastern European populations [39,40] due to the large intake compared with individuals living in Southern European countries, such as France, Spain and Italy [41–43]. Coffee drinking has been associated with positive health outcomes [44]. Regarding espresso coffee, despite it being reported to provide an important antioxidant capacity within the context of a common diet [45,46], results regarding its effects on health are varied, ranging from positive [47–49] to negative [50–52]. In general, scientific literature on espresso coffee is scarce, and further research is needed to test the impact of this beverage on human health.

Regarding alcoholic beverage consumption, women almost reached the same intake as men (3.0% vs. 3.5%) in contrast with previous studies in which men had, in some cases, double the consumption of women [32]. Regular and moderate daily alcohol consumption is a typical pattern of the Mediterranean diet, with wine being the most consumed type of alcoholic beverage [53]. This habit is especially rooted in the elderly, as confirmed by our analysis stratified by age groups. Furthermore, a small correlation has been found between alcohol beverages and polyphenols. The caloric contribution of alcohol beverages was 3%; the downside of the non-negligible caloric intake of alcoholic beverages could be softened by the benefits of moderate alcohol use. In fact, there is evidence that dietary polyphenols may exert beneficial effect toward human health [54,55]. It has been established that alcohol has a protective effect at low doses, in particular, for red wine in regard to cardiovascular diseases, and the presence of polyphenols contained in such beverages has been proposed as one of the main contributors to this effect [56,57]. Another source of polyphenols is tea, as remarked by our correlation analysis. However, its consumption was relatively low in our sample, comprising 2% of total water weight consumed, with a popularity of only 30% of the population. Finally, the least popular beverage was soy milk, which was highly correlated with phytoestrogen intake. Soy foods and beverages are hardly consumed in the Mediterranean area compared to Asian countries [58], but evidence suggests that phytoestrogens, such as isoflavones, may exert beneficial effects on health [59]. A previous study involving the present cohort showed certain positive associations between phytoestrogen consumption and hypertension despite the low consumption [34], suggesting that this beverage has the potential for dietary recommendation in Mediterranean countries and could be taken into account for future dietary strategies. Besides polyphenols, antioxidant vitamins were correlated with total water intake, and specifically with water from food. This suggests that foods with a high content of water, like fruits and some kinds of vegetables, are the main source of these substances [60–62]. As expected, correlations between vitamin C and fruit juices, and vitamin B12 and milk were found, suggesting that such beverages are among the major sources of these vitamins.

Beverages' contribution to total energy intake was 9%, less than the 10% suggested by EFSA and WHO (World Health Organization) [4,63]. It has been recently discussed worldwide whether energy intake from beverages could have a role in metabolic disorders such as obesity [64–67]. According to recent scientific literature, there is a wide difference in beverage energy contribution between countries, ranging from around 5–10% in Italy and Spain, to 16% in the UK and 21% in the US [30–32,68]. The habit of drinking sugar-sweetened beverages is not common in the context of a Mediterranean diet pattern, as reported in our results (sugar-sweetened beverages accounted for only 1.3% of total caloric intake), as well as findings from other Italian and Spanish studies (0.4–2%) [30,31]. There is evidence from this cohort that traditional dietary patterns may be associated with a lower likelihood of having metabolic disorders [69–71]. In contrast, studies conducted in the UK and the US reported alarming trends in sugar-sweetened beverage consumption, which have been ascribed as being potentially responsible for the rise in metabolic disorders in these areas [32,68].

The main limitation of this study was the lack of a hydration biomarker that could definitely correlate fluid intake with the hydration levels of the individuals involved in the survey. Second, the cross-sectional nature of the study design and the use of a FFQ to estimate dietary information may lead to recall bias, with some overestimations (for instance on water intakes) and underestimations (alcohol beverages).

5. Conclusions

In conclusion, the results of the present study show that our sample population had adequate intake of TWI in accordance with EFSA reference values. Caloric beverages did not have a big impact on total caloric intake among the sample population, entering the boundaries of EFSA and WHO recommendation limits. Some beverages, like fruit juices, can cause a significant intake of certain vitamins and could be included in specific recommendations to avoid nutritional deficiencies. A small number of studies have investigated hydration status on a population level, thus further investigations are needed to identify trends and issues that may require specific health and nutrition policies or targeted interventions.

Author Contributions: Marina Marranzano conceived and designed the experiments; Armando Platania performed the experiments; Armando Platania and Dario Sinatra analyzed the data; Armando Platania wrote the paper; Dora Castiglione and Maurizio D' Urso provided data and clinical revision.

Conflicts of Interest: The authors declare no conflict of interest.

References

1. Arnaud, M.J. *Hydration Throughout Life: International Conference, Vittel, France, June 9–12, 1998*; John Libbey Eurotext: Montrouge, France, 1998.
2. Watson, P.; Whale, A.; Mears, S.A.; Reyner, L.A.; Maughan, R.J. Mild hypohydration increases the frequency of driver errors during a prolonged, monotonous driving task. *Physiol .Behav.* **2015**, *147*, 313–318. [CrossRef] [PubMed]
3. Maughan, R.J. Impact of mild dehydration on wellness and on exercise performance. *Eur. J. Clin. Nutr.* **2003**, *57* (Suppl. 2), S19–S23. [CrossRef] [PubMed]
4. European Food Safety Authority (EFSA) Panel on Dietetic Products, Nutrition and Allergies. Scientific opinion on dietary reference values for water. *EFSA J.* **2010**, *8*, 1459.
5. Nissensohn, M.; Castro-Quezada, I.; Serra-Majem, L. Beverage and water intake of healthy adults in some european countries. *Int. J. Food Sci. Nutr.* **2013**, *64*, 801–805. [CrossRef] [PubMed]
6. Imamura, F.; O'Connor, L.; Ye, Z.; Mursu, J.; Hayashino, Y.; Bhupathiraju, S.N.; Forouhi, N.G. Consumption of sugar sweetened beverages, artificially sweetened beverages, and fruit juice and incidence of type 2 diabetes: Systematic review, meta-analysis, and estimation of population attributable fraction. *BMJ* **2015**, *351*, 3576. [CrossRef] [PubMed]
7. Xi, B.; Huang, Y.; Reilly, K.H.; Li, S.; Zheng, R.; Barrio-Lopez, M.T.; Martinez-Gonzalez, M.A.; Zhou, D. Sugar-sweetened beverages and risk of hypertension and CVD: A dose-response meta-analysis. *Br. J. Nutr.* **2015**, *113*, 709–717. [CrossRef] [PubMed]
8. Ruanpeng, D.; Thongprayoon, C.; Cheungpasitporn, W.; Harindhanavudhi, T. Sugar and artificially sweetened beverages linked to obesity: A systematic review and meta-analysis. *QJM* **2017**, *110*, 513–520. [CrossRef] [PubMed]
9. Larsson, S.C.; Crippa, A.; Orsini, N.; Wolk, A.; Michaelsson, K. Milk consumption and mortality from all causes, cardiovascular disease, and cancer: A systematic review and meta-analysis. *Nutrients* **2015**, *7*, 7749–7763. [CrossRef] [PubMed]
10. Guo, J.; Astrup, A.; Lovegrove, J.A.; Gijsbers, L.; Givens, D.I.; Soedamah-Muthu, S.S. Milk and dairy consumption and risk of cardiovascular diseases and all-cause mortality: Dose-response meta-analysis of prospective cohort studies. *Eur. J. Epidemiol.* **2017**, *32*, 269–287. [CrossRef] [PubMed]
11. Grosso, G.; Micek, A.; Godos, J.; Sciacca, S.; Pajak, A.; Martinez-Gonzalez, M.A.; Giovannucci, E.L.; Galvano, F. Coffee consumption and risk of all-cause, cardiovascular, and cancer mortality in smokers and non-smokers: A dose-response meta-analysis. *Eur. J. Epidemiol.* **2016**, *31*, 1191–1205. [CrossRef] [PubMed]
12. Marventano, S.; Salomone, F.; Godos, J.; Pluchinotta, F.; Del Rio, D.; Mistretta, A.; Grosso, G. Coffee and tea consumption in relation with non-alcoholic fatty liver and metabolic syndrome: A systematic review and meta-analysis of observational studies. *Clin. Nutr.* **2016**, *35*, 1269–1281. [CrossRef] [PubMed]
13. Yang, J.; Mao, Q.X.; Xu, H.X.; Ma, X.; Zeng, C.Y. Tea consumption and risk of type 2 diabetes mellitus: A systematic review and meta-analysis update. *BMJ Open* **2014**, *4*, e005632. [CrossRef] [PubMed]
14. Tang, J.; Zheng, J.S.; Fang, L.; Jin, Y.; Cai, W.; Li, D. Tea consumption and mortality of all cancers, CVD and all causes: A meta-analysis of eighteen prospective cohort studies. *Br. J. Nutr.* **2015**, *114*, 673–683. [CrossRef] [PubMed]
15. Zhang, C.; Qin, Y.Y.; Wei, X.; Yu, F.F.; Zhou, Y.H.; He, J. Tea consumption and risk of cardiovascular outcomes and total mortality: A systematic review and meta-analysis of prospective observational studies. *Eur. J. Epidemiol.* **2015**, *30*, 103–113. [CrossRef] [PubMed]
16. Bagnardi, V.; Rota, M.; Botteri, E.; Tramacere, I.; Islami, F.; Fedirko, V.; Scotti, L.; Jenab, M.; Turati, F.; Pasquali, E.; et al. Alcohol consumption and site-specific cancer risk: A comprehensive dose-response meta-analysis. *Br. J. Cancer* **2015**, *112*, 580–593. [CrossRef] [PubMed]
17. Praud, D.; Rota, M.; Rehm, J.; Shield, K.; Zatonski, W.; Hashibe, M.; La Vecchia, C.; Boffetta, P. Cancer incidence and mortality attributable to alcohol consumption. *Int. J. Cancer* **2016**, *138*, 1380–1387. [CrossRef] [PubMed]
18. Rosado, C.I.; Marin, A.L.V.; Martinez, J.A.; Cabrerizo, L.; Gargallo, M.; Lorenzo, H.; Quiles, J.; Planas, M.; Polanco, I.; de Avila, D.R.; et al. Importance of water in the hydration of the spanish population: Fesnad 2010 document. *Nutr. Hosp.* **2011**, *26*, 27–36.

19. Popkin, B.M.; D'Anci, K.E.; Rosenberg, I.H. Water, hydration, and health. *Nutr. Rev.* **2010**, *68*, 439–458. [CrossRef] [PubMed]
20. Grosso, G.; Marventano, S.; D'Urso, M.; Mistretta, A.; Galvano, F. The mediterranean healthy eating, ageing, and lifestyle (meal) study: Rationale and study design. *Int. J. Food Sci. Nutr.* **2017**, *68*, 577–586. [CrossRef] [PubMed]
21. Craig, C.L.; Marshall, A.L.; Sjostrom, M.; Bauman, A.E.; Booth, M.L.; Ainsworth, B.E.; Pratt, M.; Ekelund, U.; Yngve, A.; Sallis, J.F.; et al. International physical activity questionnaire: 12-country reliability and validity. *Med. Sci. Sports Exerc.* **2003**, *35*, 1381–1395. [CrossRef] [PubMed]
22. Mistretta, A.; Marventano, S.; Platania, A.; Godos, J.; Galvano, F.; Grosso, G. Metabolic profile of the mediterranean healthy eating, lifestyle and aging (meal) study cohort. *Mediterr. J. Nutr. Metab.* **2017**, *10*, 131–140. [CrossRef]
23. World Health Organization. *Obesity: Preventing and Managing the Global Epidemic*; Report of a Who Consultation Presented at the World Health Organization; June 3–5, 1997; World Health Organization: Geneva, Switzerland, 1997.
24. Buscemi, S.; Rosafio, G.; Vasto, S.; Massenti, F.M.; Grosso, G.; Galvano, F.; Rini, N.; Barile, A.M.; Maniaci, V.; Cosentino, L.; et al. Validation of a food frequency questionnaire for use in italian adults living in sicily. *Int. J. Food Sci. Nutr.* **2015**, *66*, 426–438. [CrossRef] [PubMed]
25. Marventano, S.; Mistretta, A.; Platania, A.; Galvano, F.; Grosso, G. Reliability and relative validity of a food frequency questionnaire for italian adults living in sicily, southern italy. *Int. J. Food Sci. Nutr.* **2016**, *67*, 857–864. [CrossRef] [PubMed]
26. Marletta, L.; Carnovale, E. *Tabelle di Composizione Degli Alimenti*; Istituto Nazionale di Ricerca per gli Alimenti e la Nutrizione: Milano, Italy, 2000.
27. Neveu, V.; Perez-Jiménez, J.; Vos, F.; Crespy, V.; Du Chaffaut, L.; Mennen, L.; Knox, C.; Eisner, R.; Cruz, J.; Wishart, D.; et al. Phenol-explorer: An online comprehensive database on polyphenol contents in foods. *Database* **2010**. [CrossRef] [PubMed]
28. Godos, J.; Marventano, S.; Mistretta, A.; Galvano, F.; Grosso, G. Dietary sources of polyphenols in the mediterranean healthy eating, aging and lifestyle (meal) study cohort. *Int. J. Food Sci. Nutr.* **2017**, 1–7. [CrossRef] [PubMed]
29. Willett, W.C. Reproducibility and validity of food frequency questionnaire. In *Nutritional Epidemiology*, 2nd ed.; Oxford University Press: Oxford, UK, 1998.
30. Nissensohn, M.; Sanchez-Villegas, A.; Ortega, R.M.; Aranceta-Bartrina, J.; Gil, A.; Gonzalez-Gross, M.; Varela-Moreiras, G.; Serra-Majem, L. Beverage consumption habits and association with total water and energy intakes in the spanish population: Findings of the anibes study. *Nutrients* **2016**, *8*, 232. [CrossRef] [PubMed]
31. Mistura, L.; D'Addezio, L.; Turrini, A. Beverage consumption habits in italian population: Association with total water intake and energy intake. *Nutrients* **2016**, *8*. [CrossRef] [PubMed]
32. Gibson, S.; Shirreffs, S.M. Beverage consumption habits "24/7" among british adults: Association with total water intake and energy intake. *Nutr. J.* **2013**, *12*, 9. [CrossRef] [PubMed]
33. Grosso, G.; Marventano, S.; Giorgianni, G.; Raciti, T.; Galvano, F.; Mistretta, A. Mediterranean diet adherence rates in sicily, southern italy. *Public Health Nutr.* **2014**, *17*, 2001–2009. [CrossRef] [PubMed]
34. Marventano, S.; Godos, J.; Platania, A.; Galvano, F.; Mistretta, A.; Grosso, G. Mediterranean diet adherence in the mediterranean healthy eating, aging and lifestyle (meal) study cohort. *Int. J. Food Sci. Nutr.* **2018**, *69*, 100–107. [CrossRef] [PubMed]
35. Bonaccorsi, G.; Lorini, C.; Santomauro, F.; Sofi, F.; Vannetti, F.; Pasquini, G.; Macchi, C.; Mugello Study, G. Adherence to mediterranean diet and nutritional status in a sample of nonagenarians. *Exp. Gerontol.* **2018**, *103*, 57–62. [CrossRef] [PubMed]
36. De Lorenzo, A.; Noce, A.; Bigioni, M.; Calabrese, V.; Della Rocca, D.G.; Di Daniele, N.; Tozzo, C.; Di Renzo, L. The effects of italian mediterranean organic diet (IMOD) on health status. *Curr. Pharm. Des.* **2010**, *16*, 814–824. [CrossRef] [PubMed]
37. Mistretta, A.; Marventano, S.; Antoci, M.; Cagnetti, A.; Giogianni, G.; Nolfo, F.; Rametta, S.; Pecora, G.; Marranzano, M. Mediterranean diet adherence and body composition among southern italian adolescents. *Obes. Res. Clin. Pract.* **2017**, *11*, 215–226. [CrossRef] [PubMed]

38. Kremer, J.I.; Gompel, K.; Bakuradze, T.; Eisenbrand, G.; Richling, E. Urinary excretion of niacin metabolites in humans after coffee consumption. *Mol. Nutr. Food Res.* **2018**, e1700735. [CrossRef] [PubMed]
39. Grosso, G.; Stepaniak, U.; Topor-Madry, R.; Szafraniec, K.; Pajak, A. Estimated dietary intake and major food sources of polyphenols in the polish arm of the hapiee study. *Nutrition* **2014**, *30*, 1398–1403. [CrossRef] [PubMed]
40. Ovaskainen, M.L.; Torronen, R.; Koponen, J.M.; Sinkko, H.; Hellstrom, J.; Reinivuo, H.; Mattila, P. Dietary intake and major food sources of polyphenols in finnish adults. *J. Nutr.* **2008**, *138*, 562–566. [CrossRef] [PubMed]
41. Tresserra-Rimbau, A.; Medina-Remon, A.; Perez-Jimenez, J.; Martinez-Gonzalez, M.A.; Covas, M.I.; Corella, D.; Salas-Salvado, J.; Gomez-Gracia, E.; Lapetra, J.; Aros, F.; et al. Dietary intake and major food sources of polyphenols in a spanish population at high cardiovascular risk: The predimed study. *Nutr. Metab. Cardiovasc. Dis.* **2013**, *23*, 953–959. [CrossRef] [PubMed]
42. Perez-Jimenez, J.; Neveu, V.; Vos, F.; Scalbert, A. Identification of the 100 richest dietary sources of polyphenols: An application of the phenol-explorer database. *Eur. J. Clin. Nutr.* **2010**, *64* (Suppl. 3), S112–S120. [CrossRef]
43. Godos, J.; Rapisarda, G.; Marventano, S.; Galvano, F.; Mistretta, A.; Grosso, G. Association between polyphenol intake and adherence to the mediterranean diet in sicily, southern Italy. *NFS J.* **2017**, *8*, 1–7. [CrossRef]
44. Grosso, G.; Godos, J.; Galvano, F.; Giovannucci, E.L. Coffee, caffeine, and health outcomes: An umbrella review. *Annu. Rev. Nutr.* **2017**, *37*, 131–156. [CrossRef] [PubMed]
45. Caprioli, G.; Cortese, M.; Maggi, F.; Minnetti, C.; Odello, L.; Sagratini, G.; Vittori, S. Quantification of caffeine, trigonelline and nicotinic acid in espresso coffee: The influence of espresso machines and coffee cultivars. *Int. J. Food Sci. Nutr.* **2014**, *65*, 465–469. [CrossRef] [PubMed]
46. Caprioli, G.; Cortese, M.; Sagratini, G.; Vittori, S. The influence of different types of preparation (espresso and brew) on coffee aroma and main bioactive constituents. *Int. J. Food Sci. Nutr.* **2015**, *66*, 505–513. [CrossRef] [PubMed]
47. Godos, J.; Sinatra, D.; Blanco, I.; Mule, S.; La Verde, M.; Marranzano, M. Association between dietary phenolic acids and hypertension in a mediterranean cohort. *Nutrients* **2017**, *9*. [CrossRef]
48. Pounis, G.; Tabolacci, C.; Costanzo, S.; Cordella, M.; Bonaccio, M.; Rago, L.; D'Arcangelo, D.; Di Castelnuovo, A.F.; de Gaetano, G.; Donati, M.B.; et al. Reduction by coffee consumption of prostate cancer risk: Evidence from the Moli-sani cohort and cellular models. *Int. J. Cancer* **2017**, *141*, 72–82. [CrossRef] [PubMed]
49. Solfrizzi, V.; Panza, F.; Imbimbo, B.P.; D'Introno, A.; Galluzzo, L.; Gandin, C.; Misciagna, G.; Guerra, V.; Osella, A.; Baldereschi, M.; et al. Coffee consumption habits and the risk of mild cognitive impairment: The Italian longitudinal study on aging. *J. Alzheimers Dis.* **2015**, *47*, 889–899. [CrossRef] [PubMed]
50. Parodi, S.; Merlo, F.D.; Stagnaro, E. Working Group for the Epidemiology of Hematolymphopoietic Malignancies in, I. Coffee consumption and risk of non-hodgkin's lymphoma: Evidence from the Italian multicentre case-control study. *Cancer Causes Control* **2017**, *28*, 867–876. [CrossRef] [PubMed]
51. Grioni, S.; Agnoli, C.; Sieri, S.; Pala, V.; Ricceri, F.; Masala, G.; Saieva, C.; Panico, S.; Mattiello, A.; Chiodini, P.; et al. Espresso coffee consumption and risk of coronary heart disease in a large Italian cohort. *PLoS ONE* **2015**, *10*, e0126550. [CrossRef] [PubMed]
52. Filiberti, R.A.; Fontana, V.; De Ceglie, A.; Blanchi, S.; Grossi, E.; Della Casa, D.; Lacchin, T.; De Matthaeis, M.; Ignomirelli, O.; Cappiello, R.; et al. Association between coffee or tea drinking and barrett's esophagus or esophagitis: An Italian study. *Eur. J. Clin. Nutr.* **2017**, *71*, 980–986. [CrossRef] [PubMed]
53. Giacosa, A.; Barale, R.; Bavaresco, L.; Faliva, M.A.; Gerbi, V.; La Vecchia, C.; Negri, E.; Opizzi, A.; Perna, S.; Pezzotti, M.; et al. Mediterranean way of drinking and longevity. *Crit. Rev. Food Sci. Nutr.* **2016**, *56*, 635–640. [CrossRef] [PubMed]
54. Grosso, G.; Godos, J.; Lamuela-Raventos, R.; Ray, S.; Micek, A.; Pajak, A.; Sciacca, S.; D'Orazio, N.; Del Rio, D.; Galvano, F. A comprehensive meta-analysis on dietary flavonoid and lignan intake and cancer risk: Level of evidence and limitations. *Mol. Nutr. Food Res.* **2017**, *61*. [CrossRef] [PubMed]
55. Grosso, G.; Micek, A.; Godos, J.; Pajak, A.; Sciacca, S.; Galvano, F.; Giovannucci, E.L. Dietary flavonoid and lignan intake and mortality in prospective cohort studies: Systematic review and dose-response meta-analysis. *Am. J. Epidemiol.* **2017**, *185*, 1304–1316. [CrossRef] [PubMed]

56. Chiva-Blanch, G.; Arranz, S.; Lamuela-Raventos, R.M.; Estruch, R. Effects of wine, alcohol and polyphenols on cardiovascular disease risk factors: Evidences from human studies. *Alcohol Alcohol.* **2013**, *48*, 270–277. [CrossRef] [PubMed]
57. Arranz, S.; Chiva-Blanch, G.; Valderas-Martinez, P.; Medina-Remon, A.; Lamuela-Raventos, R.M.; Estruch, R. Wine, beer, alcohol and polyphenols on cardiovascular disease and cancer. *Nutrients* **2012**, *4*, 759–781. [CrossRef] [PubMed]
58. Mocciaro, G.; Ziauddeen, N.; Godos, J.; Marranzano, M.; Chan, M.Y.; Ray, S. Does a mediterranean-type dietary pattern exert a cardio-protective effect outside the mediterranean region? A review of current evidence. *Int. J. Food Sci. Nutr.* **2017**, 1–12. [CrossRef] [PubMed]
59. Godos, J.; Bergante, S.; Satriano, A.; Pluchinotta, F.R.; Marranzano, M. Dietary phytoestrogen intake is inversely associated with hypertension in a cohort of adults living in the mediterranean area. *Molecules* **2018**, *23*. [CrossRef] [PubMed]
60. Olza, J.; Aranceta-Bartrina, J.; Gonzalez-Gross, M.; Ortega, R.M.; Serra-Majem, L.; Varela-Moreiras, G.; Gil, A. Reported dietary intake and food sources of zinc, selenium, and vitamins A, E and C in the spanish population: Findings from the anibes study. *Nutrients* **2017**, *9*. [CrossRef] [PubMed]
61. Dominguez-Perles, R.; Mena, P.; Garcia-Viguera, C.; Moreno, D.A. Brassica foods as a dietary source of vitamin C: A review. *Crit. Rev. Food Sci. Nutr.* **2014**, *54*, 1076–1091. [CrossRef] [PubMed]
62. Marranzano, M.; Godos, J.; Sumantra, R.; Galvano, F. Association between dietary flavonoids intake and obesity in a cohort of adults living in the Mediterranean area. *Int. J. Food Sci. Nutr.* **2018**, ahead of print. [CrossRef] [PubMed]
63. World Health Organization. *Diet, Nutrition and the Prevention of Chronic Diseases*; Report No. 916; World Health Organization: Geneva, Switzerland, 2002.
64. Lustig, R.H.; Schmidt, L.A.; Brindis, C.D. Public health: The toxic truth about sugar. *Nature* **2012**, *482*, 27–29. [CrossRef] [PubMed]
65. Johnson, R.J.; Segal, M.S.; Sautin, Y.; Nakagawa, T.; Feig, D.I.; Kang, D.H.; Gersch, M.S.; Benner, S.; Sanchez-Lozada, L.G. Potential role of sugar (fructose) in the epidemic of hypertension, obesity and the metabolic syndrome, diabetes, kidney disease, and cardiovascular disease. *Am. J. Clin. Nutr.* **2007**, *86*, 899–906. [PubMed]
66. Johnson, R.K.; Appel, L.J.; Brands, M.; Howard, B.V.; Lefevre, M.; Lustig, R.H.; Sacks, F.; Steffen, L.M.; Wylie-Rosett, J. Dietary sugars intake and cardiovascular health: A scientific statement from the American Heart Association. *Circulation* **2009**, *120*, 1011–1020. [CrossRef] [PubMed]
67. Malik, V.S.; Popkin, B.M.; Bray, G.A.; Despres, J.P.; Hu, F.B. Sugar-sweetened beverages, obesity, type 2 diabetes mellitus, and cardiovascular disease risk. *Circulation* **2010**, *121*, 1356–1364. [CrossRef] [PubMed]
68. Drewnowski, A.; Rehm, C.D.; Constant, F. Water and beverage consumption among adults in the United States: Cross-sectional study using data from NHANES 2005–2010. *BMC Public Health* **2013**, *13*, 1068. [CrossRef] [PubMed]
69. La Verde, M.; Mule, S.; Zappala, G.; Privitera, G.; Maugeri, G.; Pecora, F.; Marranzano, M. Higher adherence to the Mediterranean diet is inversely associated with having hypertension: Is low salt intake a mediating factor? *Int. J. Food Sci. Nutr.* **2018**, *69*, 235–244. [CrossRef] [PubMed]
70. Platania, A.; Zappala, G.; Mirabella, M.U.; Gullo, C.; Mellini, G.; Beneventano, G.; Maugeri, G.; Marranzano, M. Association between mediterranean diet adherence and dyslipidaemia in a cohort of adults living in the Mediterranean area. *Int. J. Food Sci. Nutr.* **2017**, 1–11. [CrossRef] [PubMed]
71. Zappala, G.; Buscemi, S.; Mule, S.; La Verde, M.; D'Urso, M.; Corleo, D.; Marranzano, M. High adherence to Mediterranean diet, but not individual foods or nutrients, is associated with lower likelihood of being obese in a Mediterranean cohort. *Eat. Weight Disord.* **2017**. [CrossRef] [PubMed]

14

Extraction of Antioxidant Phenolic Compounds from Brewer's Spent Grain: Optimization and Kinetics Modeling

Ramiro A. Carciochi [1,2,*], Carlos A. Sologubik [1], María B. Fernández [1,3], Guillermo D. Manrique [1] and Leandro Galván D'Alessandro [2]

1 Faculty of Engineering, Universidad Nacional del Centro de la Provincia de Buenos Aires, Av. del Valle 5737, Olavarría 7400, Argentina; csologubik@gmail.com (C.A.S.); mbfernan@fio.unicen.edu.ar (M.B.F.); gmanrique@fio.unicen.edu.ar (G.D.M.)
2 ISA, Univ. Lille 1, INRA, Univ. Artois, Univ. Littoral Côte d'Opale, EA 7394-ICV-Institut Charles Viollette, 48 Boulevard Vauban, F-59000 Lille, France; leandro.galvan@yncrea.fr
3 Centro de Investigación en Física e Ingeniería del Centro de la Provincia de Buenos Aires-CIFICEN (UNCPBA-CICPBA-CONICET), Tandil 7000, Argentina
* Correspondence: ramiro.carciochi@polytech-lille.fr

Abstract: The kinetics of polyphenol extraction from brewer's spent grain (BSG), using a batch system, ultrasound assistance, and microwave assistance and the evolution of antioxidant capacity of these extracts over time, were studied. The main parameters of extraction employed in the batch system were evaluated, and, by applying response surface analysis, the following optimal conditions were obtained: Liquid/solid ratio of 30:1 mL/g at 80 °C, using 72% (*v*/*v*) ethanol:water as the solvent system. Under these optimized conditions, ultrasound assistance demonstrated the highest extraction rate and equilibrium yield, as well as shortest extraction times, followed by microwave assistance. Among the mathematical models used, Patricelli's model proved the most suitable for describing the extraction kinetics for each method tested, and is therefore able to predict the response values and estimate the extraction rates and potential maximum yields in each case.

Keywords: brewer's spent grain; extraction; polyphenols; optimization; modeling

---

1. Introduction

Brewer's spent grain (BSG) is the solid fraction that remains following wort production, which is the first step of the brewing process. BSG is the main by-product from breweries, representing about 20 kg per hectoliter of beer produced [1]. In addition, this source is rich in oligo- and polysaccharides, as well as in polyphenols, which are widely recognized as having antioxidant and antiradical properties [2]. Since it is mainly used as animal feed or fertilizer, BSG can be considered a valuable and underexploited source of bioactive compounds, with potential application in the cosmetic, pharmaceutical and food industries [3].

Extraction is the initial and most important step in the recovery and purification of bioactive compounds from plant materials. Many factors such as solvent composition, extraction temperature and solvent-to-solid ratio, may significantly influence the extraction efficiency, antioxidant activity and phenolic content. Hence, it is necessary to optimize the extraction conditions to improve phenolic recovery and antioxidant activity. The traditional method of optimization (OVAT, one variable at a time) is laborious and time-consuming, since only a single factor at a time is taken into consideration. In this method, the interactions among factors are ignored, hence the chances of obtaining the true optimum conditions are dubious [4]. To overcome this difficulty, a statistical optimization procedure in the form of response surface methodology (RSM) is used.

The conventional solid-liquid extraction method is made in a batch system (BE), however some assistance from emerging technologies, such as ultrasound (UAE) and microwave (MAE), may be conveniently applied during extraction due to their simple, effective and inexpensive natures. In addition, these green methodologies increase extraction yields and decrease extraction times. In order to evaluate the effect of each one of these methods on extraction, a comparison of the kinetics of the processes under the same operational conditions should be performed. Mathematical modeling is a useful tool that facilitates the design, optimization and control of the studied process. In solid–liquid extraction of bioactive substances from plant materials, several theoretical, empirical and semi-empirical models have been successfully employed [5–7].

The objective of this work was to study the effects of different extraction methods on the extraction kinetics of phenolic compounds from BSG. The first aim was to optimize the operational extraction conditions of such compounds in a batch system to subsequently evaluate the UAE and MAE processes under optimized conditions. Finally, several mathematical models were tested in order to select one that can be used to accurately describe the extraction process.

2. Materials and Methods

2.1. Materials

Brewer's spent grain from pale barley malt (Pilsen type) was supplied by a local microbrewery in Buenos Aires (Argentina). Folin–Ciocalteau reagent, 2,2-diphenyl-1-picrylhydrazyl (DPPH), and gallic acid were supplied by Sigma-Aldrich Chemical Co. (St. Louis, MO, USA). All other chemicals and reagents were of analytical grade.

2.2. Methods

2.2.1. Optimization of Polyphenols Extraction in Batch System

Batch extraction optimization was performed using a central composite face-centered design by varying the following extraction parameters: temperature of extraction (X1; 40, 60 and 80 (°C)), ethanol content (X2; 60, 70 and 80 (%, *v*/*v*)), and liquid/solid (L/S) ratio (X3; 10:1, 20:1 and 30:1 (mL/g)). These conditions and a fixed extraction time (60 min) were selected as a result of preliminary experiments evaluating one factor-at-a-time approach (data not shown). The experimental design conditions are shown in Table 1. Total phenolic compounds (TPC) and DPPH radical scavenging were determined as response variables of the experimental design. For each response, a quadratic equation model was obtained. Regression analysis was conducted, and the response surfaces were plotted using Statgraphics Centurion XVI (version 16.1.18; StatPoint Technologies Inc., Warrenton, VA, USA). The fit of the models to the experimental data was given by the coefficient of determination (R^2). In addition, each model was validated by calculating the value of the lack of fit test, in which a *p*-value higher than 0.05 indicates that the model was adequate to predict the response values [8].

Prior to extraction, BSG was oven-dried at 60 °C for 24 h and subsequently milled and sieved to obtain particle size less than 0.5 mm. Then, according to each run (Table 1), the BSG powder sample (3, 4.5, or 9 g) was suspended in the specific solvent media (60, 70, or 80% ethanol in water (*v*/*v*); 90 mL final volume) and then submitted to different extraction conditions for 60 min in a batch system of 150 mL capacity with magnetic stirring (300 rpm) coupled to an external circulating water bath connected to a thermostat. Afterwards, samples were centrifuged at 10,677 g for 10 min (Sorvall Legend X1, Thermo Scientific, Waltham, MA, USA) and the supernatant was carefully removed for further analyses.

Table 1. Experimental design of three tested variables with the observed responses values for total phenolic content (TPC) and DPPH radical scavenging.

Run	Temperature (°C; X1)	Ethanol Concentration (%; *v*/*v*; X2)	Liquid/Solid Ratio (mL/g; X3)	TPC (mg GAE/g DW)	DPPH Inhibition (%)
1	40 (−1)	60 (−1)	10:1 (−1)	2.15	1.86
2	80 (+1)	60 (−1)	10:1 (−1)	2.33	2.23
3	40 (−1)	80 (+1)	10:1 (−1)	1.59	3.17
4	80 (+1)	80 (+1)	10:1 (−1)	2.34	5.68
5	40 (−1)	60 (−1)	30:1 (+1)	2.67	8.40
6	80 (+1)	60 (−1)	30:1 (+1)	3.57	10.99
7	40 (−1)	80 (+1)	30:1 (+1)	2.02	7.40
8	80 (+1)	80 (+1)	30:1 (+1)	3.16	11.93
9	40 (−1)	70 (0)	20:1 (0)	2.41	6.50
10	80 (+1)	70 (0)	20:1 (0)	3.19	7.59
11	60 (0)	60 (−1)	20:1 (0)	2.85	5.70
12	60 (0)	80 (+1)	20:1 (0)	2.28	7.85
13	60 (0)	70 (0)	10:1 (−1)	2.59	2.61
14	60 (0)	70 (0)	30:1 (+1)	3.07	9.87
15	60 (0)	70 (0)	20:1 (0)	2.74	7.11
16	60 (0)	70 (0)	20:1 (0)	2.89	6.95
17	60 (0)	70 (0)	20:1 (0)	2.83	6.56
18	60 (0)	70 (0)	20:1 (0)	2.89	6.56

2.2.2. Ultrasound and Microwave Assisted Extraction Methods

Under optimal conditions found for BE, extraction kinetics were performed for all three tested methods, taking samples at regular time intervals until 120 min, which were then centrifuged under the above mentioned conditions. Sonication in UAE was applied using an ultrasound probe (VCX500, Sonics & Materials Inc., Newtown, CT, USA) operating in continuous mode at a wave amplitude of 50%, frequency of 20 KHz and ultrasound power of 45 W. MAE was performed in an open-system microwave oven (MPD8520 model, Philco, Ushuaia, Argentina) operating in continuous mode at a frequency of 2.45 GHz and 800 W of microwave power. To avoid solvent loss, a reflux system was connected to the extraction flask.

2.2.3. Total Phenolic Content (TPC) and Antioxidant Capacity Determination

TPC assay in extracts was performed using Folin Ciocalteau reagent under the same conditions described in a previous work [9]. Briefly, 0.1 mL extracts were mixed with 0.1 mL of 2 N Folin–Ciocalteau reagent and 0.3 mL of 20% sodium carbonate solution. The volume of the mixture was adjusted to 2 mL with distilled water and incubated in the dark for 2 h. Subsequently, the absorbance of the samples was measured spectrophotometrically at 765 nm. Results were expressed as gallic acid equivalents (GAE) in mg per g of BSG on a dry weight (DW) basis.

Antioxidant capacity was determined by measuring the ability of the extracts to scavenge the free radical 2,2-diphenyl-1-picrylhydrazyl (DPPH). For the reactions, 50 μL of each extract was added to 1950 μL of DPPH solution (60 μM prepared in methanol) and allowed to stand for 30 min in darkness at room temperature before measuring the absorbance at 517 nm. Results were expressed as a percentage of radical scavenging, as previously described by Meneses [10].

2.2.4. Modeling of Kinetics Profile and Statistical Analysis

The extraction kinetics curves obtained for TPC and DPPH assays for each of the extraction methods tested (BE, UAE and MAE) were fitted to three equations, with the aim of finding the most appropriate model for the experimental data. These have been successfully applied to model the kinetics of polyphenol extraction and extensively cited in the bibliography, such as Peleg, Page, and Patricelli (Equations (1)–(3), Table 2). The fitting process was carried out using Statgraphics Centurion XVI (version 16.1.18; StatPoint Technologies Inc., Warrenton, VA, USA) by a nonlinear, least squares regression method. The concordance between the experimental data and calculated value was established by the coefficient of determination (R^2), adjusted coefficient of determination (adj R^2), root mean squared error (RMSE), and percentage average absolute relative deviation (%AARD), according to Equations (4)–(7), shown in Table 3.

Table 2. Equations of mathematical models employed.

Name	Model	Equation
Peleg	$C(t) = \frac{t}{k_1 + k_2 \times t}$	(1)
Page	$C(t) = \exp\left(-k_1 \times t^{k_2}\right)$	(2)
Patricelli	$C(t) = C_1(1 - \exp(-k_1 \times t)) + C_2(1 - \exp(-k_2 \times t))$	(3)

$C(t)$ is the concentration of polyphenols (mg GAE/g DW) at t time (min); k_1, and k_2 are constants; C_1 and C_2 are the yields at equilibrium for washing and diffusion steps, respectively.

Table 3. Equations of statistical parameters employed.

Statistical Parameters	Equation
$R^2 = 1 - \frac{\sum_{i=1}^{n}(Y_i - \hat{Y}_i)^2}{\sum_{i=1}^{n}(Y_i - \overline{Y})^2}$	(4)
$adjR^2 = 1 - (1 - R^2)\frac{n-1}{n-m}$	(5)
$RMSE = \sqrt{\frac{\sum_{i=1}^{n}(Y_i - \hat{Y}_i)^2}{n-m}}$	(6)
$\%AARD = \frac{100}{n}\sum_{i}^{n}\frac{\lvert Y_i - \hat{Y}_i \rvert}{Y_i}$	(7)

Y_i and $\hat{Y}_i$ are the experimental and calculated values of yield, respectively; $\overline{Y}$ is the arithmetic average value of the experimental points; n is the number of the experimental points; m is the number of parameters of the regression model.

3. Results and Discussion

3.1. Extraction Optimization in Batch System

The effects of three independent variables on the yields of TPC and DPPH radical scavenging values of extracts are shown in Table 1. Phenolic compounds extracted from BSG ranged from 1.59 to 3.57 mg GAE/g, whereas antioxidant activity varied between 1.86 and 11.93% of DPPH radical inhibition. These values are comparable to those reported by other authors [10,11], whose results ranged from 1.26 to 7.13 mg GAE/g DW and 12.02 to 16.91% inhibition, for TPC and DPPH assays, respectively. A value of 20 mg GAE/g DW for TPC assay was reported by Moreira [1] using an optimized microwave-assisted method under alkaline conditions, thus showing an advantage of these novel extraction techniques compared to conventional ones.

For each response, regression equations evaluating the effects of each factor and their interactions were obtained. After subsequent statistical analysis by the ANOVA test (Table 4), the predictive fitted equation models and significant terms ($p > 0.05$) were obtained (Table 5).

The corresponding coefficients of determination (R^2) of the models were 0.9701, and 0.9864 for TPC and antioxidant activity, respectively. These values showed that more than 97.01% of the total variation in the response was explained by the models. Additionally, the very low p-values (<0.0001) in each evaluated response indicated the significance of the model terms. In addition, the non-significant value of lack of fit ($p > 0.05$) showed that the models could be used to predict the results. Finally, response surface plots were established using the fitted models in order to determine the optimal levels of the evaluated variables on extraction of phenolic compounds and antioxidant activity.

Table 4. Analysis of variance (ANOVA) for the fitted quadratic polynomial model for optimization of extraction parameters.

Source	TPC (R^2 = 0.9701)					DPPH (R^2 = 0.9864)				
	DF	SS	MS	F-Value	p-Value	DF	SS	MS	F-Value	p-Value
Model	6	3.83	0.64	59.49	<0.0001	7	134.34	19.19	103.33	<0.0001
Lack of Fit	8	0.10	0.01	2.62	0.2300	7	1.62	0.23	2.90	0.2056
Pure Error	3	0.015	0.005			3	0.239	0.080		

DF, degree of freedom; SS, sum of squares; MS, mean square.

Table 5. Predictive model equations of the experimental response variables.

Response	Polynomial Equation	
TPC (mg GAE/g DW)	$y = 2.83 + 0.38X_1 - 0.22X_2 + 0.35X_3 + 0.10X_1X_2 + 0.14X_1X_3 - 0.33X_2^2$	(8)
DPPH radical scavenging (%)	$y = 6.85 + 1.11X_1 + 0.69X_2 + 3.30X_3 + 0.51X_1X_2 + 0.53X_1X_3 - 0.60X_2X_3 - 0.44X_3^2$	(9)

3.2. Effect of Extraction Conditions on TPC Yield

Figure 1 presents the response surface plots for the influence of extraction parameters on TPC yield. An increased extraction yield was observed when the liquid/solid (L/S) ratio increased from 10:1 to 30:1 mL/g (Figure 1A). This is concordant with mass transfer principles, since a higher L/S ratio implies higher concentration gradient between the solid and the bulk of the liquid, resulting in a greater driving force for diffusion of compounds to the solvent. This effect was further improved by increasing extraction temperature from 40 to 80 °C (Figure 1B), showing a considerable positive interaction between these variables. It is true that greater temperatures generally improve the solubility and diffusivity of compounds, thus increasing the mass transfer between the plant matrix and bulk solvent [5]. Regarding the effect of solvent composition, TPC yield slightly increased with an increase in ethanol concentration from 60% to about 68%, whilst ethanol concentrations greater than this led to a gradual decrease in TPC yields (Figure 1C). This could be explained by different ethanol:water ratios modifying the polarity of the solvent system, thereby altering the solubility of different phenolic compounds and consequently determining which will be extracted [12]. Thus, the conditions that maximized Equation (8) (Table 5) in a BE process were: a 30:1 mL/g liquid/solid ratio, a temperature of 80 °C, and an ethanol concentration of 66.7% in the solvent system.

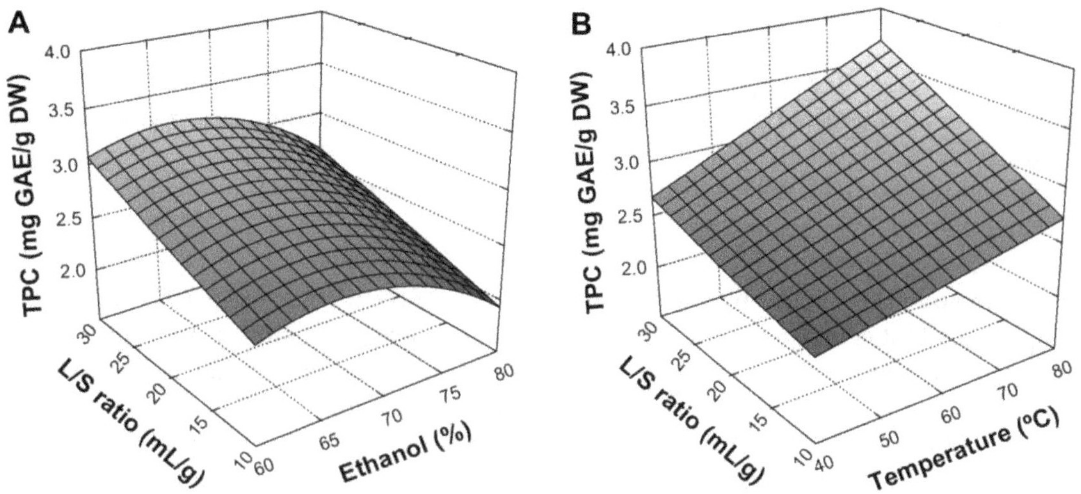

Figure 1. *Cont.*

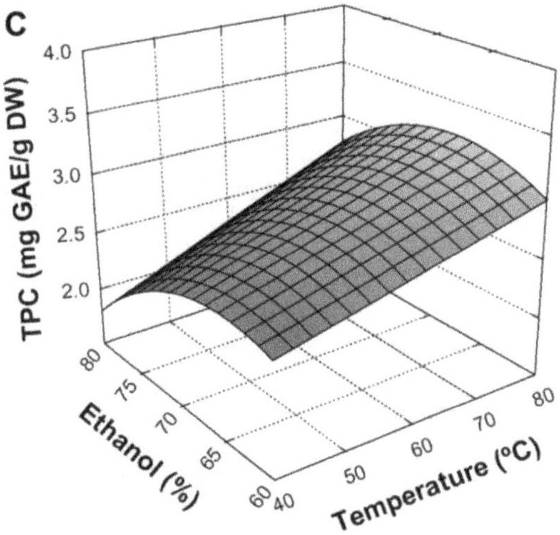

Figure 1. Response surface plots showing the effects of ethanol concentration and liquid/solid ratio (**A**), extraction temperature and liquid/solid ratio (**B**), and extraction temperature and ethanol concentration (**C**) on the extraction yield of TPC in BSG extracts. The missed variable in each graph was kept at the centre point.

3.3. Effect of Extraction Conditions on DPPH Radical Scavenging

According to Equation (9) (Table 5), the liquid/solid ratio was the variable that had the greatest effect ($p < 0.05$) on DPPH radical scavenging of extracts. This was followed by temperature, which had a lesser impact. The influence of extraction parameters on DPPH radical scavenging is shown in Figure 2. Similarly to TPC, DPPH inhibition increased when the L/S ratio increased from 10:1 to 30:1 mL/g and temperature increased from 40 to 80 °C (Figure 2A,B, respectively). Furthermore, the interaction between these variables was significant ($p < 0.05$), with positive effects on DPPH radical scavenging (Figure 2B). Regarding the solvent effect, Figure 2C shows that an increase in ethanol concentration from 60 to 80% produced a positive, linear effect on antioxidant activity. Similarly, the interaction between the solvent system and temperature also produced a positive and statistically-significant ($p < 0.05$) effect. According to these results, maximum DPPH radical scavenging in BE was be achieved under the following conditions: an L/S ratio of 30:1 mL/g at 80 °C, using 80% ethanol as a solvent system.

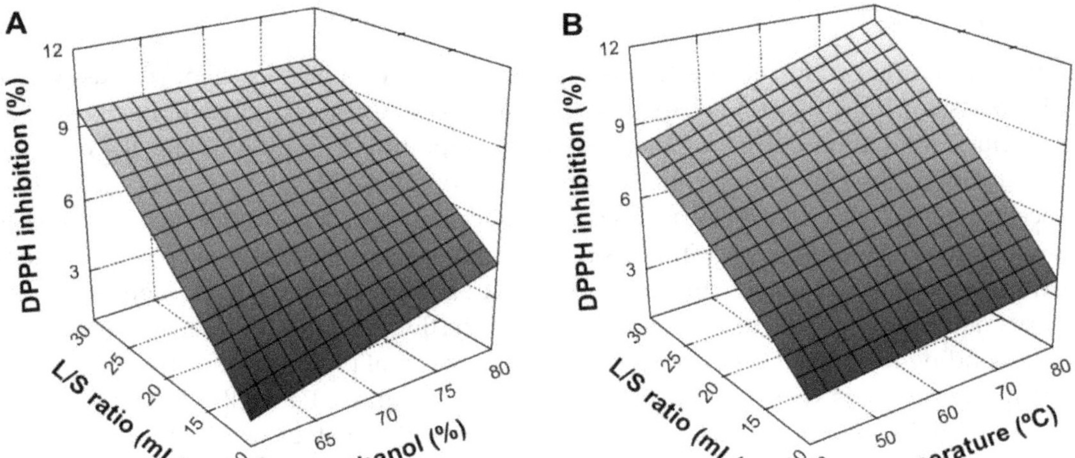

Figure 2. *Cont.*

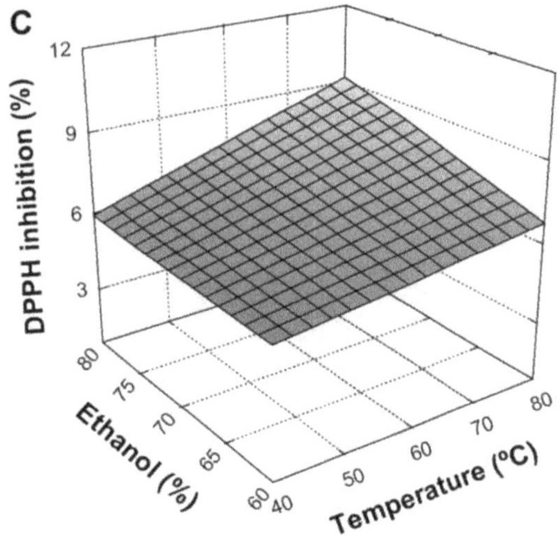

Figure 2. Response surface plots showing the effects of ethanol concentration and liquid/solid ratio (**A**), extraction temperature and liquid/solid ratio (**B**), and extraction temperature and ethanol concentration (**C**) on DPPH inhibition (%) of BSG extracts. The missed variable in each graph was kept at the center point.

3.4. Optimization of the Extraction Conditions

To optimize the process with two or more output responses, a multiresponse analysis was carried out using the desirability function in the chosen statistical software. The target was to obtain a BSG extract with a high content of phenolic compounds and antioxidant activity. Thus, through maximizing both responses, optimum extraction conditions were obtained: L/S ratio of 30:1 mL/g, 80 °C, and 72% ethanol concentration. Experimental verification of these conditions was performed in quintuplicate, obtaining values of 3.57 ± 0.08 mg GAE/g and 11.55 ± 0.08% DPPH inhibition, for TPC and DPPH assay, respectively. These values confirm the predicted values (3.59 mg GAE/g and 11.55% DPPH radical scavenging) within a 95% confidence level. Hence, under the aforementioned conditions, a BSG extract rich in antioxidant phenolic compounds was obtained.

3.5. Extraction Kinetics Study

Extraction under optimized conditions was performed for a batch system (BE) as well as for assisted processes using ultrasound (UAE) and microwaves (MAE), in order to determine the influence of each extraction method on the yield of phenolic compounds (Figure 3A), and the evolution of extract antioxidant capacity versus time (Figure 3B). Both figures showed a clear, positive effect of assistance techniques, however this was more pronounced for ultrasound assistance than microwave assistance. The mean comparison by Tukey's test showed significant differences ($p < 0.05$) among the three extraction techniques from 10 to 50 min of extraction for TPC yields. In addition, the kinetics of each extraction method for both responses were fitted to the three equation models presented in Table 2. The corresponding results of nonlinear regression and statistical parameters for BA, UAE and MAE fitted by all three models are shown in Table 6. For both responses, Patricelli's model was the most accurate fit, with the highest coefficient of determination and adjusted coefficient of determination, and the lowest root mean squared error (RMSE) and percentage average absolute relative deviation (%AARD), compared to Peleg and Page models.

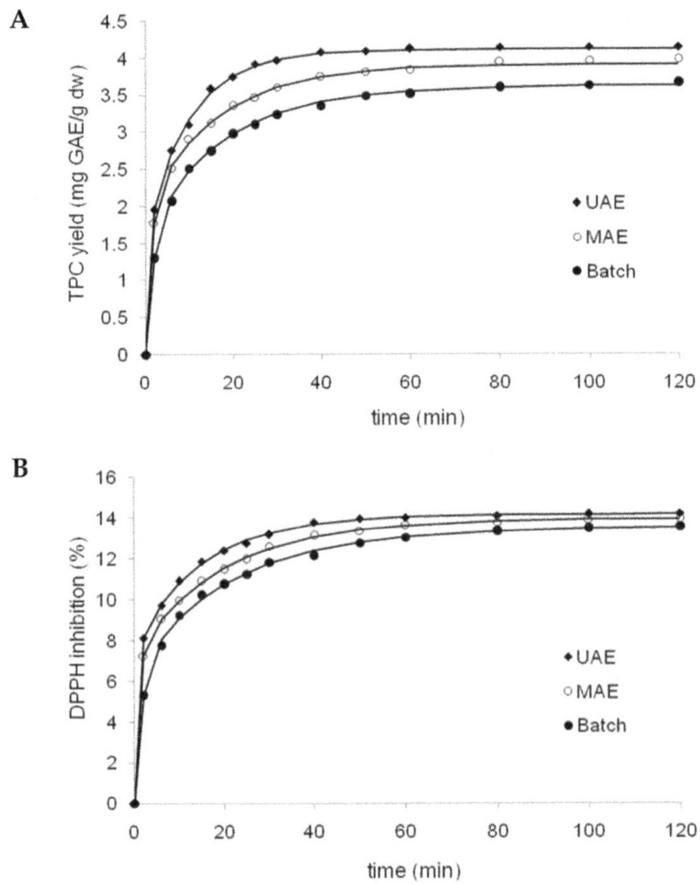

Figure 3. Kinetics profiles of polyphenols extraction (**A**) and antioxidant activity (**B**) of extracts obtained by three tested methods (batch system, ultrasound and microwave assistance) from brewer's spent grain (BSG) fitted by patricelli's model. Symbols: Experimental data; lines: Model fitting curves.

The empirical model proposed by Patricelli [13] involves two simultaneous processes with different kinetics coefficients: a washing stage and a diffusion stage (Equation (3), Table 2). The total amount of extracted solute (equilibrium yield) is equal to the sum of the amounts extracted during both stages. An estimate of the initial extraction rate is given by the first derivative of the equation when $t = 0$ [14]. Thus, according to Patricelli's model, the equilibrium yields of TPC are 4.11, 3.91, and 3.62 mg GAE/g for UAE, MAE and BE, respectively. These results showed that UAE and MAE significantly increased polyphenol extraction relative to BE, with increases of 13% and 8% for equilibrium conditions, respectively. Additionally, polyphenol extraction was faster using UAE and MAE, according to higher extraction rates (2.42 and 1.66 mg/g/min, respectively) in comparison to BE (0.98 mg/g/min). The observed increase in polyphenol extraction could be due to mechanical effects induced on BSG cell walls, produced during the collapse of the cavitation bubbles (shockwave-induced damage and microjet impact on the surface of the solid material), in relation to MAE where the extraction principle is based on the synergistic combination of heat and mass transfers working from the inside to the outside of the solid sample (in contrast to conventional extraction, in which both transport phenomena occur in different directions) [15,16].

According to transfer coefficients calculated for Patricelli's model (Table 6), the coefficients of the washing stage (k1) for both responses (TPC and DPPH radical scavenging) were much greater than those of the diffusion stage (k2) for all extraction methods tested. As can be seen in Figure 3A,B, all extraction methods showed a quick extraction rate at the outset which was subsequently reduced. This is explained well by Patricelli's model, since the washing stage allows for quick dissolution of the target components located both at the surface and within broken matrix cells. On the other hand, the diffusion stage is slower due to mass transfer limitations, where the remaining active compounds diffuse from the interior of intact cells into the solvent [5,14]. In addition, a comparison of k values among three methods (Table 6) evidenced greater coefficients for assisted methods relative to BE, mainly in relation to the washing stage. Thus, the assistance of microwaves and especially ultrasound greatly accelerated the washing phase of extraction.

Table 6. Coefficients and statistical parameters of extraction modelling for all models ($p < 0.05$).

Response Variable	Model	Extraction Method	Coefficient				Statistical Parameter			
			K1	K2	C1	C2	RMSE	R^2	adjR^2	%AARD
TPC	Peleg	BE	1.28	0.27	-	-	0.168	0.939	0.936	2.389
		UAE	0.68	0.23	-	-	0.298	0.825	0.817	7.520
		MAE	0.84	0.25	-	-	0.193	0.919	0.916	3.147
	Page	BE	−0.62	0.17	-	-	0.330	0.796	0.788	9.216
		UAE	−0.90	0.11	-	-	0.310	0.808	0.800	8.120
		MAE	−0.78	0.13	-	-	0.278	0.836	0.829	6.539
	Patricelli	BE	0.53	0.06	1.64	1.98	0.115	0.968	0.967	0.915
		UAE	1.34	0.10	1.63	2.48	0.100	0.954	0.952	0.689
		MAE	0.79	0.06	1.95	1.96	0.105	0.970	0.968	0.770
DPPH	Peleg	BE	0.33	0.07	-	-	0.210	0.993	0.993	3.718
		UAE	0.15	0.07	-	-	0.221	0.988	0.987	4.131
		MAE	0.20	0.07	-	-	0.243	0.988	0.987	5.017
	Page	BE	−1.85	0.08	-	-	0.275	0.988	0.987	6.411
		UAE	−2.13	0.05	-	-	0.226	0.987	0.987	4.323
		MAE	−2.01	0.06	-	-	0.218	0.990	0.989	4.029
	Patricelli	BE	0.61	0.05	6.56	6.93	0.125	0.997	0.996	1.076
		UAE	1.47	0.07	7.72	6.40	0.083	0.997	0.996	0.478
		MAE	1.15	0.05	7.34	6.56	0.070	0.996	0.996	0.342

4. Conclusions

In this study, optimal extraction conditions for antioxidant polyphenols from BSG in a batch system were obtained using an L/S ratio of 30:1 mL/g, temperature of 80 °C, and 72% ethanol concentration solvent system. Under these experimental conditions, it was clearly shown that ultrasound and, to a lesser extent, microwave assistance increased the extraction rate, equilibrium yield and decreased extraction time. Of the mathematical models describing extraction kinetics tested, Patricelli's model proved the highest quality fit and was the most suitable for simulating the extraction methods tested. The results of this work could contribute to the optimization and simulation of green extraction process for valorization of agri-food wastes.

Acknowledgments: Authors would like to thank to CONICET (Argentina) for providing financial support to this project (Postdoctoral fellowship granted to Carciochi).

Author Contributions: Ramiro A. Carciochi, Carlos A. Sologubik and Leandro Galván D'Alessandro conceived, designed and performed the experiments. María B. Fernández and Guillermo D. Manrique participated in the analysis of the data and contributed intellectually to the manuscript.

Conflicts of Interest: The authors declare no conflict of interest.

References

1. Moreira, M.M.; Morais, S.; Carvalho, D.O.; Barros, A.A.; Delerue-Matos, C.; Guido, L.F. Brewer's spent grain from different types of malt: Evaluation of the antioxidant activity and identification of the major phenolic compounds. *Food Res. Int.* **2013**, *54*, 382–388. [CrossRef]
2. Mussato, S.I. Biotechnological potential of brewing industry by-products. In *Biotechnology for Agro-Industrial Residues Utilisation*, 1st ed.; Singh-Nee Nigam, P., Pandey, A., Eds.; Springer: Dordrecht, The Netherlands, 2009; pp. 313–326. ISBN 978-1-4020-9941-0.
3. Guo, M.; Du, J.; Zhang, Z.; Zhang, K.; Jin, Y. Optimization of brewer's spent grain-enriched biscuits processing formula. *J. Food Process Eng.* **2014**, *37*, 122–130. [CrossRef]

4. Liyana-Pathirana, C.; Shahidi, F. Optimization of extraction of phenolic compounds from wheat using response surface methodology. *Food Chem.* **2005**, *93*, 47–56. [CrossRef]
5. Chan, C.-H.; Yusoff, R.; Ngoh, G.-C. Modeling and kinetics study of conventional and assisted batch solvent extraction. *Chem. Eng. Res. Des.* **2014**, *92*, 1169–1186. [CrossRef]
6. Xi, J.; He, L.; Yan, L. Kinetic modeling of pressure-assisted solvent extraction of polyphenols from green tea in comparison with the conventional extraction. *Food Chem.* **2015**, *166*, 287–291. [CrossRef] [PubMed]
7. Tušek, A.J.; Benković, M.; Cvitanović, A.B.; Valinger, D.; Jurina, T.; Kljusurić, J.G. Kinetics and thermodynamics of the solid-liquid extraction process of total polyphenols, antioxidants and extraction yield from *Asteraceae* plants. *Ind. Crops Prod.* **2016**, *91*, 205–214. [CrossRef]
8. Carciochi, R.A.; Manrique, G.D.; Dimitrov, K. Optimization of antioxidant phenolic compounds extraction from quinoa (*Chenopodium quinoa*) seeds. *J. Food Sci. Technol.* **2015**, *52*, 4396–4404. [CrossRef] [PubMed]
9. Carciochi, R.A.; D'Alessandro, L.G.; Manrique, G.D. Effect of roasting conditions on the antioxidant compounds of quinoa seeds. *Int. J. Food Sci. Technol.* **2016**, *51*, 1018–1025. [CrossRef]
10. Meneses, N.G.T.; Martins, S.; Teixeira, J.A.; Mussatto, S.I. Influence of extraction solvents on the recovery of antioxidant phenolic compounds from brewer's spent grains. *Sep. Purif. Technol.* **2013**, *108*, 152–158. [CrossRef]
11. McCarthy, A.L.; O'Callaghan, Y.C.; Neugart, S.; Piggott, C.O.; Connolly, A.; Jansen, M.A.K.; Krumbein, A.; Schreiner, M.; Fitzgerald, R.J.; O'Brien, N.M. The hydroxycinnamic acid content of barley and brewers' spent grain (BSG) and the potential to incorporate phenolic extracts of BSG as antioxidants into fruit beverages. *Food Chem.* **2013**, *141*, 2567–2574. [CrossRef] [PubMed]
12. D'Alessandro, L.G.; Kriaa, K.; Nikov, I.; Dimitrov, K. Ultrasound assisted extraction of polyphenols from black chokeberry. *Sep. Purif. Technol.* **2012**, *93*, 42–47. [CrossRef]
13. Patricelli, A.; Assogna, A.; Casalaina, A.; Emmi, E.; Sodini, G. Fattori che influenzano l'estrazione dei lipidi da semi decorticati di girasole. *Riv. Ital. Sostanze Grasse* **1979**, *56*, 136–142.
14. Mustapa, A.N.; Martin, A.; Gallego, J.R.; Mato, R.B.; Cocero, M.J. Microwave-assisted extraction of polyphenols from *Clinacanthus nutans* Lindau medicinal plant: Energy perspective and kinetics modeling. *Chem. Eng. Process.* **2015**, *97*, 66–74. [CrossRef]
15. Chemat, F.; Huma, Z.; Khan, M.K. Applications of ultrasound in food technology: Processing, preservation and extraction. *Ultrason. Sonochem.* **2011**, *18*, 813–835. [CrossRef] [PubMed]
16. Veggi, P.C.; Martinez, J.; Meireles, M.A.A. Fundamentals of microwave extraction. In *Microwave-Assisted Extraction for Bioactive Compounds: Theory and Practice*, 1st ed.; Chemat, F., Cravotto, G., Eds.; Springer: New York, NY, USA, 2013; pp. 15–52. ISBN 978-1-4899-7361-0.

15

The Extract of *D. dasycarpus* Ameliorates Oxazolone-Induced Skin Damage in Mice by Anti-Inflammatory and Antioxidant Mechanisms

Tsong-Min Chang [1], Ting-Ya Yang [2], Yu-Lin Niu [3] and Huey-Chun Huang [2,*]

[1] Department of Applied Cosmetology and Master Program of Cosmetic Sciences, Hungkuang University, Taichung 43302, Taiwan; ctm@sunrise.hk.edu.tw
[2] Department of Medical Laboratory Science and Biotechnology, College of Medicine, China Medical University, No. 91 Hsueh-Shih Road, Taichung 40402, Taiwan; tyyang@mail.cmu.edu.tw
[3] Niuer International Skincare Science Research Institute, 9F, No. 266, Ruiguang Rd., Neihu Dist., Taipei 11491, Taiwan; niuer80@gmail.com
* Correspondence: lchuang@mail.cmu.edu.tw

Abstract: *Dictamni dasycarpus* is a type of Chinese medicine made from the root bark of *D. dasycarpus*. It has been reported to show a wide spectrum of biological and pharmacological effects, for example, it has been used widely for the treatment of rheumatism, nettle rash, itching, jaundice, chronic hepatitis and skin diseases. In the current study, *D. dasycarpus* extract was investigated for its antioxidant and anti-inflammatory effects, as well as its capability to alleviate oxazolone-induced skin damage in mice. The possible anti-inflammatory mechanism of *D. dasycarpus* extract against oxidative challenge was elucidated by measuring the levels of reactive oxygen species (ROS) production, interleukin-6, Tumor necrosis factor-α, NLRP3 (NACHT, LRR and PYD domains-containing protein 3 (NALP3)) inflammasome and interleukin-1β in HaCaT cells. *D. dasycarpus* extract did not affect cell viability in basal conditions. The extract significantly reduced oxazolone-induced epidermal swelling compared to untreated animal in the hairless albino mice (ICR mice) model. At the molecular level, Western blot assays indicated that the *D. dasycarpus* extract attenuated oxazolone-induced activation of apoptosis-associated speck-like protein containing CARD (ASC), procaspase-1, NF-κB and mitogen-activated protein kinase (MAPKs) such as c-Jun N-terminal protein kinase (JNK) and p38. This study demonstrates that *D. dasycarpus* extract could protect skin cells against oxidative and inflammatory insult by modulating the intracellular levels of ROS, TNF-α, interleukin-1, interleukin-6, NLR family pyrin domain containing 3 (NLRP3) inflammasome generation, antioxidant enzyme activity and cell signaling pathways. *D. dasycarpus* extract also attenuated the expression of NF-κB in HaCaT keratinocytes and thereby effectively downregulated inflammatory responses in the skin. Furthermore, *D. dasycarpus* extract alleviated oxazolone-induced damage in mice. Our results suggest the potential application of *D. dasycarpus* extract in preventing inflammatory processes in dermatitis.

Keywords: *D. dasycarpus*; ROS; interleukin-1β; interleukin-6; tumor necrosis factor-α; NF-κB; inflammasome

---

1. Introduction

Traditional Chinese medicine (TCM) therapy used in Taiwan has been enrolled in the National Health Insurance Research Database since 2002 [1,2]. Herbal formulas and single herbs, such as Fang-Feng (*Saposhnikovia divaricate*) and Bai-Xian-Pi (*Dictamni dasycarpus; D. dasycarpus*), were prescribed for treating dermatitis [3]. *D. dasycarpus* has been found to possess many interesting pharmacological and physiological activities in the treatment of skin diseases in clinic, although it lacks the mechanistic evidence [4,5]. Phytochemicals such as polyphenols or flavonoids are the most abundant naturally occurring anti-inflammation compounds and have anti-oxidative properties [6,7]. In this study, we studied the protective mechanisms of *D. dasycarpus* against inflamed dermatitis.

The hapten oxazolone-induced dermatitis in mice has been developed as the model for experimental atopic dermatitis or contact dermatitis. Repeated oxazolone applications provoke a pruritic dermatosis with epidermal hyperplasia, erythematous and edematous dermatosis [8,9]. The T cells in the skin tissue sensitize and elicit a hypersensitive inflammation reaction [10], whereas skin keratinocytes provide pro-inflammatory cytokines to initiate and maintain the T cell-mediated immune responses in inflammatory lesions [11,12]. To go through various stages is very important for epidermal keratinocytes to induce adaptive immunity, antigen presentation, keratinocyte activation, and the expression of adhesion molecules. In addition, keratinocytes also act as a potent source of cytokines and chemokines, which result in a particular dialogue between keratinocytes and activated immune cells [13]. In addition, the keratinocytes act as innate immune sensors that synergistically induce of additional inflammation [14,15]. Inflammasomes are multiprotein complexes that assemble in the cytosol after exposure to pathogen-associated molecular patterns (PAMPs) or danger-associated molecular patterns (DAMPs) and result in the activation of caspase-1 and subsequent cleavage of pro-inflammatory cytokines interleukin (IL)-1β and IL-18 [16]. The dysregulated inflammasome activity is associated with numerous skin inflammatory syndromes and skin cancer predisposition [17]. Therefore, attenuating inflammasome activation may provide a valuable therapeutic strategy in treating various inflammation-related disorders [18].

The goal of this study was to investigate the effect of *D. dasycarpus* extract on inflammatory mediators and cellular signaling pathways in oxazolone-challenged mice and HaCaT cells. The topical application of *D. dasycarpus* extract inhibited oxazolone-induced expression of inflammatory mediators. The activation of NF-κB signaling pathways was also investigated. Furthermore, we also elucidated the effect of *D. dasycarpus* extract on oxazolone-mediated NLRP3 activation.

2. Materials and Methods

2.1. Herb Extraction and Chemicals

The herbs were purchased from Sun Ten Pharmaceutical Co., Ltd. (New Taipei City, Taiwan). *Periostracum cicadae* (PC) and *D. dasycarpus* (DD) were extracted with 50% *v*/*v* ethanol as previously reported [19]. All dried extract was weighed and re-constituted in 0.1% dimethyl sulfoxide (DMSO) containing culture medium to 1 mg/mL. All other chemicals and solvents were obtained from Sigma-Aldrich Inc. (St. Louis, MO, USA).

2.2. Animals and Treatments

Mice experiments were conducted in accordance with the International Standards on Animal Welfare and in accordance with the ethical standards of the Laboratory Animal Service Center of China Medical University (Affidavit of Approval of Animal Use Protocol No. 2017-090). Repeated topical application of oxazolone over an extended period was used to induce allergic contact dermatitis in hairless male ICR mice (BioLASCO Taiwan Co., Ltd., Taipei, Taiwan). The mice were subdivided into groups based on their latest body weight (five mice in each group) using a stratified randomization method. Animals were sensitized once with 5% (*w*/*v*) 4-ethoxymethylene-2-phenyl-2-oxazolin-5-one (oxazolone) and dissolved 3:1 in acetone and olive oil (150 μL) on the shaved back. After 3 days, the mice were challenged with 1% oxazolone every other day for 10 days. For the experimental group animals, 5 mg/kg of *P. cicadae* or *D. dasycarpus* was applied onto the mice backs at the day interval. On the other hand, the control group animals were treated with ethanol at the same day interval. All mice were sacrificed and sampled on day 24 [20,21].

2.3. Specimens and Immunohistochemistry

After the 24 days of treatment, pentobarbital was administered to all mice (200 mg/kg, IP), and 1 cm^2 skin tissues were then quickly removed. The skin samples were fixed in 4% buffered neutral formalin solution for 24 h at room temperature, and paraffin was embedded. Serial sections were floated in warm water containing 2% gelatin to prevent peeling off of the sample. The sections were deparaffinized, rehydrated, and stained with hematoxylin and eosin (H&E) for immunohistochemistry. Deparaffinization, re-hydration and, quenching of endogenous peroxidase of the 5 mm paraffin cross-sections were evaluated by 30 min incubation in 0.3% H_2O_2 and incubation with 0.5 mg/mL of anti-cyclooxygenase (COX)-2, anti-CD3, anti-CD45 antibodies or control IgG overnight, followed by incubation with biotinylated secondary Abs and developed with the Vectastain Elite ABC kit (Vector) with 3,3-diaminobenzidine (DAB) as a substrate. Examination was done by light microscopy at 200× magnifications.

HaCaT cells were fixed with 4% paraformaldehyde in 250 mM Hepes, pH 7.4, freshly diluted from 16% stocks stored at −20 °C. After standing at room temperature for 5 min, the cells were washed with phosphate-buffered saline (PBS) and treated with blocking solution (PBST, 1% fetal bovine serum, FBS) at 4 °C for 1 h. Cells were incubated with an NLRP3 Ab in blocking solution at 4 °C overnight in a wet chamber. After washing in PBST, the cells were incubated with the appropriate secondary antibody mixtures in blocking solution for at least 1 h at room temperature. The cells were washed three times in PBS and mounted in gold antifade reagent with DAPI (Molecular Probes, Eugene, OR, USA). Confocal analysis was performed using a Leica TCS SP2 confocal microscope: 10 horizontal scans using a 63× (1.3 NA) oil immersion objective were recorded for each image with the imaging software (exported as a TIFF file).

2.4. Cell Culture

HaCaT cells were maintained in Dulbecco's Modified Eagle Medium (DMEM, HyClone; GE Healthcare Life Sciences, Marlborough, MA, USA) supplemented with 10% fetal bovine serum and 1% antibiotics at standard cell culture conditions (37 °C, 5% CO_2 in a humidified incubator).

2.5. Cytokines Measurement

Supernatant obtained from the HaCaT cell culture in the various treatment groups were analysed for interleukin IL-1β, IL-6, IL-8, tumor necrosis factor (TNF)-α with enzyme-linked immunosorbent assay (ELISA) kit (eBioscience, San Diego, CA, USA), according to the manufacturer's instructions.

2.6. Reactive Oxygen Species (ROS) Measurement

HaCaT cells were seeded in 96-well plates at a concentration of 1×10^5 cells/mL. Cells were treated with oxazolone (50 μM), subsequently washed twice with PBS and incubated with 20 μg/mL of *P. cicadae* or *D. Dasycarpus* for 24 h. After being treated with 10 μM 2,7-dichlorofluorescein diacetate (DCFH-DA; Sigma-Aldrich) in PBS for 30 min, the media was discarded, and the cells were washed twice with PBS. The ROS fluorescence were monitored by fluorescence microscopy (Olympus IX71). The mitochondrial ROS (mito ROS) were detected by the Mito SOX^{TM} Red Mitochondrial Superoxide Indicator (Invitrogen, Carlsbad, CA, USA) and monitored by fluorescence microscopy.

2.7. Western Blot Analysis

Cells were lysed in PBS containing 1% nonidet P-40, 0.5% sodium deoxycholate, 0.1% sodium dodecyl sulfate (SDS), 5 μg/mL aprotinin, 100 μg/mL phenylmethylsulfonyl fluoride, 1 μg/mL pepstatin A, and 1 mM ethylenediaminetetraacetic acid (EDTA) at 4 °C for 20 min. Total lysates were quantified using a microBCA kit (Thermo Fisher Scientific, Waltham, MA, USA). Proteins (10 μg) were resolved by SDS-polyacrylamide gel electrophoresis and electrophoretically transferred to a PVDF (poly(vinylidene fluoride)) membrane. The membrane was blocked in 5% fat-free milk in

PBST (PBS with 0.05% Tween-20), followed by incubation overnight with the following primary antibodies diluted in PBST: JNK Ab, p-JNK Ab, p38 Ab, p-P38 Ab, ASC Ab, procaspase-1 Ab (diluted to 1:1000, all from Santa Cruz Biotech (Dallas, TX, USA)), p65 Ab (Genetex, Taiwan) and NLRP3 Ab (Adipogen, San Diego, CA, USA). The primary antibodies were removed, and the membrane was washed extensively in PBST. Subsequent incubation with horseradish peroxidase-conjugated goat anti-rabbit antibodies (1:20,000, Santa Cruz Biotech) was performed at room temperature for 2 h. The membrane was washed extensively in PBST to remove any excess secondary antibodies, and the blot was visualized with enhanced chemiluminescence reagent (GE Healthcare, South Jakarta, Indonesia).

2.8. Statistical Analysis

Statistical analyses were carried out using Student's *t*-test (sigma plot 10.0. Systat Software, Inc., San Jose, CA, USA) * $p < 0.05$ was considered significant, ** $p < 0.01$, *** $p < 0.001$.

3. Results

Mouse dorsal skin was sensitized with 5% oxazolone on day 1 and challenged with 1% oxazolone for an additional week at 2-day intervals to develop the acute allergic contact dermatitis. Topical exposure to oxazolone induced a significant skin swelling response and inflammation erythema. The recruitment of inflammatory cells ($CD3^+$, $CD45^+$ cells) was significantly increased in oxazolone-exposed skin sites. The expression of COX-2, an important mediator of acute phase reactions, was also significantly increased compared with control mice after oxazolone treatment. Histologic evaluation showed keratosis in the stratum corneum and an erosive change in epidermis, mild acanthosis and remarkable loss of hair follicles (epilation), loss of blood vessels and remarkable loss hair of follicles and hypertrophic fat cells, as well as remarkable muscle atrophy compared with the intact structure of the whole skin with no treatment (Figure 1A). Prominent epidermal hyperplasia with abnormal keratinization and hyperkeratosis was quantitated in Figure 1B. The results showed that the oxazolone-treated group had a significantly higher level of skin thickness. The *D. dasycarpus*-treated group showed remarkably decreased oxazolone-induced swelling and erythematic intensity. Similarly, the *P. cicadae* treated group completely prevented UVB-induced damages in the epidermal. In addition, the dermal-epidermal junction returned to near-normal levels compared to that of the control group as noted by the well-marked appearance of dermal papillae and epidermal rete ridges. Moreover, the upper portion of the dermis showed an ordered arrangement of hair follicles. These results indicated that topical administrated *D. dasycarpus* and *P. cicadae* alleviate oxazolone-induced dermatitis at the relative low dose of 5 mg/kg.

The cultured HaCaT cells were treated with *D. dasycarpus* and *P. cicadae* followed by oxazolone exposure to evaluate the possible mechanism of action of these two Chinese herbs in intracellular stress (Figure 2). The cellular oxygen levels were dramatically increased in the oxazolone-treated cells, whereas the ROS levels were significantly reduced in cells treated with *D. dasycarpus* and *P. cicadae.* In addition, ROS levels in cytoplasm were higher compared to the ROS in mitochondria after treatment with the two herb medicines. These results demonstrated that *D. dasycarpus* and *P. cicadae* can effectively scavenge ROS induced by oxazolone in HaCaT cells.

To elucidate the protective mechanism of *D. dasycarpus* and *P. cicadae* on oxazolone-induced allergic contact dermatitis, HaCaT cells were challenged with oxazolone followed by incubation with *D. dasycarpus* and *P. cicadae*. It was found that *D. dasycarpus* and *P. cicadae* showed marked activity against oxazolone-induced expression of p65, procaspase-1 and ASC at 24 h (Figure 3). The inhibitory effect of *D. dasycarpus* was more potent than the effects of *P. cicadae* on p65 production, even though *P. cicadae* has been reported to be an effective inflammatory inhibitor. We examined the effects of *P. cicadae* and *D. dasycarpus* on the activation of the master regulators of antioxidant response, JNK and p38. The results shown in Figure 3 reveal that the inflammation resulted in phosphorylation of the stress-activated MAP kinases p38 and JNK. Cells treated with *P. cicadae* and *D. dasycarpus* exhibited decreased phosphorylation of JNK and p38 compared to cells treated only with oxazolone. The results showed that both herbal medicines reduced the inflammation response of oxazolone-stimulated HaCaT cells through p38 and JNK signaling, which could subsequently decrease IL-6 production.

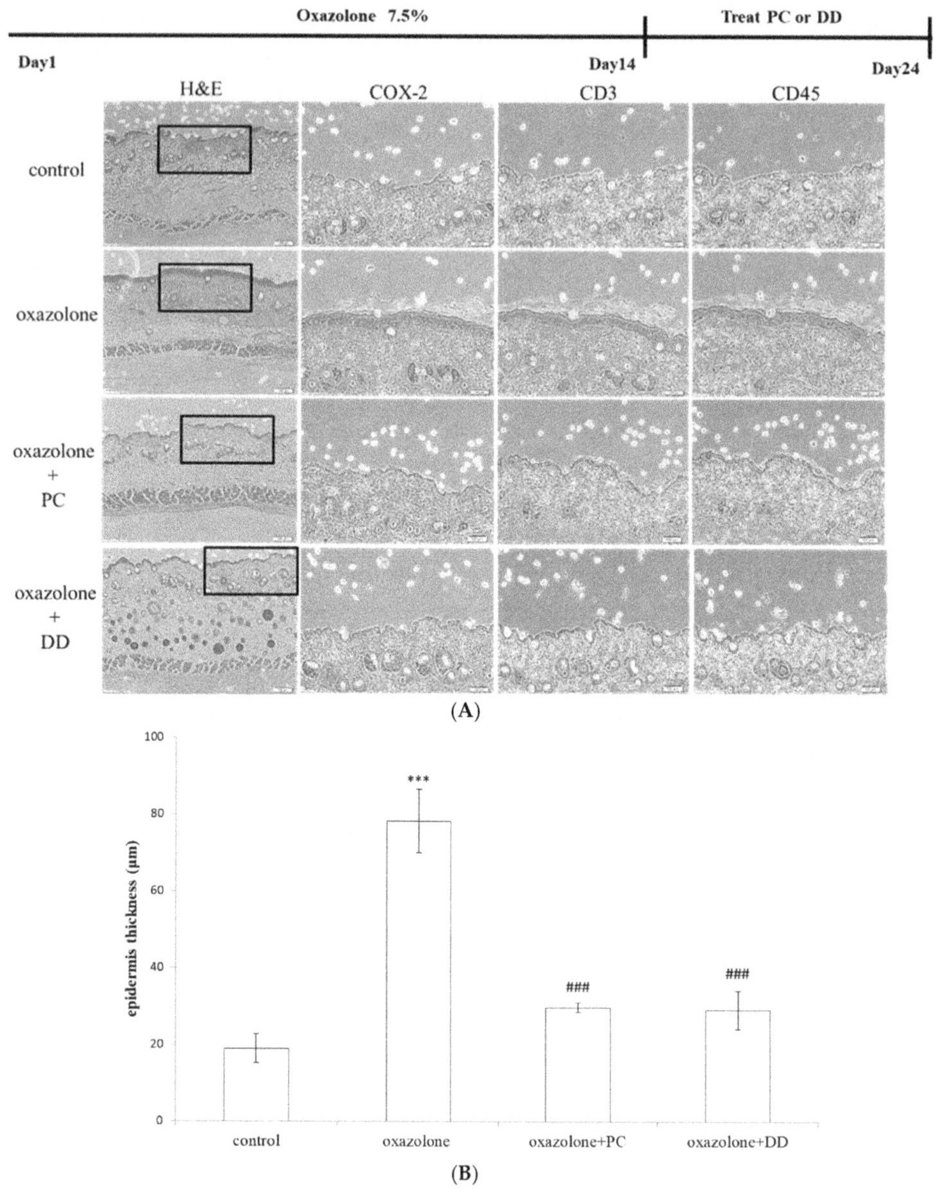

Figure 1. The effect of *P. cicadae* (PC) and *D. dasycarpus* (DD) on oxazolone-induced skin edema. (**A**) Representative scheme showing the treatment of the dermatitis mouse. Histopathological images of *P. cicadae* or *D. dasycarpus* of oxazolone-induced mouse dermatitis. Five-percent oxazolone was applied onto mice back every 2 days, for 10 days. The control group was treated with ethanol instead of oxazolone. Mouse skin was excised after the last application, and a representative section of H&E staining from five mice is shown. Topical treatment 5 mg/kg of *P. cicadae* or *D. dasycarpus* inhibited oxazolone-induced extensive structural damage in both the epidermis and dermis (magnification, 40×). Infiltration of $CD3^+$ or $CD45^+$ lymphocytes into the dermis and the development of pro-inflammatory component COX-2 were remarkably alleviated in the *P. cicadae* and *D. dasycarpus* treated group. (**B**) Epidermal thickness (μm) was measured histopathologically by H&E staining. Data represents of mean ± SD of three different animals; *** $p < 0.001$, significant when oxazolone-treated group was compared with control; ### $p < 0.001$, significant when PC/CD^+ oxazolone-treated group was compared to oxazolone only group; COX: cyclooxygenase; CD: cluster of differentiation.

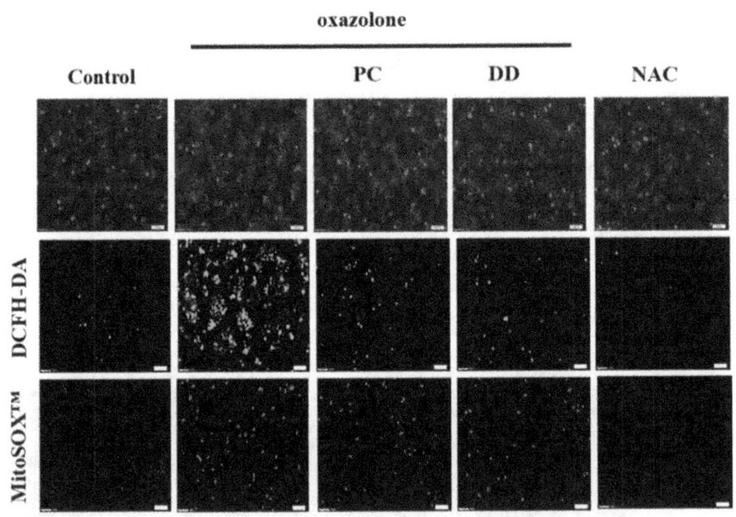

Figure 2. The effect of *P. cicadae* and *D. dasycarpus* on the oxidative levels of HaCaT cells exposed to oxazolone. HaCaT cells were sensitized with oxazolone and treated with *P. cicadae* or *D. dasycarpus*. The generation of cellular ROS were measured by the 2′,7′-dichlorofluorescin diacetate (DCFH-DA), whereas mitochondrial superoxide generation was analyzed by using MitoSOX™ Red as a probe. *N*-acetylcysteine (NAC) was used as an antioxidant control. Representative micrographs (40×) demonstrating. *P. cicadae* and *D. dasycarpus* effectively prevented oxazolone-produced cellular and mitochondrial superoxide in HaCaT cells.

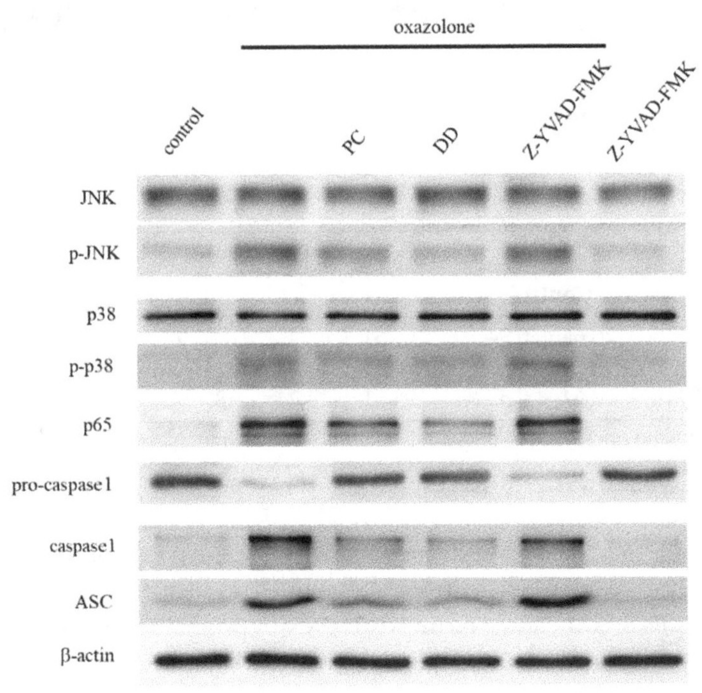

Figure 3. Effects of *P. cicadae* and *D. dasycarpus* on oxazolone-irritated inflammation in HaCaT cells. The HaCaT cells stimulated by oxazolone were cultured with either *P. cicadae* or *D. dasycarpus*. The relative activation of JNK and p38 was determined by Western blotting, and the levels of JNK and p38 were used as an indication of equal loading. Caspase-1, procaspase-1, ASC and p65 expression in HaCaT cells lysates was measured by immunoblotting, whereas β-actin was used as a loading control.

Mitochondria are potential organelles for NLRP3 inflammasome activation because of their vital role in the production of ROS. Western blotting analysis revealed that the 20 kDa form of caspase-1 was present in cell lysates after an overnight treatment with oxazolone. Our results further confirmed that oxazolone could activate the NLRP3 inflammasome and stimulate the maturation of procaspase-1. The *D. dasycarpus* downregulated the capacity of oxazolone, including the inhibition of the expression of procaspase-1 and ASC. The confocal results showed NLRP3 dispersed over the cytoplasm (Figure 4), and the activation state was also confirmed by abundant IL-1β secretion from the same set of cells (Table 1). It was also found that *D. dasycarpus* effectively blocks NLRP3 generation induced by oxazolone.

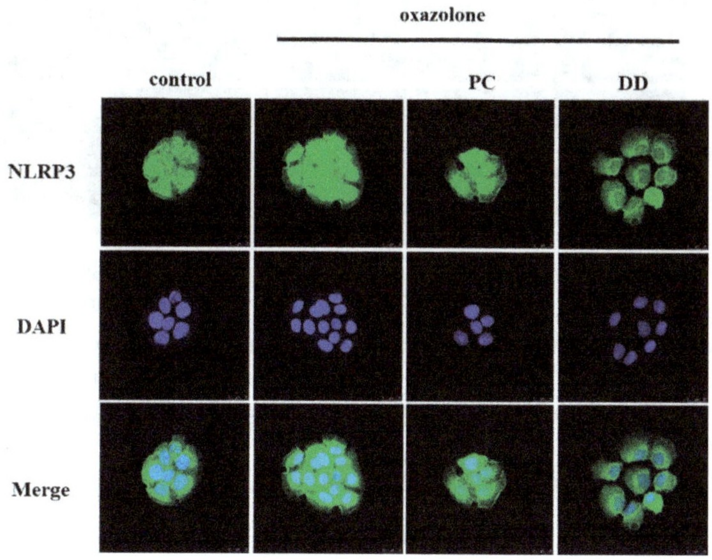

Figure 4. Fluorescent confocal microscopic images showing the localization of inflammasome components NLRP3 (green) in HaCaT cells.

Table 1. Cytokine levels in oxazolone-treated HaCaT cells and PC/DD + oxazolone-treated cells.

		Oxazolone		
	Control		PC	DD
TNF-α pg/mL	20.64 ± 0.94	96.51 ± 9.74	87.97 ± 2.35	71.85 ± 4.95 [a]
IL-6 pg/mL	13.20 ± 2.87	27.40 ± 1.19	14.20 ± 2.43 [b]	12.30 ± 2.17 [b]
IL-8 pg/mL	20.64 ± 0.57	198.51 ± 14.24	87.97 ± 3.75 [b]	51.85 ± 5.21 [b]

Compared to oxazolone-only group, [a] $p < 0.01$; [b] $p < 0.001$; TNF: Tumor Necrosis Factor; IL-6: Interleukin 6.

IL-6 is a marker of activated keratinocytes. As shown in Table 1, oxazolone resulted in dramatic increases in IL-6 protein levels in HaCaT cells. In contrast, treatment with oxazolone plus *P. cicadae* or *D. dasycarpus* significantly reduced IL-6 expression. We further examined the effect of *P. cicadae* and *D. dasycarpus* on IL-8 and TNF-α expression by ELISA. Treatment with *P. cicadae* and *D. dasycarpus* markedly inhibited oxazolone-mediated cytokine expression. The increased levels of IL-1β following oxazolone stress were decreased by pretreatment with the irreversible caspase-1 inhibitor Z-YVAD-FMK (Z-Tyr-Val-Ala-Asp fluoromethylketone). Treatment with *D. dasycarpus* prevented IL-1β expression and *D. dasycarpus* exerted a stronger inhibitory effect than *P. cicadae* (Table 2). Hence, our results demonstrate that the NLRP3 inflammasome is associated with the production of IL-1β after oxazolone stimulation, and *D. dasycarpus* plays a role in a decrease in IL-1β secretion in HaCaT cells treated with oxazolone.

Table 2. ELISA analysis showing oxazolone-induced increase in IL-1βproduction in the absence and presence of Z-YVAD-FMK in HaCaT cells. *P. cicadae* and *D. dasycarpus* abolished oxazolone–induced increase in IL-1β.

	Oxazolone					
	Control		PC	DD	Z-YVAD-FMK	Z-YVAD-FMK
IL-1β pg/mL	25.24 ± 0.57	180.11 ± 14.24	87.67 ± 4.95 [a]	72.65 ± 7.21 [a]	57.34 ± 4.54 [b]	28.84 ± 0.27 [b]

Fold of oxazolone, [a] $p < 0.01$; [b] $p < 0.001$.

4. Discussion

In this study, we investigated the anti-inflammatory activity of *D. dasycarpus*, including the inhibition of the generation of cytokines and the inflammasome, as well as the downregulation of the oxazolone-induced p38 and NF-κB. *D. dasycarpus* displayed in vivo activity at a concentration of 5 mg/kg against oxazolone-induced dermatitis. These results suggest that the *D. dasycarpus* could cease inflammation, which could be achieved via the depletion of ROS and its downstream signaling pathways.

Several compounds have been identified in *D. dasycarpus* extract by pressurized liquid extraction followed by high-performance liquid chromatography [22]. Among these compounds, limonoid and obacunone are the top two abundant triterpenoids, which are well known to possess anti-inflammation beneficial properties [23,24]. In addition, a wide variety of phenylalkylketone compounds derived from herbal products activate potent antioxidant activities, which may also contribute to the dermaprotective effects of *D. dasycarpus* extract on the skin [25].

Oxazolone has been used to induce colitis and contact dermatitis in mice [26]. Our results showed that oxazolone provoked various chemical mediators such as TNF-α, IL-1β, and prostaglandin E2 in the mice skin. In HaCaT cells, oxazolone-induced irritant effects triggered ROS generation and mitochondrial oxidative stress. Recently, oxidative stress has been proposed to play an important role in the activation of the inflammasome [27,28]. Accordingly, ROS are required for NLRP3 inflammasome activation [29,30]. Activation of NLRP3 by extracellular inflammatory insults results in the transcriptional regulation and post-translational modifications of license receptor activation. The indirect immunofluorescence staining of the NLRP3 protein shows a significant overlap of NLRP3 with the endoplasmic reticulum (ER) under non-stimulatory conditions. *D. dasycarpus* could downregulate NLRP3 activation through scavenging ROS, suppressing the expression of ASC, and localizing resting NLRP3 to endoplasmic reticulum structures (Figure 4). Therefore, *D. dasycarpus* limited the assembly of NLRP3 inflammasome, thus preventing procaspase-1 progression, caspase-1 activation and the maturation IL-1β.

The inhibition of pro-inflammatory cytokine expression has been reported to improve dermatitis in terms of protection from extended adaptive immunity. We confirmed that oxazolone exhibited dermatitis symptoms, such as erythema and desquamation in the dorsal skin, and has successfully prevented this cutaneous damage in mice by topical administration of *P. cicadae*, as well as *D. dasycarpus*. *P. cicadae* and *D. dasycarpus* also diminished oxazolone-induced inflammation by decreasing the levels of pro-inflammatory cytokines including IL-6, IL-8, and TNF-α and exhibited signaling regulatory effects in HaCaT cells. *D. dasycarpus* treatment antagonized NF-κB-dependent inflammatory mediators such as IL-1β, IL-6, IL-8, and COX-2 at a protein level since the NF-κB responsive elements have been defined [31–33]. Furthermore, our results also showed that *D. dasycarpus* reduced inflammation activity via down-regulation of the p38 and JNK pathways, which could subsequently decrease IL-6 production [34]. *D. dasycarpus* displayed better anti-inflammatory bioactivity than the same concentration of *P. cicadae* upon oxazolone-stimulated in in vivo and in vitro models [19]. Hence, we propose that *D. dasycarpus* could be an antioxidant for therapy against skin exposure to oxazolone (Figure 5).

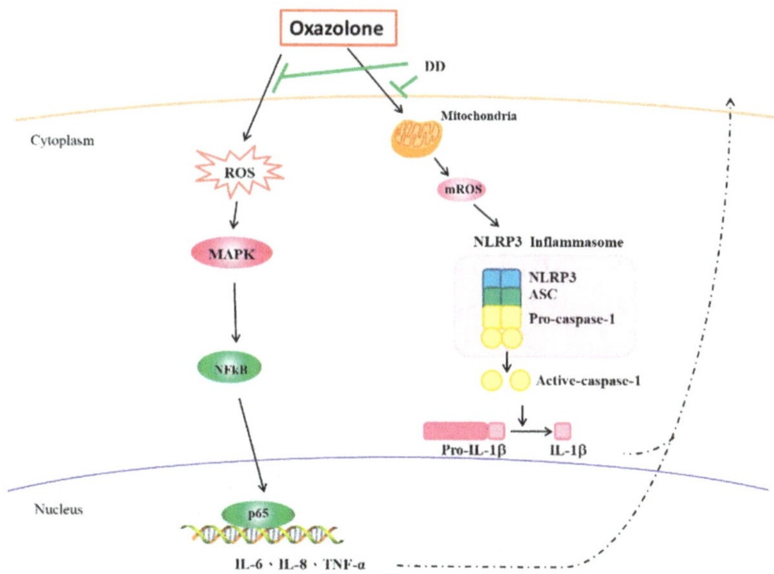

Figure 5. Proposed mechanism by which *D. dasycarpus* abolishes oxazolone-stimulated cytokines production, as well as diminishes NLRP3 inflammasome activation in HaCaT cells.

5. Conclusions

We demonstrated both in vivo and in vitro that *D. dasycarpus* protection may involve silencing NLRP3 inflammasome activities and alleviating inflammatory responses. The underlying mechanism was associated with the NF-κB and p38 signaling pathways.

Author Contributions: Conceptualization, H.-C.H.; Formal analysis, T.-Y.Y. and H.-C.H.; Funding acquisition, T.-M.C.; Investigation, T.-M.C., Y.L.N. and H.-C.H.; Methodology, T.-M.C., T.-Y.Y. and H.-C.H.; Project administration, T.-M.C. and H.-C.H.; Resources, Y.-L.N. and H.-C.H.; Software, T.-Y.Y. and Y.-L.N.; Writing–original draft, H.-C.H.; Writing–review & editing, T.-M.C.

Funding: This research was funded by Ministry of Science and Technology, Taiwan: MOST 104-2213-B-241-001 and MOST 106-2622-8-214-002-TB1.

Acknowledgments: This study was financially supported by the Ministry of Science and Technology, Taiwan, under Grant No. MOST 104-2213-B-241-001 and MOST 106-2622-8-214-002-TB1.

Conflicts of Interest: The authors declare that they have no competing interests.

References

1. Chen, F.-P.; Chen, T.-J.; Kung, Y.-Y.; Chen, Y.-C.; Chou, L.-F.; Chen, F.-J.; Hwang, S.-J. Use frequency of traditional Chinese medicine in Taiwan. *BMC Health Serv. Res.* **2007**, *7*, 26. [CrossRef] [PubMed]
2. Weng, S.-W.; Chen, B.-C.; Wang, Y.-C.; Liu, C.-K.; Sun, M.-F.; Chang, C.-M.; Lin, J.-G.; Yen, H.-R. Traditional Chinese medicine use among patients with psoriasis in Taiwan: A nationwide population-based study. *Evid. Based Complement. Altern. Med.* **2016**, *2016*, 13. [CrossRef] [PubMed]
3. Lin, J.-F.; Liu, P.-H.; Huang, T.-P.; Lien, A.S.-Y.; Ou, L.-S.; Yu, C.-H.; Yang, S.-L.; Chang, H.-H.; Yen, H.-R. Characteristics and prescription patterns of traditional Chinese medicine in atopic dermatitis patients: Ten-year experiences at a Medical Center in Taiwan. *Complement. Ther. Med.* **2014**, *22*, 141–147. [CrossRef] [PubMed]
4. Wu, T.-S.; Wang, M.-L.; Shyur, H.-J.; Leu, Y.-L.; Chan, Y.-Y.; Teng, C.-M.; Kuo, S.-C. Chemical constituents and bioactive principles from the root bark of *Dictamnus dasycarpus+*. *Chin. Pharm. J.* **1994**, *46*, 447–455.
5. Yang, B.; Lee, H.-B.; Kim, S.; Park, Y.C.; Kim, K.; Kim, H. Decoction of *Dictamnus Dasycarpus* Turcz. Root Bark Ameliorates Skin Lesions and Inhibits Inflammatory Reactions in Mice with Contact Dermatitis. *Pharmacogn. Mag.* **2017**, *13*, 483–487. [PubMed]

6. Gasparrini, M.; Forbes-Hernandez, T.Y.; Afrin, S.; Reboredo-Rodriguez, P.; Cianciosi, D.; Mezzetti, B.; Quiles, J.L.; Bompadre, S.; Battino, M.; Giampieri, F. Strawberry-based cosmetic formulations protect human dermal fibroblasts against UVA-induced damage. *Nutrients* **2017**, *9*, 605. [CrossRef] [PubMed]
7. Rodrigues, K.C.M.; Chibli, L.A.; Santos, B.C.S.; Temponi, V.S.; Pinto, N.C.C.; Scio, E.; Del-Vechio-Vieira, G.; Alves, M.S.; Sousa, O.V. Evidence of bioactive compounds from *Vernonia polyanthes* leaves with topical anti-inflammatory potential. *Int. J. Mol. Sci.* **2016**, *17*, 1929. [CrossRef] [PubMed]
8. Man, M.-Q.; Hatano, Y.; Lee, S.H.; Man, M.; Chang, S.; Feingold, K.R.; Leung, D.Y.M.; Holleran, W.; Uchida, Y.; Elias, P.M. Characterization of a hapten-induced, murine model with multiple features of atopic dermatitis: Structural, immunologic, and biochemical changes following single versus multiple oxazolone challenges. *J. Investig. Dermatol.* **2008**, *128*, 79–86. [CrossRef] [PubMed]
9. Saint-Mezard, P.; Krasteva, M.; Chavagnac, C.; Bosset, S.; Akiba, H.; Kehren, J.; Nicolas, J.F.; Berard, F.; Kanitakis, J.; Kaiserlian, D. Afferent and efferent phases of allergic contact dermatitis (ACD) can be induced after a single skin contact with haptens: Evidence using a mouse model of primary ACD. *J. Investig. Dermatol.* **2003**, *120*, 641–647. [CrossRef] [PubMed]
10. Pasparakis, M.; Haase, I.; Nestle, F.O. Mechanisms regulating skin immunity and inflammation. *Nat. Rev. Immunol.* **2014**, *14*, 289. [CrossRef] [PubMed]
11. Andor, P.; Istvan, N.; Lajos, K. Innate immunity in the skin: How keratinocytes fight against pathogens. *Curr. Immunol. Rev.* **2005**, *1*, 29–42.
12. McKenzie, R.C.; Sauder, D.N. Keratinocyte cytokines and growth factors. Functions in skin immunity and homeostasis. *Dermatol. Clin.* **1990**, *8*, 649–661. [PubMed]
13. Ansel, J.; Perry, P.; Brown, J.; Damm, D.; Phan, T.; Hart, C.; Luger, T.; Hefeneider, S. Cytokine modulation of keratinocyte cytokines. *J. Investig. Dermatol.* **1990**, *94*, s101–s107. [CrossRef]
14. Feldmeyer, L.; Keller, M.; Niklaus, G.; Hohl, D.; Werner, S.; Beer, H.D. The inflammasome mediates UVB-induced activation and secretion of interleukin-1β by keratinocytes. *Curr. Biol.* **2007**, *17*, 1140–1145. [CrossRef] [PubMed]
15. Feldmeyer, L.; Werner, S.; French, L.E.; Beer, H.D. Interleukin-1, inflammasomes and the skin. *Eur. J. Cell Biol.* **2010**, *89*, 638–644. [CrossRef] [PubMed]
16. Broz, P.; Dixit, V.M. Inflammasomes: Mechanism of assembly, regulation and signalling. *Nat. Rev. Immunol.* **2016**, *16*, 407–420. [CrossRef] [PubMed]
17. Zhong, F.L.; Mamai, O.; Sborgi, L.; Boussofara, L.; Hopkins, R.; Robinson, K.; Szeverenyi, I.; Takeichi, T.; Balaji, R.; Lau, A.; et al. Germline NLRP1 mutations cause skin inflammatory and cancer susceptibility syndromes via inflammasome activation. *Cell* **2016**, *167*, 187–202. [CrossRef] [PubMed]
18. Yamanashi, T.; Iwata, M.; Kamiya, N.; Tsunetomi, K.; Kajitani, N.; Wada, N.; Iitsuka, T.; Yamauchi, T.; Miura, A.; Pu, S.; et al. Beta-hydroxybutyrate, an endogenic NLRP3 inflammasome inhibitor, attenuates stress-induced behavioral and inflammatory responses. *Sci. Rep.* **2017**, *7*, 7677. [CrossRef] [PubMed]
19. Chang, T.M.; Tsen, J.H.; Yen, H.; Yang, T.Y.; Huang, H.C. Extract from *Periostracum cicadae* inhibits oxidative stress and inflammation induced by ultraviolet B irradiation on HaCaT keratinocytes. *Evid. Based Complement. Altern. Med.* **2017**, *2017*, 8325049. [CrossRef] [PubMed]
20. Chapman, J.; Ruben, Z.; Butchko, G. Histology of and quantitative assays for oxazolone-induced allergic contact dermatitis in mice. *Am. J. Dermatopathol.* **1986**, *8*, 130–138. [CrossRef] [PubMed]
21. Petersen, T.K. In vivo pharmacological disease models for psoriasis and atopic dermatitis in drug discovery. *Basic Clin. Pharmacol. Toxicol.* **2006**, *99*, 104–115. [CrossRef] [PubMed]
22. Jiang, Y.; Li, S.P.; Chang, H.T.; Wang, Y.T.; Tu, P.F. Pressurized liquid extraction followed by high-performance liquid chromatography for determination of seven active compounds in Cortex Dictamni. *J. Chromatogr. A* **2006**, *1108*, 268–272. [CrossRef] [PubMed]
23. Liu, S.J.; Zhou, L.; Zhang, J.; Yu, B.Y.; Li, C.Y.; Liu, Z.X.; Ju, W.Z. Determination of limonin in dog plasma by liquid chromatography–tandem mass spectrometry and its application to a pharmacokinetic study. *Biomed. Chromatogr.* **2013**, *27*, 515–519. [CrossRef] [PubMed]
24. Patlolla, J.M.; Rao, C.V. Triterpenoids for cancer prevention and treatment: Current status and future prospects. *Curr. Pharm. Biotechnol.* **2012**, *13*, 147–155. [CrossRef] [PubMed]
25. Radice, M.; Manfredini, S.; Ziosi, P.; Dissette, V.; Buso, P.; Fallacara, A.; Vertuani, S. Herbal extracts, lichens and biomolecules as natural photo-protection alternatives to synthetic UV filters. A systematic review. *Fitoterapia* **2016**, *114*, 144–162. [CrossRef] [PubMed]

26. Itani, S.; Watanabe, T.; Nadatani, Y.; Sugimura, N.; Shimada, S.; Takeda, S.; Otani, K.; Hosomi, S.; Nagami, Y.; Tanaka, F. NLRP3 inflammasome has a protective effect against oxazolone-induced colitis: A possible role in ulcerative colitis. *Sci. Rep.* **2016**, *6*, 39075. [CrossRef] [PubMed]
27. Fabio, M. Signaling by ROS drives inflammasome activation. *Eur. J. Immunol.* **2010**, *40*, 616–619.
28. He, Y.; Hara, H.; Núñez, G. Mechanism and regulation of NLRP3 inflammasome activation. *Trends Biochem. Sci.* **2016**, *41*, 1012–1021. [CrossRef] [PubMed]
29. Abais, J.M.; Xia, M.; Zhang, Y.; Boini, K.M.; Li, P.-L. Redox regulation of NLRP3 inflammasomes: ROS as trigger or effector? *Antioxid. Redox Signal.* **2015**, *22*, 1111–1129. [CrossRef] [PubMed]
30. Tschopp, J.; Schroder, K. NLRP3 inflammasome activation: The convergence of multiple signalling pathways on ROS production? *Nat. Rev. Immunol.* **2010**, *10*, 210–215. [CrossRef] [PubMed]
31. Mukaida, N.; Okamoto, S.; Ishikawa, Y.; Matsushima, K. Molecular mechanism of interleukin-8 gene expression. *J. Leukoc. Biol.* **1994**, *56*, 554–558. [CrossRef] [PubMed]
32. Tak, P.P.; Firestein, G.S. NF-κB: A key role in inflammatory diseases. *J. Clin. Investig.* **2001**, *107*, 7–11. [CrossRef] [PubMed]
33. Xia, J.; Song, X.; Bi, Z.; Chu, W.; Wan, Y. UV-induced NF-κB activation and expression of IL-6 is attenuated by (-)-epigallocatechin-3-gallate in cultured human keratinocytes in vitro. *Int. J. Mol. Med.* **2005**, *16*, 943–950. [CrossRef] [PubMed]
34. Yang, J.-H.; Yoo, J.-M.; Lee, E.; Lee, B.; Cho, W.-K.; Park, K.-I.; Yeul Ma, J. Anti-inflammatory effects of Perillae Herba ethanolic extract against TNF-α/IFN-γ-stimulated human keratinocyte HaCaT cells. *J. Ethnopharmacol.* **2018**, *211*, 217–223. [CrossRef] [PubMed]

Permissions

All chapters in this book were first published in ANTIOXIDANTS, by MDPI; hereby published with permission under the Creative Commons Attribution License or equivalent. Every chapter published in this book has been scrutinized by our experts. Their significance has been extensively debated. The topics covered herein carry significant findings which will fuel the growth of the discipline. They may even be implemented as practical applications or may be referred to as a beginning point for another development.

The contributors of this book come from diverse backgrounds, making this book a truly international effort. This book will bring forth new frontiers with its revolutionizing research information and detailed analysis of the nascent developments around the world.

We would like to thank all the contributing authors for lending their expertise to make the book truly unique. They have played a crucial role in the development of this book. Without their invaluable contributions this book wouldn't have been possible. They have made vital efforts to compile up to date information on the varied aspects of this subject to make this book a valuable addition to the collection of many professionals and students.

This book was conceptualized with the vision of imparting up-to-date information and advanced data in this field. To ensure the same, a matchless editorial board was set up. Every individual on the board went through rigorous rounds of assessment to prove their worth. After which they invested a large part of their time researching and compiling the most relevant data for our readers.

The editorial board has been involved in producing this book since its inception. They have spent rigorous hours researching and exploring the diverse topics which have resulted in the successful publishing of this book. They have passed on their knowledge of decades through this book. To expedite this challenging task, the publisher supported the team at every step. A small team of assistant editors was also appointed to further simplify the editing procedure and attain best results for the readers.

Apart from the editorial board, the designing team has also invested a significant amount of their time in understanding the subject and creating the most relevant covers. They scrutinized every image to scout for the most suitable representation of the subject and create an appropriate cover for the book.

The publishing team has been an ardent support to the editorial, designing and production team. Their endless efforts to recruit the best for this project, has resulted in the accomplishment of this book. They are a veteran in the field of academics and their pool of knowledge is as vast as their experience in printing. Their expertise and guidance has proved useful at every step. Their uncompromising quality standards have made this book an exceptional effort. Their encouragement from time to time has been an inspiration for everyone.

The publisher and the editorial board hope that this book will prove to be a valuable piece of knowledge for researchers, students, practitioners and scholars across the globe.

List of Contributors

Eric Pace, Amy Clemens, Tennille Crossman and H.P. Vasantha Rupasinghe
Department of Plant, Food, and Environmental Sciences, Faculty of Agriculture, Dalhousie University, Truro, NS B2N 5E3, Canada

Yuanyuan Jiang
Department of Plant, Food, and Environmental Sciences, Faculty of Agriculture, Dalhousie University, Truro, NS B2N 5E3, Canada
College of Science, Sichuan Agricultural University, Yaan 625014, China

Thomas Nury, Anne Vejux and Gérard Lizard
Team Bio-PeroxIL, Biochemistry of the Peroxisome, Inflammation and Lipid Metabolism (EA7270)/ University Bourgogne Franche-Comté/Inserm, 21000 Dijon, France

Wiem Meddeb
Team Bio-PeroxIL, Biochemistry of the Peroxisome, Inflammation and Lipid Metabolism (EA7270)/ University Bourgogne Franche-Comté/Inserm, 21000 Dijon, France
Department of Biotechnology, Institut Préparatoire aux Etudes Scientifiques et Techniques (IPEST), La Marsa 2070, Tunisia
Laboratory Matériaux, Molécules et Applications (LMMA), University of Carthage, La Marsa, Tunis 2078, Tunisia
Faculty of Science of Bizerte, Zarzouna, Bizerte 7021, Tunisia

Leila Rezig
Food Conservation and Valorization Laboratory, High Institute of Food Industries, 58 Avenue Alain Savary, El Khadra City, Tunis 1003, Tunisia

Amira Zarrouk
Lab. NAFS, Nutrition—Functional Food & Vascular Diseases LR12-ES-05, University of Monastir, Monastir 5000, Tunisia
Faculty of Medicine, University of Sousse, Sousse 4002, Tunisia

Michel Prost
Laboratoire Spiral, 21560 Couternon, France

Lionel Bretillon
Eye & Nutrition Research Group, CSGA, UMR 1324 INRA, 6265 CNRS, 21000 Dijon, France

Mondher Mejri
Department of Biotechnology, Institut Préparatoire aux Etudes Scientifiques et Techniques (IPEST), La Marsa 2070, Tunisia
Laboratory Matériaux, Molécules et Applications (LMMA), University of Carthage, La Marsa, Tunis 2078, Tunisia
Department of Biotechnology, University of Jendouba, Jendouba 8100, Tunisia

Maria Graça Miguel
Faculdade de Ciências e Tecnologia, MeditBio, Universidade do Algarve, Campus de Gambelas, 8005-139 Faro, Portugal

Alessandro Pinto
Department of Experimental Medicine, Sapienza University of Rome, 00161 Roma, Italy

Alessio Bonucci, Elisa Maggi, Mariangela Corsi and Rita Businaro
Department of Medico-Surgical Sciences and Biotechnologies, Sapienza University of Rome, 04100 Latina, Italy

Hamid Arazi and Abbas Asadi
Department of Exercise Physiology, Faculty of Sports Sciences, University of Guilan, Rasht 1438, Iran

Katsuhiko Suzuki
Faculty of Sport Sciences, Waseda University, Tokorozawa 359-1192, Japan

John Mark Cline and Greg Dugan
Department of Pathology, Section on Comparative Medicine, Wake Forest University School of Medicine, Medical Center Boulevard, Winston-Salem, NC 27157-1040, USA

John Daniel Bourland
Department of Radiation Oncology, Wake Forest University School of Medicine, Medical Center Boulevard, Winston-Salem, NC 27157-1040, USA

Donna L. Perry
Department of Pathology, Section on Comparative Medicine, Wake Forest University School of Medicine, Medical Center Boulevard, Winston-Salem, NC 27157-1040, USA

Integrated Research Facility, Division of Clinical Research, National Institute of Allergy and Infectious Disease, National Institutes of Health, Frederick, MD 21702, USA

Joel D. Stitzel and Ashley A. Weaver
Department of Biomedical Engineering, Wake Forest University School of Medicine, Biotech Place, 575 N. Patterson Ave., Winston-Salem, NC 21701, USA

Chen Jiang and Kouros Owzar
Department of Biostatistics and Bioinformatics, Duke University Medical Center, Durham, NC 27708, USA

Artak Tovmasyan and Ines Batinic-Haberle
Department of Radiation Oncology, Duke University Medical Center, Durham, NC 27708, USA

Ivan Spasojevic
Department of Medicine Duke University Medical Center, Durham, NC 27708, USA
Duke Cancer Institute, Pharmaceutical Research Shared Resource, PK/PD Core Laboratory, Duke University Medical Center, Durham, NC 27708, USA

Zeljko Vujaskovic
Department of Radiation Oncology, Duke University Medical Center, Durham, NC 27708, USA
Department of Radiation Oncology, University of Maryland School of Medicine, 655 W. Baltimore Street, Baltimore, MD 21201, USA

Twinkle Chowdhury, Matthew F. Allen, Trista L. Thorn, Yan He and Sandra J. Hewett
Department of Biology, Program in Neuroscience, Syracuse University, Syracuse, NY 13210, USA

Nor Helwa Ezzah Nor Azman, Jo Aan Goon, Siti Madiani Abdul Ghani and Wan Zurinah Wan Ngah
Department of Biochemistry, Faculty of Medicine, Universiti Kebangsaan Malaysia, Jalan Yaacob Latif, Kuala Lumpur 56000, Malaysia

Zalina Hamid
Sime Darby Foods and Beverages Marketing Sdn. Bhd, Petaling Jaya 47301, Selangor, Malaysia

Vasily N. Manskikh
A.N. Belozersky Institute of Physico-Chemical Biology, Lomonosov Moscow State University, 119992 Moscow, Russia

Irina B. Pevzner, Ljubava D. Zorova, Denis N. Silachev and Dmitry B. Zorov
A.N. Belozersky Institute of Physico-Chemical Biology, Lomonosov Moscow State University, 119992 Moscow, Russia
V.I. Kulakov National Medical Research Center of Obstetrics, Gynecology and Perinatology, 117997 Moscow, Russia

Egor Y. Plotnikov
A.N. Belozersky Institute of Physico-Chemical Biology, Lomonosov Moscow State University, 119992 Moscow, Russia
V.I. Kulakov National Medical Research Center of Obstetrics, Gynecology and Perinatology, 117997 Moscow, Russia
Institute of Molecular Medicine, Sechenov First Moscow State Medical University, 119991 Moscow, Russia

Anna A. Brezgunova
Biological Faculty, Lomonosov Moscow State University, 119992 Moscow, Russia

Vasily A. Popkov
A.N. Belozersky Institute of Physico-Chemical Biology, Lomonosov Moscow State University, 119992 Moscow, Russia
V.I. Kulakov National Medical Research Center of Obstetrics, Gynecology and Perinatology, 117997 Moscow, Russia
Faculty of Bioengineering and Bioinformatics, Lomonosov Moscow State University, 119992 Moscow, Russia

James Friel and Chenxi Cai
Department of Food and Human Nutritional Sciences, University of Manitoba, Winnipeg, MB R3T 2N2, Canada

Wafaa Qasem
Food and Nutrition Administration, Ministry of Health, Safat 13041, Kuwait

Jahaun Azadmanesh
Department of Biochemistry and Molecular Biology, 985870 Nebraska Medical Center, Omaha, NE 68198-5870, USA

Gloria E. O. Borgstahl
Department of Biochemistry and Molecular Biology, 985870 Nebraska Medical Center, Omaha, NE 68198-5870, USA
Eppley Institute for Cancer and Allied Diseases, 986805 Nebraska Medical Center, Omaha, NE 68198-6805, USA

Sophie C. Broome and Jonathan S. T. Woodhead
Discipline of Nutrition, Faculty of Medical and Health Sciences, The University of Auckland, Auckland 1023, New Zealand

Troy L. Merry
Discipline of Nutrition, Faculty of Medical and Health Sciences, The University of Auckland, Auckland 1023, New Zealand
Maurice Wilkins Centre for Molecular Biodiscovery, The University of Auckland, Auckland 1023, New Zealand

Armando Platania, Dora Castiglione, Dario Sinatra and Marina Marranzano
Department of Medical and Surgical Sciences and Advanced Technologies "G.F. Ingrassia", University of Catania, 95123 Catania, Italy

Maurizio D' Urso
Provincial Health Authority of Catania, 95127 Catania, Italy

Carlos A. Sologubik and Guillermo D. Manrique
Faculty of Engineering, Universidad Nacional del Centro de la Provincia de Buenos Aires, Av. del Valle 5737, Olavarría 7400, Argentina

Leandro Galván D'Alessandro
ISA, Univ. Lille 1, INRA, Univ. Artois, Univ. Littoral Côte d'Opale, EA 7394-ICV-Institut Charles Viollette, 48 Boulevard Vauban, F-59000 Lille, France

Ramiro A. Carciochi
Faculty of Engineering, Universidad Nacional del Centro de la Provincia de Buenos Aires, Av. del Valle 5737, Olavarría 7400, Argentina
ISA, Univ. Lille 1, INRA, Univ. Artois, Univ. Littoral Côte d'Opale, EA 7394-ICV-Institut Charles Viollette, 48 Boulevard Vauban, F-59000 Lille, France

María B. Fernández
Faculty of Engineering, Universidad Nacional del Centro de la Provincia de Buenos Aires, Av. del Valle 5737, Olavarría 7400, Argentina
Centro de Investigación en Física e Ingeniería del Centro de la Provincia de Buenos Aires-CIFICEN (UNCPBA-CICPBA-CONICET), Tandil 7000, Argentina

Tsong-Min Chang
Department of Applied Cosmetology and Master Program of Cosmetic Sciences, Hungkuang University, Taichung 43302, Taiwan

Ting-Ya Yang and Huey-Chun Huang
Department of Medical Laboratory Science and Biotechnology, College of Medicine, China Medical University, No. 91 Hsueh-Shih Road, Taichung 40402, Taiwan

Yu-Lin Niu
Niuer International Skincare Science Research Institute, 9F, No. 266, Ruiguang Rd., Neihu Dist., Taipei 11491, Taiwan

Index

www.ingramcontent.com/pod-product-compliance
Lightning Source LLC
LaVergne TN
LVHW060545210926
848485LV00005B/1262